Treatment of Peritoneal Metastasis

Editor

EDWARD A. LEVINE

SURGICAL ONCOLOGY CLINICS OF NORTH AMERICA

www.surgonc.theclinics.com

Consulting Editor
TIMOTHY M. PAWLIK

July 2018 • Volume 27 • Number 3

ELSEVIER

1600 John F. Kennedy Boulevard ● Suite 1800 ● Philadelphia, Pennsylvania, 19103-2899

http://www.theclinics.com

SURGICAL ONCOLOGY CLINICS OF NORTH AMERICA Volume 27, Number 3
July 2018 ISSN 1055-3207, ISBN-13: 978-0-323-61082-7

Editor: John Vassallo (j.vassallo@elsevier.com)
Developmental Editor: Sara Watkins

Surgical Oncology Clinics of North America (ISSN 1055-3207) is published quarterly by Elsevier Inc., 360 Park Avenue South, New York, NY 10010-1710. Months of publication are January, April, July, and October. Business and Editorial Offices: 1600 John F. Kennedy Blvd., Ste. 1800, Philadelphia, PA 19103-2899. Customer Service Office: 3251 Riverport Lane, Maryland Heights, MO 63043. Periodicals postage paid at New York, NY and additional mailing offices. Subscription prices are $296.00 per year (US individuals), $505.00 (US institutions) $100.00 (US student/resident), $337.00 (Canadian individuals), $638.00 (Canadian institutions), $205.00 (Canadian student/resident), $418.00 (foreign individuals), $638.00 (foreign institutions), and $205.00 (foreign student/resident). Foreign air speed delivery is included in all *Clinics* subscription prices. All prices are subject to change without notice. **POSTMASTER:** Send address changes to *Surgical Oncology Clinics of North America*, Elsevier Health Science Division, Subscription Customer Service, 3251 Riverport Lane, Maryland Heights, MO 63043. **Customer Service: 1-800-654-2452 (US and Canada). 314-447-8871 (outside US and Canada). Fax: 314-447-8029. E-mail: journalscustomerservice-usa@elsevier.com (for print support); journalsonline support-usa@elsevier.com (for online support).**

Reprints. For copies of 100 or more, of articles in this publication, please contact the Commercial Reprints Department, Elsevier Inc., 360 Park Avenue South, New York, New York 10010-1710. Tel. 212-633-3874; Fax: 212-633-3820; E-mail: reprints@elsevier.com.

Surgical Oncology Clinics of North America is covered in *MEDLINE/PubMed (Index Medicus) and EMBASE/ Excerpta Medica, Current Contents/Clinical Medicine, and ISI/BIOMED.*

Contributors

CONSULTING EDITOR

TIMOTHY M. PAWLIK, MD, MPH, PhD, FACS, FRACS (Hon)
Professor and Chair, Department of Surgery, The Urban Meyer III and Shelley Meyer Chair
for Cancer Research, Professor of Surgery, Oncology, Health Services Management and
Policy, The Ohio State University, Wexner Medical Center, Columbus, Ohio, USA

EDITOR

EDWARD A. LEVINE, MD
Chief, Surgical Oncology Service, Professor of Surgery, Department of General Surgery,
Wake Forest School of Medicine, Winston-Salem, North Carolina, USA

AUTHORS

NITA AHUJA, MD, MBA, FACS
Department of Surgery, Cancer Biology, Department of Oncology, The Sidney
Kimmel Comprehensive Cancer Center, Johns Hopkins Medical Institute, Baltimore,
Maryland, USA; Chair, Department of Surgery, Yale School of Medicine, New Haven,
Connecticut, USA

H. RICHARD ALEXANDER Jr, MD
Chief Surgical Officer, Rutgers Cancer Institute of New Jersey, Professor, Department
of Surgery, Rutgers Robert Wood Johnson Medical School, New Brunswick,
New Jersey, USA

OSCAR ALONSO-CASADO, MD, PhD
Hepatobiliary and Pancreatic Surgery, Department of Surgical Oncology, MD Anderson
Cancer Center, Madrid, Spain; Associate Professor, Department of Surgical Oncology,
Division of Surgery, The University of Texas MD Anderson Cancer Center, Houston,
Texas, USA

DARIO BARATTI, MD
Ss Tumori Peritoneali, Fondazione IRCCS Istituto Nazionale dei Tumori di Milano, Milano,
Milan, Italy

ROBERT M. BARONE, MD
Department of Surgical Oncology, Sharp Memorial Hospital, San Diego, California, USA

LUIGI BATTAGLIA, MD
Sc Chirurgia Colonrettale, Fondazione IRCCS Istituto Nazionale dei Tumori di Milano,
Milano, Milan, Italy

LÉONOR BENHAIM, MD, PhD
Department of Visceral and Oncological Surgery, Gustave Roussy, Villejuif, France

CHARLOTTE CARLIER, MS
Department of Surgery, Ghent University, Cancer Research Institute Ghent (CRIG), Ghent, Belgium

WIM P. CEELEN, MD, PhD, FACS
Department of Surgery, Ghent University, Cancer Research Institute Ghent (CRIG), Ghent, Belgium

FADI S. DAHDALEH, MD
Fellow, Complex General Surgical Oncology, Section of General Surgery/Surgical Oncology, The University of Chicago Medicine, Chicago, Illinois, USA

MARCELLO DERACO, MD
Ss Tumori Peritoneali, Fondazione IRCCS Istituto Nazionale dei Tumori di Milano, Milan, Milano, Milan, Italy

MATTHIEU FARON, MD
Department of Visceral and Oncological Surgery, Gustave Roussy, Villejuif, France

KEITH F. FOURNIER, MD
Associate Professor, Department of Surgical Oncology, The University of Texas MD Anderson Cancer Center, Houston, Texas, USA

JAVIER GALIPIENZO-GARCÍA, MD, PhD
Attending Anesthesiologist, Department of Anesthesiology and Pain Management, MD Anderson Cancer Center, Madrid, Spain

MAXIMILIANO GELLI, MD
Department of Visceral and Oncological Surgery, Gustave Roussy, Villejuif, France

DIANE GOÉRÉ, MD, PhD
Department of Visceral and Oncological Surgery, Gustave Roussy, Villejuif, France

SANTIAGO GONZÁLEZ-MORENO, MD, PhD
Medical Director, Chairman, Department of Surgical Oncology, Peritoneal Surface Oncology Program, MD Anderson Cancer Center, Madrid, Spain; Adjunct Professor, Department of Surgical Oncology, Division of Surgery, The University of Texas MD Anderson Cancer Center, Houston, Texas, USA

TRAVIS E. GROTZ, MD
Department of Surgical Oncology, The University of Texas MD Anderson Cancer Center, Houston, Texas, USA; Senior Associate Consultant, Division of Hepatobiliary and Pancreas Surgery, Mayo Clinic, Rochester, Minnesota, USA

STEFANO GUADAGNI, MD
Department of Biotechnological and Applied Clinical Sciences, Università degli Studi dell'Aquila, L'Aquila, Italy

MARCELLO GUAGLIO, MD
Ss Tumori Peritoneali, Fondazione IRCCS Istituto Nazionale dei Tumori di Milano, Milano, Milan, Italy

RYAN J. HENDRIX, MD
Division of Surgical Oncology, Department of Surgery, University of Massachusetts Medical School, Worcester, Massachusetts, USA

CHARLES HONORÉ, MD, PhD
Department of Visceral and Oncological Surgery, Gustave Roussy, Villejuif, France

ENUSHA KARUNASENA, PhD
Department of Oncology, GI Clinical Cancer Research and Cancer Immunology, The Sidney Kimmel Comprehensive Cancer Center, Johns Hopkins Medical Institute, Baltimore, Maryland, USA

SHIGEKI KUSAMURA, MD, PhD
Ss Tumori Peritoneali, Fondazione IRCCS Istituto Nazionale dei Tumori di Milano, Milano, Milan, Italy

NICK LAGAST, MSE
Department of Surgery, Ghent University, Cancer Research Institute Ghent (CRIG), Ghent, Belgium

LAURA A. LAMBERT, MD
Clinical Professor, Surgical Oncology, Department of Surgery, Huntsman Cancer Institute, University of Utah, Salt Lake City, Utah, USA

EDWARD A. LEVINE, MD
Chief, Surgical Oncology Service, Professor of Surgery, Department of General Surgery, Wake Forest School of Medicine, Winston-Salem, North Carolina, USA

CLAIRE YUE LI, MD
NewYork-Presbyterian Hospital, New York, New York, USA

MANUEL J. LINERO-NOGUERA, MD
Chairman, Department of Anesthesiology and Pain Management, MD Anderson Cancer Center, Madrid, Spain

RUSSELL N. LOW, MD
Department of Radiology, Sharp Memorial Hospital, San Diego, California, USA

PAUL F. MANSFIELD, MD
Professor, Department of Surgical Oncology, The University of Texas MD Anderson Cancer Center, Houston, Texas, USA

KEVIN WYATT McMAHON, PhD
Department of Surgery, Johns Hopkins Medical Institute, Baltimore, Maryland, USA

ERAN NIZRI, MD, PhD
Department of General Surgery, Tel Aviv Sourasky Medical Center, Sackler Faculty of Medicine, Tel Aviv University, Tel Aviv, Israel

GLORIA ORTEGA-PÉREZ, MD
Attending Surgical Oncologist, Peritoneal Surface Oncology Program, Department of Surgical Oncology, MD Anderson Cancer Center, Madrid, Spain

DAVID SALVATIERRA-DÍAZ, MD
Attending Anesthesiologist, Department of Anesthesiology and Pain Management, MD Anderson Cancer Center, Madrid, Spain

JONATHAN SHAM, MD
Department of Surgery, Johns Hopkins Medical Institute, Baltimore, Maryland, USA

PERRY SHEN, MD
Surgical Oncology Service, Department of General Surgery, Wake Forest School of Medicine, Winston-Salem, North Carolina, USA

ALEKSANDER SKARDAL, PhD
Wake Forest Institute for Regenerative Medicine, Wake Forest School of Medicine, Winston-Salem, North Carolina, USA

ISABELLE SOURROUILLE, MD
Department of Visceral and Oncological Surgery, Gustave Roussy, Villejuif, France

PAUL H. SUGARBAKER, MD, FACS, FRCS
Program in Peritoneal Surface Oncology, Center for Gastrointestinal Malignancies, MedStar Washington Hospital Center, Washington, DC, USA

KIRAN K. TURAGA, MD, MPH
Associate Professor of Surgery, Vice Chief, Section of General Surgery/Surgical Oncology, Director of Surgical GI Cancer and Regional Therapeutics Program, Chicago, Illinois, USA

KONSTANTINOS I. VOTANOPOULOS, MD, PhD
Surgical Oncology Service, Department of General Surgery, Wake Forest School of Medicine, Winston-Salem, North Carolina, USA

Contents

The treatments for peritoneal metastases have evolved over 30 years. Now the concepts that guided clinicians are being tested in clinical trials to optimize standardized treatment regimens. The essential features of a successful management plan are cytoreductive surgery combined with cancer chemotherapy in a large volume of intraperitoneal fluid administered into the peritoneal space. The cytotoxicity of the cancer chemotherapy is maximized by moderate hyperthermia. The patients must be carefully selected using well-defined prognostic indicators. The efforts to date are multinational, with centers of excellence located throughout the world.

MRI provides considerable advantages for imaging of patients with peritoneal tumor. Its inherently superior contrast resolution compared with computed tomography allows MRI to more accurately depict small peritoneal tumors that are often missed on other imaging tests. Combining different contrast mechanisms, including diffusion-weighted MRI and gadolinium-enhanced MRI, provides a powerful tool for preoperative and surveillance imaging in patients being considered for cytoreductive surgery and heated intraperitoneal chemotherapy.

The peritoneal malignancies span the biologic spectrum of aggressiveness from the indolent growth pattern and superficial nature of well-differentiated mucinous appendiceal adenocarcinoma to the rapidly growing and invasive nature of poorly differentiated signet ring cell adenocarcinomas of the appendix, colon, and stomach. An understanding of the biology, distribution, and volume of disease is critical to appropriately selecting patients for cytoreduction and hyperthermic intraperitoneal chemotherapy (HIPEC) with the goal of long-term survival. Herein the authors discuss the appropriate evaluation and selection of patients with peritoneal surface malignancies for cytoreduction and HIPEC.

tutor-based training program has been implemented in Europe. This initiative will improve the standardization of the combined procedure and improve quality of services across the continent.

Gastric cancer (GC) has a predilection to metastasize to the peritoneum, denoting a poor prognosis. Treatment strategies available for advanced GC have significantly evolved over time and can be categorized into systemic, regional, and surgical. Although systemic therapies have been the mainstay for the treatment of advanced GC, their ability in achieving long-term survival in patients with peritoneal involvement is modest at best. This article describes advances in combined modality treatment of peritoneal metastases, specifically with an emphasis on peritoneal-directed therapies.

Diffuse malignant peritoneal mesothelioma (MPM) is a rare cancer that is ultimately fatal in almost all afflicted individuals. Morbidity and mortality from MPM is due to its propensity to progress locoregionally within the abdominal cavity. Patients with MPM most commonly present with nonspecific abdominal symptoms that usually lead to diagnosis when the condition is relatively advanced. MPM is considered a chemotherapy-resistant malignancy.

The early symptoms of appendiceal cancer may mimic the clinical picture of appendicitis. Most patients are diagnosed incidentally during surgical exploration or late when peritoneal or systemic dissemination has already occurred, as colonoscopy rarely diagnoses an appendiceal cancer. Systemic/extraperitoneal metastases are distinctly unusual for appendiceal mucinous lesions.

Peritoneal metastases are the third most common site of recurrence of colorectal cancer. Diagnosis is difficult and often made at an advanced stage even on imaging. Curative treatment relies on complete cytoreductive surgery plus hyperthermic intraperitoneal chemotherapy (HIPEC), which dramatically improves survival in select patients. Main prognostic factors are based on the extent of the peritoneal disease and the completeness of surgery. Therefore, identifying patients at high risk of developing peritoneal metastases with the aim of diagnosing and treating patients at an early stage appears crucial. Proactive attitude and prophylactic treatment based on HIPEC are being evaluated on clinical trials.

Despite advances in the management of peritoneal carcinomatosis, morbidity remains high with survival often measured in weeks to months. Patients are often subjected to symptoms and complications that affect quality of life. Much of the management revolves around palliation of symptoms and providing support and resources to address emotional and existential concerns. This article reviews surgical and nonsurgical palliative treatments for the symptoms and complications associated with advanced, incurable peritoneal carcinomatosis. It is important that providers caring for patients with peritoneal carcinomatosis be knowledgeable in the palliative management of this condition, including the usefulness of early palliative care referral.

SURGICAL ONCOLOGY CLINICS OF NORTH AMERICA

THE CLINICS ARE AVAILABLE ONLINE!
Access your subscription at:
www.theclinics.com

Foreword

Peritoneal Malignancies

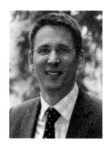

Timothy M. Pawlik, MD, MPH, PhD, FACS, RACS (Hon)
Consulting Editor

This issue of *Surgical Oncology Clinics of North America* is devoted to the diagnosis and treatment of peritoneal surface malignances. Over the last two decades, there has been a marked increase in our knowledge and treatment of peritoneal malignancies. In fact, while cytoreductive surgery and intraperitoneal chemotherapy were relegated to only a handful of centers in the 1990s and early 2000s, now virtually every major cancer center has a peritoneal surface program. In turn, our understanding of the many different cancers that can manifest as peritoneal disease has expanded and has led to refinements in patient selection, timing of surgery, as well as the operative approach. The role of cytoreductive surgery alone relative to cytoreductive surgery combined with intraperitoneal chemotherapy, as well as what disease (eg, appendiceal, mesotheioloma, gastric, colon cancer) consistutes an optimal indication for cytoreductive surgery, have been topics of ongoing debate. In addition, much has been learned about the pharmokinetics of intraperitoneal drug delivery.

To address the important topic of peritoneal surface malignancies, guest editor Edward A. Levine, Professor of Surgery and Chief of Surgical Oncology Services at Wake Forest University, relied on an incredible group of expert authors. Dr Levine himself is an international expert in the field of peritoneal surface malignancies and cytoreductive surgery. Dr Levine has over three decades of experience treating patients with peritoneal surface malignancies and is widely considered a leader in the field. In fact, Dr Levine and his colleagues at Wake Forest have one of the largest surgical experiences with cytoreductive surgery in the United States. Not only has Dr Levine and his group at Wake Forest published over 100 articles on the topic but also the Wake Forest group has participated in the training of many residents and fellows in the treatment of patients with this challenging disease. As such, Dr Levine is ideally suited to be the guest editor of this important issue of the *Surgical Oncology Clinics of North America*.

The issue covers a number of important topics, including such interesting matters as patient selection, genomics, imaging, as well as palliative management of advanced

Surg Oncol Clin N Am 27 (2018) xiii–xiv
https://doi.org/10.1016/j.soc.2018.03.002
1055-3207/18/© 2018 Published by Elsevier Inc.

peritoneal carcinomatosis. The issue specifically covers evolving treatment strategies for cytoreductive surgery and intraperitoneal chemotherapy for patients with gastric cancer, as well as peritoneal metastasis from malignant mesothelioma, appendiceal cancer, and colorectal cancer. Expert surgeons in the field who are internationally recognized for their contributions to the field of peritoneal malignancies handle each topic beautifully. In sum, this is a fantastic, comprehensive, and thorough state-of-the-art review on a wide range of topics relevant to peritoneal malignancies. I would like to thank Dr Levine and his amazing group of colleagues for an excellent issue of the *Surgical Oncology Clinics of North America* and for taking on such an important topic.

Timothy M. Pawlik, MD, MPH, PhD, FACS, RACS (Hon)
Department of Surgery
Oncology, Health Services Management
and Policy
The Ohio State University
Wexner Medical Center
395 West 12th Avenue, Suite 670
Columbus, OH 43210, USA

E-mail address:
Tim.Pawlik@osumc.edu

Preface

Current Management of Peritoneal Surface Malignancy

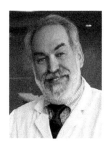

Edward A. Levine, MD
Editor

This issue of the *Surgical Oncology Clinics of North America* represents the third issue dedicated to diagnosis and treatment of peritoneal surface malignancy. The first, volume 12, issue 3, was guest edited by Paul Sugarbaker in 2003,[1] and the second, volume 21, issue 4, was guest edited by Jesus Esquivel in 2012.[2] While both issues are excellent, much has been learned and has changed since the previous issues.

Traditionally, the approach to isolated peritoneal metastases was nihilistic and involved delivering palliative chemotherapy and eventually preparing of the patient for hospice care. This is in stark contrast to the approach to isolate single-system metastases to the liver, lung, adrenal, brain, and lymph nodes from solid tumors, which frequently relies upon surgical resection, with other ablative modalities playing a supporting role. The outcomes for completely resected metastases to the liver or peritoneum from colon cancer, for example, are remarkably similar, yet the utilization of cytoreductive surgery lags far behind the rate of liver resections. Much of the initial resistance from our oncologic colleagues was due to the lack of prospective randomized trials. However, two such trials have been completed for colorectal cancer, both of which strongly support the utility of cytoreductive surgery and hyperthermic intraperitoneal chemotherapy (HIPEC) as clearly improving survival.

There has been a remarkable proliferation of centers treating patients with cytoreductive surgery and intraperitoneal chemotherapy over the past decade. This has been fueled by increasing experience with cytoreductive techniques and HIPEC, which shows outcomes far superior to that achieved with systemic chemotherapy alone. Dr Paul Sugarbaker's lead article recounts the history of this emerging modality and highlights the roles of surgeons and centers' pioneering efforts.

The other articles in this issue cover a variety of related topics. Patient selection for this frequently formidable procedure is crucial for best outcomes. Consequently, several articles have been dedicated to these selection issues: imaging for peritoneal

Surg Oncol Clin N Am 27 (2018) xv–xvi
https://doi.org/10.1016/j.soc.2018.03.001
1055-3207/18/© 2018 Published by Elsevier Inc.

surgonc.theclinics.com

metastases, genomics of peritoneal malignancies, and patient selection for cytoreductive surgery. Understanding the pharmacokinetic implications of intracavitary drug delivery is background that needs to be understood by oncologists of all types and is explained in the article by Dr Wim Ceelen. Similarly, the techniques and safety issues involved as well as the long learning curves associated with these procedures are addressed and should be of interest to those considering starting a new program.

The more common indications for cytoreductive surgery and HIPEC are discussed in the articles on mesothelioma, colorectal, appendiceal, and gastric cancers. Despite our best efforts, many of these ailments will recur, and many patients will eventually succumb to their disease. Therefore, a new article in this issue relates to palliative management of advanced peritoneal disease by Dr Laura A. Lambert.

The authors of this issue represent many of the leaders from preeminent international centers. The consistency of the data from the experienced centers underscores that, in this approach to the problem, it is the biology of the disease and the condition of the patient that determine the outcome. Interest in more aggressive approaches to peritoneal metastases is clearly expanding, supported by meetings such as the Regional Cancer Therapies Symposium and the Peritoneal Surface Oncology Group International. Furthermore, the significant increase in the quality of the applied translational science as well as the significant increase in the number of prospective randomized trials implies that improvement in our ability to care for our patients is on the horizon. Clearly, as this issue illustrates, the era of approaching our patients with peritoneal surface malignancy with therapeutic nihilism is over.

Edward A. Levine, MD
Surgical Oncology Service
Department of General Surgery
Wake Forest University
Wake Forest University Medical Center Boulevard
Winston Salem, NC 27157, USA

E-mail address:
elevine@wakehealth.edu

REFERENCES

1. Sugarbaker PH. Management of peritoneal surface malignancy. Preface. Surg Oncol Clin N Am 2003;12:xxi–xxv.
2. Esquivel J. Treatment of peritoneal surface malignancies. Surg Oncol Clin N Am 2012;21:xv–xviii.

Peritoneal Metastases, a Frontier for Progress

Paul H. Sugarbaker, MD, FACS, FRCS

KEYWORDS

- HIPEC • Intraperitoneal chemotherapy • Appendiceal mucinous neoplasms
- Pseudomyxoma peritonei • Colorectal cancer • Hyperthermia

KEY POINTS

- Peritoneal metastases has been an unsolved problem in oncology, causing progressive disease in a large proportion of patients with gastric, colorectal, and pancreas cancers.
- The current standard of care for success in management of peritoneal metastases from gastrointestinal cancer combines complete cytoreductive surgery, perioperative intraperitoneal chemotherapy, and intraperitoneal hyperthermia.
- Peritonectomy and visceral resections are used to surgically eliminate all visible evidence of peritoneal metastases so that hyperthermic intraperitoneal chemotherapy can eliminate microscopic disease.
- Efforts to develop treatments that show success in the cure of peritoneal surface malignancy have been combined multinational initiatives in Europe, the United States, Japan, and Australia.

INTRODUCTION

There is a glimmer of hope that a major enemy of the success in a cure of gastrointestinal and gynecologic malignancy may be brought under control. This consistent cause of treatment failure is peritoneal metastases. However, now we are learning how to use peritonectomy and visceral resections to achieve a complete visible clearing of the abdominal and pelvic space. In addition, we are learning how to use cancer chemotherapy as an integral part of this surgical intervention. There is now a combined management strategy, perhaps not perfect, but safe enough and effective enough to become a standard of care for selected patients with appendiceal peritoneal metastases, colorectal peritoneal metastases, and peritoneal mesothelioma.[1] The possibilities for prevention and treatment strategies for gastrointestinal and gynecologic malignancy may be nothing short of spectacular!

Financial Disclosure: The author has nothing to disclose.
Program in Peritoneal Surface Oncology, Center for Gastrointestinal Malignancies, MedStar Washington Hospital Center, 106 Irving Street, Northwest, Suite 3900, Washington, DC 20010, USA
E-mail address: Paul.Sugarbaker@medstar.net

Surg Oncol Clin N Am 27 (2018) 413–424
https://doi.org/10.1016/j.soc.2018.02.001
1055-3207/18/© 2018 Elsevier Inc. All rights reserved.

Where did the combined treatment strategies get started? Who made them work? How has it grown so definitively to bring us all together here this evening? I hope this article can answer some of these questions. This is peritoneal metastases, a frontier for progress.

WHY STUDY PERITONEAL METASTASES?

People ask why spend so much time and effort dedicated to the study of peritoneal metastases. For Francois Gilly, that answer was easy. This is a terrible problem in oncology that, in the past, had no reasonable treatments. The French multi-institutional prospective study, EVOCAPE 1 (Evolution of Peritoneal Carcinomatosis), was designed to establish the natural history of peritoneal metastases in patients with gastric cancer, colorectal cancer, and pancreas cancer.[2] The data collected were even more shocking than previously expected. It was gathered from the time of diagnosis of the primary cancer with peritoneal seeding in 212 patients and from 158 patients when peritoneal seeding was diagnosed in follow-up. The median survival of 125 patients with gastric cancer with peritoneal seeding was 3.1 months. The median survival of 118 patients with colorectal cancer with peritoneal seeding was 5.2 months, and for patients with pancreas cancer it was only 2.1 months.

Also, the data showed that the extent of disease was an important determinant of survival. Peritoneal metastases should not be recorded, as in the past, as present versus absent but the disease should be quantitated. EVOCAPE data showed that patients with cancerous nodules less than 5 mm lived significantly longer than patients with nodules greater than 5 mm. The answer to this question, "Why study carcinomatosis?" is that this is a terrible problem in oncology—something needed to be done!

INTRAPERITONEAL CANCER CHEMOTHERAPY

Perhaps we will never know who first infused cancer chemotherapy into the peritoneal space in a patient with peritoneal metastases. However, it is clear that Dedrick and colleagues[3] at the American National Cancer Institute provided a rationale for direct intraperitoneal administration. Dedrick and coworkers discovered that the rate at which anticancer drugs leave the peritoneal space is considerably slower than the rate at which the body metabolizes or excretes the drug. This results in a marked increased concentration of cancer chemotherapy at the peritoneal surface and also at the surface of a peritoneal cancer nodule as compared with the concentration in the bloodstream and bone marrow. Dedrick and coworkers' data showed that intraperitoneal instillation would produce greater local efficacy but less systemic toxicity. Mitomycin C is a common drug now used for intraperitoneal instillation in patients with peritoneal metastases (**Fig. 1**). In this pharmacologic study, on the vertical axis the concentration of the drug is plotted. The time over a period of 90 minutes is shown on the horizontal axis. At all points in time the intraperitoneal concentration of mitomycin C is much greater than in the blood. Mathematically, the exposure of a cancer nodule is more than 27 times greater than the exposure of bone marrow cells.[4] Intraperitoneal instillation of selected cancer chemotherapy agents may cause greater efficacy within the peritoneal space and less toxicity to the body.

HEAT ALONE IN THE PERITONEAL SPACE

The use of heat to fight cancer is as old as Greek medicine. Hippocrates said, "Those diseases which medicines do not cure, the knife cures; those which the knife cannot cure, fire cures; and those which fire cannot cure, are to be reckoned wholly incurable."[5] The use of intraperitoneal heat alone to help control cancer was not described

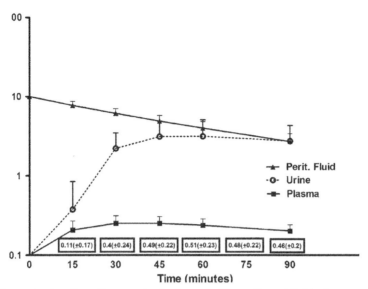

Fig. 1. Concentration times time graph of mitomycin C in peritoneal fluid, plasma, and urine in 145 patients. The area under the curve ratio of peritoneal fluid to plasma was 26.6 ± 7.1. Peak plasma concentration was 0.25 ± 0.06 μg/mL at 30 minutes. Also shown are the total milligrams of mitomycin C excreted in the urine at 15-minute intervals. (*From* Van der Speeten K, Stuart OA, Chang D, et al. Changes induced by surgical and clinical factors in the pharmacology of intraperitoneal mitomycin C in 145 patients with peritoneal carcinomatosis. Cancer Chemother Pharmacol 2011;68:150; with permission.)

until 1995. Shiu and Fortner[6] at Memorial Sloan Kettering Cancer Center devised an apparatus that looks similar to a modern hyperthermic intraperitoneal chemotherapy (HIPEC) machine. There was a water bath, a heat exchanger, a thermometer, and a pump to maintain a closed circuit for warm saline. In one of the experiments, rats were treated for 4 days after intraperitoneal injection of cancer cells. The treatment was for 30 minutes and the temperature was 43°C. Data show the percentage of experimental animals surviving the peritoneal metastases over time when heat was administered 4 days after cancer cells were injected intraperitoneally. The survival of heat-treated rats was 65%. The survival of the control rats was 5%. In these and several other experiments, intraperitoneal heat significantly improved the survival of rats inoculated with intraperitoneal cancer.

THE FIRST HYPERTHERMIC INTRAPERITONEAL CHEMOTHERAPY

There can be no doubt that John Spratt was the first to bring these laboratory observations together as a clinical experiment. A delivery system for hyperthermic intraperitoneal chemotherapy was created. He called the apparatus the "thermal infusion filtration system or TIFS." The apparatus was originally described as a master's thesis at the University of Missouri.[7] After Dr Spratt moved to Louisville, Kentucky, he treated a 33-year-old man with pseudomyxoma peritonei. First, he performed surgical resection and this was followed by intraperitoneal heated thiotepa at 42°C for 90 minutes. In the article published in *Cancer Research*, no adverse events were recorded and the procedure was repeated with methotrexate 8 days later.[8] The long-term outcome of this clinical research is not known.

HYPERTHERMIC INTRAPERITONEAL CHEMOTHERAPY GOES TO JAPAN

Curiously, the HIPEC technology described by Spratt was not further developed in the United States or Europe. However, the Japanese were quick to see the possible application of heated intraperitoneal chemotherapy to treat or prevent peritoneal metastases from gastric cancer. In 1984, Koga and coworkers[9] in Yonago, Japan, took Spratt's concept back to the animal laboratory. They treated rats by continuous hyperthermic peritoneal perfusion, introducing a new Japanese drug, mitomycin C. Donryu rats inoculated intraperitoneally with an ascites hepatoma survived longer when treated with heat plus mitomycin C versus heat alone or mitomycin C alone ($P<.05$).

Also, Koga and his team reported in 1988 a study to prevent peritoneal metastases in serosal-positive patients with gastric cancer treated with mitomycin C.[10] The historical control and randomized studies were both positive. This study was the first effort to use an adjuvant HIPEC. It was the forerunner of the current prospective and randomized study, GASTRICHIP.[11]

Fujimoto and colleagues[12,13] from Chiba, Japan, published a series of articles on the treatment of peritoneal metastases and the prevention of peritoneal metastases from gastric cancer, which included randomized studies.

Fujimura, Yonemura, and others from Kanazawa, Japan, introduced cisplatin at 300 mg and mitomycin C at 30 mg as a HIPEC solution to prevent peritoneal metastases.[14] In his 58 randomized patients, heated intraperitoneal chemotherapy was more effective than normothermic intraperitoneal chemotherapy and the control patients has the poorest survival ($P<.01$).

PERITONECTOMY PROCEDURES AND PROGNOSTIC INDICATORS

The pharmacologic studies showed high concentrations of chemotherapy in the peritoneal space but limited penetration into the cancer nodule. Chemotherapy entered the cancer nodule only by simple diffusion. Also, data showed no long-term survival if intraperitoneal chemotherapy was used in patients with visible cancer. Nodules needed to be extremely small, preferably microscopic in size. To treat peritoneal metastases, the peritonectomy procedures were developed.[15] A fixed retractor, proper patient position, and high-voltage electrosurgery along with a generous amount of patience and persistence were necessary to achieve a complete visible resection of peritoneal metastases and involved viscera.

An observation not uncommon to cancer treatments was that not all patients benefitted. As larger numbers of patients were treated, the clinical features and histopathology could be analyzed and the prognostic features of peritoneal metastases patients could be determined.[16] This makes it possible to select patients most likely to benefit.

Sugarbaker and Jablonski[17] reported that (1) patients with appendiceal malignancy survived better than patients with colon cancer, (2) complete cytoreduction was far superior to incomplete, and (3) a small or moderate volume of peritoneal metastases showed improved survival as compared with gross disease. After the peritoneal cancer index (**Fig. 2**) became available, quantitating the extent of disease became necessary in all patients.[18]

HYPERTHERMIC INTRAPERITONEAL CHEMOTHERAPY RETURNS TO EUROPE AND THE UNITED STATES

In the early 1990s, heated intraperitoneal chemotherapy returned from Japan to both Europe and the United States. Francois Gilly and Annie Sayag reported on an experimental study in dogs, but they rapidly moved to the treatment of patients with

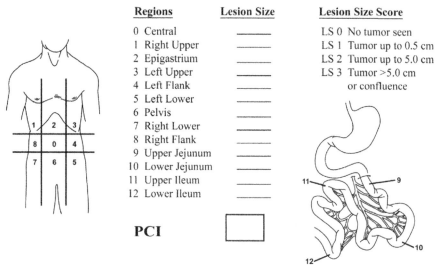

Regions	Lesion Size	Lesion Size Score
0 Central	————	LS 0 No tumor seen
1 Right Upper	————	LS 1 Tumor up to 0.5 cm
2 Epigastrium	————	LS 2 Tumor up to 5.0 cm
3 Left Upper	————	LS 3 Tumor >5.0 cm
4 Left Flank	————	or confluence
5 Left Lower	————	
6 Pelvis	————	
7 Right Lower	————	
8 Right Flank	————	
9 Upper Jejunum	————	
10 Lower Jejunum	————	
11 Upper Ileum	————	
12 Lower Ileum	————	

PCI

Fig. 2. Peritoneal cancer index (PCI). Two transverse planes and 2 sagittal planes divide the abdomen into 9 regions. The upper transverse plane is located at the lowest aspect of the costal margin and the lower transverse plane is placed at the anterior superior iliac spine. The sagittal planes divide the abdomen into 3 equal sectors. The lines define the 9 regions that are numbered in a clockwise direction with 0 at the umbilicus and 1 defining the space beneath the right hemidiaphragm. Regions 9 to 12 divide the small bowel. Lesion size score is determined after complete lysis of all adhesions and the complete inspection of all parietal and visceral peritoneal surfaces. It refers to the greatest diameter of tumor implants that are distributed on the peritoneal surfaces. Primary tumors or localized recurrences at the primary site that can be removed definitively are excluded from the lesion size assessment. If there is confluence of disease matting abdominal or pelvic structures together, this is automatically scored as L-3, even if it is a thin confluence of cancerous implants. (*Data from* Jacquet P, Sugarbaker PH. Current methodologies for clinical assessment of patients with peritoneal carcinomatosis. J Exp Clin Cancer Res 1996;15(1):49–58, and is available under a Creative Commons Attribution License 4.0.)

peritoneal metastases.[19] The goal of their efforts was to standardize an apparatus that would safely and reproducibly treat patients with peritoneal metastases using a heated chemotherapy solution with mitomycin C.

In the United States, several groups focused on the safety and efficacy of cytoreductive surgery plus perioperative heated intraperitoneal chemotherapy. However, to this point in time, no one had assessed the functional status and quality of life of these patients before and after treatment. In a National Institutes of Health-funded protocol, McQuellon and coworkers[20] studied 64 patients' function and quality of life. They used an assessment tool called Functional Assessment of Cancer Therapy for Colon Malignancy. Postoperatively, the Functional Assessment of Cancer Therapy for Colon Malignancy score decreased, by 3 months it was back to baseline, and by 6 months exceeded baseline values. The improvement in functional assessment as compared with baseline was most evident in patients who had malignant ascites.

A DUTCH RANDOMIZED TRIAL

Frans Zoetmulder has been interested in peritoneal metastases throughout his surgical career. His Dutch surgical thesis defended in 1981 was concerned with experimental peritoneal metastases. In the presence of a peritoneal wound, 10 to 100 times fewer cancer cells were needed to establish tumor growth after intraperitoneal injection compared with mice with an intact peritoneum.[21] The intact peritoneum protected mice against peritoneal metastases. He also showed that tumor cells embedded in fibrin were protected against irrigation with saline or with cytotoxic solutions. In other words, a fibrin matrix protected the cancer cells. He concluded that surgical trauma played a prominent role in peritoneal metastases with gastrointestinal malignancy. Professor Zoetmulder said, "When I heard about heated chemotherapy washing of the abdomen and pelvis after a maximal surgical effort, I felt compelled to try and prove or disprove that peritoneal metastases could be effectively treated." He did a number of things, in an orderly manner, to try and answer this question. First, he gathered together a great group of people at Antoni van Leeuwenhoek Hospital who energetically helped with this project. Second, he attempted to optimize the intraperitoneal chemotherapy used after a maximal surgical effort so that it was not only effective but also safe. His studies developed a high-dose heated mitomycin C solution given at times 0 minutes, 30 minutes, and 60 minutes for a 90-minute irrigation of the peritoneal space. This intraoperative treatment remains the standard of care in Holland. Third, after he gained considerable surgical expertise with cytoreductive surgery, a randomized trial was initiated. Patients in this trial were documented to have peritoneal metastases from colon or rectal cancer. In the experimental group, patients received a maximal cytoreductive surgery plus HIPEC. Other patients received the standard of care. After 105 patients, there was a statistically significant improvement in survival with a P-value of .032. Because of this definitive survival advantage, the ethics committee closed the study (**Fig. 3**). Cytoreductive surgery and HIPEC continues as a standard of care in Europe for patients with peritoneal metastases from colorectal cancer.

LEARNING CURVE

Moran and coworkers started performing cytoreductive surgery with perioperative chemotherapy for pseudomyxoma peritonei in 1994 and have reported on more than 1000 cases.[22] As he reviewed the first 100 consecutive patients, it became clear that there was a profound change in the outcome of this complex surgical procedure.[23] It did not seem as though there was a great difference over time with efficacy; however, there were tremendous differences over time in the safety of this procedure. He divided these first 100 patients into 3 groups. In the first group of 33 patients, the mortality was 18%, 15% underwent reoperation for bleeding, and there was a 12% incidence of anastomotic leakage. In the second group of 33 patients, the mortality decreased drastically to 3%, the operations for bleeding decreased also, as did the anastomotic leakage rate. In the final group of 34 patients, the mortality remained at 3% but there were no reoperations for bleeding and no anastomotic leakage. Moran concluded that the main components of this learning curve involved patient selection, technical factors, and an improved infrastructure involving teamwork.

MULTIINSTITUTIONAL STUDIES

Our efforts to cure peritoneal metastases would not be where they are today in the absence of multiinstitutional studies. In 2004, Glehen and colleagues[24] from 28 institutions gathered retrospectively data on 506 patients with colon or rectal cancer treated with cytoreductive surgery and perioperative intraperitoneal chemotherapy. Patients with appendiceal malignancy were excluded. The absolute requirement for complete cytoreduction was confirmed. The 5-year survival for patients having a complete cytoreduction was 31%. In the multivariate analysis, significant variables were

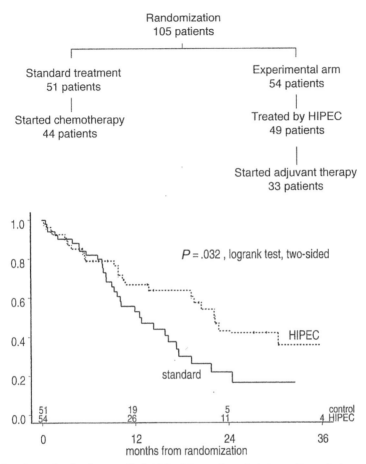

Fig. 3. Dutch randomized controlled trial of hyperthermic intraperitoneal chemotherapy (HIPEC) versus standard of care. (*From* Verwaal VJ, van Ruth S, de Bree E, et al. Randomized trial of cytoreduction and hyperthermic intraperitoneal chemotherapy versus systemic chemotherapy and palliative surgery in patients with peritoneal carcinomatosis of colorectal cancer. J Clin Oncol 2003;21(20):3741; with permission.)

completeness of cytoreduction, second-look surgery, extent of peritoneal metastases by the peritoneal cancer index, lymph node involvement, age, tumor differentiation, and synchronous resection of liver metastases (**Table 1**).

FRENCH MULTIINSTITUTIONAL STUDIES

The next multiinstitutional study was from French-speaking institutions. It was a monumental effort first reported at the 110 Congress of French Surgeons and then at the 8th Biennial Peritoneal Surface Oncology Group International (PSOGI) meeting in 2008 in Lyon. These data were published as a monograph in French, but then as separate articles in high-impact journals in English.[25] The graph on the overall survival of 1290 patients showed that cure was a reasonable goal in all diseases treated, including pseudomyxoma peritonei, appendix cancer, colorectal cancer, gastric cancer, and malignant peritoneal mesothelioma. These authors produced data showing

Table 1
International multiinstitutional study of hyperthermic intraperitoneal chemotherapy in colorectal peritoneal metastases

Variable	Cox Coefficient	P
Completeness of cytoreduction	0.71	<.0001
Treatment with second procedure	−1.10	<.001
Carcinomatosis extent	0.51	<.001
Lymph node involvement	0.23	.002
Age	0.54	.002
Tumor differentiation	0.26	.003
Synchronous resection of liver metastasis	0.52	.004
Preoperative systemic chemotherapy	0.33	.01
Adjuvant systemic chemotherapy	−0.26	.04
Treatment with IPCH	−0.33	.07
Treatment with EPIC	−0.22	.17
Sex	0.18	.12
Synchronous resection of primary tumor	0.05	.76

A negative Cox coefficient indicates improved survival. The data are a multivariate survival analysis of 506 patients treated with cytoreductive surgery combined with perioperative intraperitoneal chemotherapy.

Abbreviations: EPIC, early postoperative intraperitoneal chemotherapy; IPCH, intraperitoneal chemohyperthermia.

From Glehen O, Kwiatkowski F, Sugarbaker PH, et al. Cytoreductive surgery combined with perioperative intraperitoneal chemotherapy for the management of peritoneal carcinomatosis from colorectal cancer: a multi-institutional study. J Clin Oncol 2004;22(16):3288; with permission.

that not only were the treatment modalities important, but the institution performing the treatments had a profound effect on outcome.[26]

Although HIPEC with mitomycin C or mitomycin C plus cisplatin was a standard of care in these multiinstitutional reports, a new and perhaps more modern HIPEC was reported by Elias and French coworkers in 2009. Carefully controlled in this study was the selection of patients.[27] With hyperthermic intraperitoneal oxaliplatin and systemic 5-fluorouracil, a 51% survival was achieved at 5 years. The standard treatment group of matched patients was 13%, and what might be expected with systemic chemotherapy only (**Fig. 4**).

PROGRESS IN EUROPE

The efforts of PSOGI since its beginning have been to promote research and to educate surgical oncologists, medical oncologists, nurses, and paramedical personnel regarding peritoneal metastases treatment and the outcomes that are expected. Our PSOGI meeting in Madrid in 2004 had 300 participants and the exchange of information resulted in a special issue of *European Journal of Surgical Oncology*. In 2006, we had the PSOGI meeting in Milan. This was a consensus meeting using the Delphi methodology. The term HIPEC was born and the many concepts for optimal treatment were standardized. A special issue of the *Journal of Surgical Oncology* was produced.[28] A special issue of *The Cancer Journal* resulted from the 2008 meeting in Lyon, France.[29] Our collaborative efforts with the European Society of Surgical Oncology to implement the European Peritoneal Surface Oncology Training Program are now available with an established curriculum.[30]

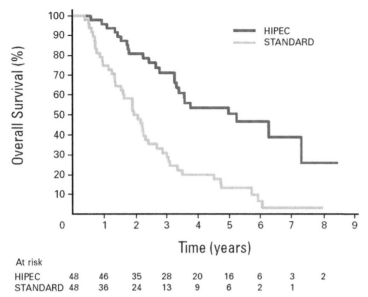

Fig. 4. French study of hyperthermic intraperitoneal chemotherapy (HIPEC) versus modern systemic chemotherapy. The overall survival of the group undergoing cytoreductive surgery, HIPEC, and systemic treatment versus those receiving standard treatment. (*From* Elias D, Lefevre JH, Chevalier J, et al. Complete cytoreductive surgery plus intraperitoneal chemohyperthermia with oxaliplatin for peritoneal carcinomatosis of colorectal origin. J Clin Oncol 2009;27(5):683; with permission.)

PROGRESS IN THE UNITED STATES

However, the efforts to share research data and educate regarding the management of peritoneal metastases has been active in the United States. The first international symposium on Regional Cancer Therapies was held in 2006 and has continued through 2016. Bartlett and coworkers have produced a special issue of *Annals of Surgical Oncology* on peritoneal metastases from each of the 11 international symposia held to date.

PROGRESS IN ASIA

The efforts to prevent or treat peritoneal metastases are active in Asia. Yonemura directs a peritoneal metastases consortium in the Osaka area, there are 4 hospitals engaged in the treatment of peritoneal metastases, especially those of appendiceal and colorectal origins. Efforts throughout Japan continue with special emphasis on the management of peritoneal metastases from gastric cancer.[31] In China, many institutions involved in peritoneal surface oncology clinical and laboratory research.[32] The outstanding efforts of Dr Li in Beijing, China, deserve special mention. David Morris and his team in Sydney, Australia, have maintained a high level of productivity.[33]

THE END OF THE BEGINNING

Currently, a lot of time and thought has been directed toward the management of ovarian cancer. Perhaps complete cytoreductive surgery with peritoneal and visceral resections along with HIPEC can bring about a significant survival benefit with this disease. There is also a focus on prevention. Will this be the greatest contribution of perioperative chemotherapy to the management of gastrointestinal cancer? Is there a new and more effective HIPEC to add to cytoreduction to preserve the surgical complete response? Maybe long-term intravenous and intraperitoneal chemotherapy will be the focus of our next clinical trials adventures.[34] We have come a long way. We have a long way to go. It is a global effort!

REFERENCES

1. O'Dwyer S, Verwaal VJ, Sugarbaker PH. Evolution of treatments for peritoneal metastases from colorectal cancer. J Clin Oncol 2015;33:2122.
2. Sadeghi B, Arvieux C, Glehen O, et al. Peritoneal carcinomatosis from non-gynecologic malignancies: results of the EVOCAPE 1 multicentric prospective study. Cancer 2000;88(2):358–63.
3. Dedrick RL, Myers CE, Bungay PM, et al. Pharmacokinetic rationale for peritoneal drug administration in the treatment of ovarian cancer. Cancer Treat Rep 1978; 62(1):1–11.
4. Van der Speeten K, Stuart OA, Chang D, et al. Changes induced by surgical and clinical factors in the pharmacology of intraperitoneal mitomycin C in 145 patients with peritoneal carcinomatosis. Cancer Chemother Pharmacol 2011;68:147–56.
5. Adams F. The genuine works of Hippocrates. New York: William Wood & Co; 1886. p. 273.
6. Shiu MH, Fortner JG. Intraperitoneal hyperthermic treatment of implanted peritoneal cancer in rats. Cancer Res 1980;40(11):4081–4.
7. Palta JR. Design and testing of a therapeutic infusion filtration system [M. S. Thesis]. Columbia (MO): University of Missouri; 1977.
8. Spratt JS, Adcock RA, Muskovin M, et al. Clinical delivery system for intraperitoneal hyperthermic chemotherapy. Cancer Res 1980;40(2):256–60.
9. Koga S, Hamazoe R, Maeta M, et al. Treatment of implanted peritoneal cancer in rats by continuous hyperthermic peritoneal perfusion in combination with an anticancer drug. Cancer Res 1984;44(5):1840–2.
10. Koga S, Hamazoe R, Meate M, et al. Prophylactic therapy for peritoneal recurrence of gastric cancer by continuous hyperthermic peritoneal perfusion with mitomycin C. Cancer 1998;61:232–7.
11. Glehen O, Passot G, Villeneuve L, et al. GASTRICHIP: D2 resection and hyperthermic intraperitoneal chemotherapy in locally advanced gastric carcinoma: a randomized and multicenter phase III study. BMC Cancer 2014;14(14):183. ClinicalTrials.gov identifier: NCT01882933.
12. Fujimoto S, Shrestha RD, Kokubun M, et al. Positive results of combined therapy of surgery and intraperitoneal hyperthermic perfusion for far-advanced gastric cancer. Ann Surg 1990;212(5):592–6.
13. Fujimoto S, Takahashi M, Mutou T, et al. Successful intraperitoneal hyperthermic chemoperfusion for the prevention of postoperative peritoneal recurrence in patients with advanced gastric carcinoma. Cancer 1998;85:529–34.
14. Fujimura T, Yonemura Y, Fushida S, et al. Continuous hyperthermic peritoneal perfusion for the treatment of peritoneal dissemination in gastric cancers and subsequent second-look operation. Cancer 1990;65(1):65–71.
15. Sugarbaker PH. Peritonectomy procedures. Ann Surg 1995;221:29–42.
16. Jacquet P, Sugarbaker PH. Current methodologies for clinical assessment of patients with peritoneal carcinomatosis. J Exp Clin Cancer Res 1996;15(1): 49–58.

17. Sugarbaker PH, Jablonski KA. Prognostic features of 51 colorectal and 130 appendiceal cancer patients with peritoneal carcinomatosis treated by cytoreductive surgery and intraperitoneal chemotherapy. Ann Surg 1995;221(2):124–32.
18. Sugarbaker PH. Successful management of microscopic residual disease in large bowel cancer. Cancer Chemother Pharmacol 1999;43(Suppl):S15–25.
19. Gilly FN, Sayag AC, Carry PY, et al. Intra-peritoneal chemo-hyperthermia (CHIP): a new therapy in the treatment of the peritoneal seedings. Preliminary report. Int Surg 1991;76(3):164–7.
20. McQuellon RP, Loggie BW, Fleming RA, et al. Quality of life after intraperitoneal hyperthermic chemotherapy (IPHC) for peritoneal carcinomatosis. Eur J Surg Oncol 2001;27(1):65–73.
21. Verwaal VJ, van Ruth S, de Bree E, et al. Randomized trial of cytoreduction and hyperthermic intraperitoneal chemotherapy versus systemic chemotherapy and palliative surgery in patients with peritoneal carcinomatosis of colorectal cancer. J Clin Oncol 2003;21(20):3737–43.
22. Ansari N, Chandrakumaran K, Dayal S, et al. Cytoreductive surgery and hyperthermic intraperitoneal chemotherapy in 1000 patients with perforated appendiceal epithelial tumours. Eur J Surg Oncol 2016;42(7):1035–41.
23. Moran BJ. Decision-making and technical factors account for the learning curve in complex surgery. J Public Health (Oxf) 2006;28(4):375–8.
24. Glehen O, Kwiatkowski F, Sugarbaker PH, et al. Cytoreductive surgery combined with perioperative intraperitoneal chemotherapy for the management of peritoneal carcinomatosis from colorectal cancer: a multi-institutional study. J Clin Oncol 2004;22(16):3284–92.
25. Glehen O, Elias D, Gilly FN. Presentation du rapport de l' Association Francaise de Chirurgie. In: Elias D, Gilly FN, Glehen O, editors. Carcinoses Peritoneales D'Origine Digestive et Primitive. France: Arnette Wolkers Kluwer; 2008. p. 101–52.
26. Glehen O, Sugarbaker PH. Special issue on management of peritoneal carcinomatosis from colorectal and appendiceal malignancy. Glehen O, Sugarbaker PH, editors. Cancer J 2009; 15(3), pp.181–254.
27. Elias D, Lefevre JH, Chevalier J, et al. Complete cytoreductive surgery plus intraperitoneal chemohyperthermia with oxaliplatin for peritoneal carcinomatosis of colorectal origin. J Clin Oncol 2009;27(5):681–5.
28. Kusamura S, Baratti D, Younan R, et al. The Delphi approach to attain consensus in methodology of local regional therapy for peritoneal surface malignancy. J Surg Oncol 2008;98(4):217–9.
29. Special issue on management of peritoneal carcinomatosis from colorectal and appendiceal malignancy. Glehen O, Sugarbaker PH, editors. Cancer J 2009; 15(3).
30. Gonzalez-Moreno S, Deraca M. European School of Peritoneal Surface Oncology and European Peritoneal Surface Oncology training program. Available at: http://www.essoweb.org/school-of-peritoneal-surface-oncology-es/; http://www.essoweb.org/european-school-of-peritoneal-surface-oncology-training-programme/. Accessed September 5, 2017.
31. Yonemura Y, Canbay E, Li Y, et al. A comprehensive treatment for peritoneal metastases from gastric cancer with curative intent. Eur J Surg Oncol 2016;42(8):1123–31.
32. Yang XJ, Huang CQ, Suo T, et al. Cytoreductive surgery and hyperthermic intraperitoneal chemotherapy improves survival of patients with peritoneal carcinomatosis from gastric cancer: final results of a phase III randomized clinical trial. Ann Surg Oncol 2011;18:1578–81.

33. Pillai K, Akhter J, Morris DL. Assessment of a novel mucolytic solution for dissolving mucus in pseudomyxoma peritonei: an *ex vivo* and *in vitro* study. Pleura and Peritoneum 2017;2:111–7. Available at: https://www.degruyter.com/downloadpdf/j/pp.2017.2.issue-2/pp-2017-0013/pp-2017-0013.pdf. Accessed March 14, 2018.
34. Chan JK, Java JJ, Fuh K, et al. The association between timing of initiation of adjuvant therapy and the survival of early stage ovarian cancer patients - an analysis of NRG Oncology/Gynecologic Oncology Group trials. Gynecol Oncol 2016; 143(3):490–5.

Imaging for Peritoneal Metastases

Russell N. Low, MD[a],*, Robert M. Barone, MD[b]

KEYWORDS

- Peritoneal tumor • Appendiceal cancer • MRI • PET-CT • Peritoneal cancer index

KEY POINTS

- Of the choices for peritoneal imaging, MRI provides superior depiction of small-volume peritoneal tumor compared with computed tomography (CT) and PET.
- The preoperative magnetic resonance peritoneal cancer index score is reasonably accurate in categorizing the volume of tumor found at surgical exploration.
- Patient selection using preoperative imaging requires accurate assessment of tumor volume and location with attention to the small bowel and mesentery.
- PET-CT is most beneficial if conventional imaging is inconclusive and there is high suspicion of disease, or to rule out extraabdominal metastases.
- Following heated intraperitoneal chemotherapy, patient surveillance with MRI can detect early tumor recurrence before an increase in serum tumor markers.

INTRODUCTION

Imaging of peritoneal metastases plays an essential role in the diagnosis and management of patients with peritoneal malignancy being considered for cytoreductive surgery (CRS) and heated intraperitoneal chemotherapy (HIPEC). Abdominal and pelvic imaging contributes valuable information to initial diagnosis, preoperative staging, patient selection, detection of postoperative complications, and patient surveillance following successful treatment.[1–10]

The combination of complex peritoneal anatomy and small size of peritoneal metastases makes peritoneal tumor imaging arguably the most difficult challenge facing the abdominal imager. Imaging options include computed tomography (CT), MRI, and PET-CT.[6,8,11–27] CT provides strictly cross-sectional anatomic imaging, whereas MRI provides a combination of cross-sectional anatomic imaging and tumor functional imaging. CT and MRI are based on uniquely different imaging principles that determine the characteristic strengths and weaknesses of each test. PET imaging of

---

[a] Department of Radiology, Sharp Memorial Hospital, 7901 Frost Street, San Diego, CA 92123, USA; [b] Department of Surgical Oncology, Sharp Memorial Hospital, 7901 Frost Street, San Diego, CA 92123, USA
* Corresponding author.
E-mail address: rlow52@yahoo.com

Surg Oncol Clin N Am 27 (2018) 425–442
https://doi.org/10.1016/j.soc.2018.02.002
1055-3207/18/© 2018 Elsevier Inc. All rights reserved.

peritoneal tumor provides functional imaging based on an assessment of the tumor's metabolism of glucose.[27]

This article discusses the technical issues surrounding peritoneal imaging, including patient preparation and (magnetic resonance) MR scanning protocols. Image interpretation in the preoperative and surveillance setting is discussed. Comparisons of MRI, CT, and PET and their clinical utility for preoperative assessment of peritoneal cancer index (PCI) and for surveillance of patients following CRS and HIPEC are described.

IMAGING CHOICE FOR PERITONEAL TUMOR IMAGING

In practice, the challenges of depicting small peritoneal metastases in the complex anatomy of the peritoneal cavity have often led to disappointing results.[1–5] In particular, the depiction of very small peritoneal tumors or subtle sheets of tumor coating the peritoneum and mesentery has been limited, leading to misdiagnosis and gross understaging. Despite preoperative imaging, open-close laparotomies continue to be a too common occurrence, highlighting the need for better anatomic and functional imaging of peritoneal metastases.

CT has superior spatial resolution and speed, producing highly detailed anatomic images of the abdomen and pelvis in a matter of seconds. In the cooperative patient, motion artifact is limited. Reformatted coronal and sagittal images allow for multiplanar imaging without any additional imaging time. However, CT is limited to assessing attenuation of x-rays by soft tissues or bone. This 1-dimensional (D) basis for image generation leads to its Achilles heel, which is a very limited soft tissue contrast resolution. The challenges of limited CT soft tissue contrast result in poor CT depiction of small peritoneal tumors, which are often indistinguishable from adjacent bowel, mesentery, ascites, and mucin.[3,5,10] The poor sensitivity of CT for detecting small peritoneal tumors limits its accuracy in determining a patient's preoperative PCI score[5] (**Fig. 1**).

MRI uses multiple contrast mechanisms to improve its sensitivity for depicting small peritoneal tumors. Initial experience confirmed that peritoneal tumors show marked enhancement on images obtained 5 minutes after administration of gadolinium contrast material.[11,12] The increased conspicuity of these enhancing peritoneal tumors improved detection of small and microscopic tumors that are often missed on CT scans and PET. The addition of diffusion MRI further improves peritoneal tumor depiction because most tumors cause restricted diffusion, producing high signal on diffusion-weighted imaging (DWI)[20–26] (**Fig. 2**).

Limitations of MR for peritoneal tumor imaging include longer examination time, which is typically 30 to 45 minutes, and increased motion artifact in the uncooperative patient. The MR examination also requires more attention to detail because it can be performed in many different ways, with different pulse sequences and parameters, which can vary results. Patient preparation with bowel contrast is an essential element, as is the use of pharmacologic agents, to decrease peristalsis. Finally, the interpretation of peritoneal MRI requires additional training for the radiologist.[10]

PET with 2-(fluorine 18 [18F]) fluoro-2-deoxy-D-glucose (FDG) localizes malignant tissue by their increased FDG tracer uptake relative to metabolically normal cells. PET equates to greater sensitivity compared with anatomic imaging techniques but has low specificity. The anatomic imaging of CT was integrated with PET's functional data to increase FDG PET-CT sensitivity and specificity compared with PET or CT alone.[27]

Peritoneal Cancer Index MRI vs CT

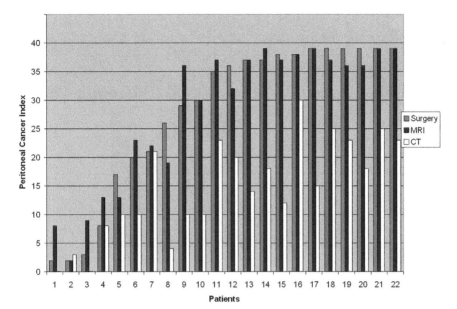

Fig. 1. Comparison of PCI from preoperative MRI, CT, and surgical PCI scores in 22 patients.

TECHNICAL CONSIDERATIONS AND PROTOCOLS FOR PERITONEAL MRI
Patient Preparation

All patients are asked not to eat or drink for the 4 hours before their MR appointment. If rectal water is to be administered, patients self-administer a Fleet enema before the examination.

Intraluminal Contrast Material

Water-soluble intraluminal contrast material is administered to distend the stomach, small bowel, and colon. Collapsed bowel can mask subtle peritoneal tumors or inflammation involving the bowel serosa, mesentery, or adjacent peritoneum. Conversely, nondistended segments of small bowel can be mistaken for an abdominal mass. Adequate bowel distention is, therefore, an essential element in the peritoneal MRI protocol that improves the accuracy and confidence on image interpretation.[17]

Water-soluble contrast material is administered orally beginning 45 minutes before the start of the MRI examination. Patients drink 1.0 to 1.5 L of oral contrast material of sufficient volume to distend the small bowel and stomach. Oral contrast agents are predominantly water with some other agents added to decrease absorption of the material through the small bowel wall. The authors currently use dilute barium sulfate suspension CT contrast material, which is 98% water. E-Z-EM Readi-CAT2 to distend the small bowel for MRI. VoLumen barium sulfate suspension, 0.1% weight to volume, 0.1% weight to weight, 450 mL is composed of sorbitol, bean gum, and water, and can also be used as an MR intraluminal agent.

Distention of the rectum and colon can be accomplished with 1 L of tap water administered through a balloon-tipped barium enema catheter. The balloon should

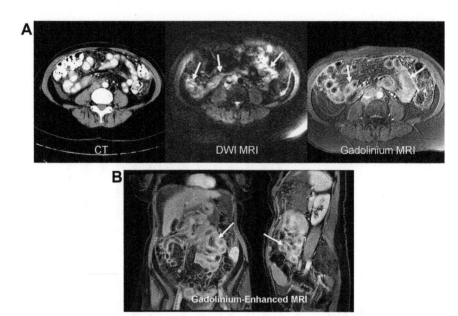

Fig. 2. Appendiceal cancer and serosal tumors: (*A*) CT scan (*left*) through the middle abdomen shows minimal ascites in the right paracolic gutter and no evidence of peritoneal or serosal tumors. DWI MRI, B-value 500 (*middle*), shows scattered and confluent serosal tumors (*arrows*). Gadolinium-enhanced MRI (*right*) shows thickened and enhancing small bowel serosal and mesenteric tumors (*arrows*). Tumors involving the small bowel and mesentery PCI areas 10 to 13 are poorly depicted on CT. MRI combining DWI and delayed gadolinium MRI depicts tumors in these areas with much better accuracy. At surgery, diffuse small bowel serosal tumors were confirmed with a surgical PCI 37 compared with CT PCI 14 and MRI PCI 39. (*B*) Coronal (*left*) and sagittal (*right*) gadolinium-enhanced 3D MRI depicts thickening and enhancement of small bowel and adjacent mesentery representing serosal tumors (*arrows*). The coronal and sagittal images are very useful to confirm small bowel tumors suspected on the transverse MRI.

be filled with water, not air, to decrease the susceptibility artifact that air would create. Although rectal water is not an absolute requirement, it can improve the depiction of subtle serosal and peritoneal tumor involving the colon and rectum.

Intravenous Contrast Agents

Intravenous gadolinium is administered using a power injector at an injection rate of 2 cc per second through an angiocatheter. We currently use a single-dose 0.1 mmol/kg of MultiHance (gadobenate dimeglumine), which may show greater enhancement of peritoneal tumors owing to its higher relaxivity.

Antiperistaltic Agents

A drug should be administered to decrease bowel peristalsis on the gadolinium-enhanced images. The 3D fast spoiled gradient-echo with Dixon water reconstruction (FSPGR) and 2D spoiled gradient-echo (SGE) images are sensitive to bowel motion, and image quality is improved by administering an antiperistaltic pharmacologic agent. Available agents include glucagon for injection, 1 mg administered intravenously at the time of gadolinium injection, Buscopan (hyoscine-N-butyl bromide), and Levsin (hyoscyamine sulfate Injection) 0.25 mg administered intravenously at the start of the examination. Before use, package inserts for all of these medications should be carefully reviewed to understand contraindications and potential drug interactions.

MAGNETIC RESONANCE HARDWARE, SCANNER, AND COILS

A high field strength MR scanner, 1.5 T or 3 T, should be used for imaging peritoneal tumors. High performance gradients (50 mT/m, 200 mT/m/s) are advantageous for high-quality DWI but are not absolutely essential. In practice, peritoneal imaging on 3.0-T MR scanners may be limited by dielectric artifact caused by the presence of ascites. An external phased array surface coil providing simultaneous coverage of the abdomen and pelvis should be used to improve signal and image quality. Typically this requires a surface coil large enough to provide at least 50 cm in the craniocaudal direction. Using the large body coil without a phased array surface coil is not an acceptable option.

MRI Peritoneal Protocol

General principles
The authors' protocol for peritoneal imaging is optimized for depicting small peritoneal tumors.[9,17,20] All images are obtained during suspended respiration to minimize breathing artifact that can obscure subtle peritoneal tumors or inflammation. Other key elements that improve tumor depiction are fat suppression and high spatial resolution. Fat suppression is used for T2-weighted imaging, DWI, and all gadolinium-enhanced images. By suppressing the high signal intensity fat, small peritoneal tumors become more conspicuous.

Table 1 lists the specific imaging parameters for the authors' current peritoneal MRI protocol. In summary, the examination includes axial dual-echo T1 SGE images, fat-suppressed T2-weighted single-shot FSE imaging, and breath hold DWI using an intermediate B-value of 800 s/mm^2. Following injection of .10 mmol/kg intravenous gadolinium, we obtain fat-suppressed 3D FSPGR images in the axial plane twice through the abdomen and pelvis. Coronal and sagittal 3D FSPGR imaging is performed. The final set of images is the axial 2D SGE with fat suppression. The authors find these images are less sensitive to breathing and motion artifact, which is common at the end of the study. The fat-suppressed 2D SGE images are obtained about 5 minutes after the injection of gadolinium when slowly enhancing peritoneal tumors are most conspicuous.[9,10]

PREOPERATIVE EVALUATION OF PATIENTS BEING CONSIDERED FOR CYTOREDUCTIVE SURGERY AND HEATED INTRAPERITONEAL CHEMOTHERAPY

Preoperative imaging has a role in several categories. Detecting systemic metastases to the liver, other solid visceral organs, bones, and pleura is important to exclude those patients from consideration for CRS and HIPEC.[3] Accurately depicting the size and location of peritoneal metastases to the 13 abdominal and pelvic regions can allow the radiologist to calculate a radiologic PCI. This assessment requires accurate imaging evaluation of the entire peritoneal cavity, including parietal peritoneal surfaces; the visceral peritoneum, including bowel serosa; and the mesentery. The peritoneal reflections and recesses surrounding the liver and other upper abdominal organs and the pelvis can present challenges owing to the complex anatomy and collapsed anatomic structures, which can obscure small peritoneal tumors.

Preoperative imaging can assess for complications of abdominal tumor, including small bowel obstruction, gastric outlet obstruction, malignant ureteral obstruction

Table 1
Peritoneal MRI protocol

Pulse Sequence	TR (ms)	TE (ms)	Matrix	NSA	Thick (mm)	Gap (mm)	FOV (cm)	FA Degrees
SSFSE	Infinite	80	320 × 226	0.6	8	0	40	90
T1 3D	172	4.4/2.2	320 × 224	1	4	−2.2	36	12
T2 SSFSE	Min	88	320 × 224	0.6	8	2	36	90
DWI	3900	Minimum	192 × 224	3	8	2	36	90
Gadolinium Injection								
3D FSPGR Dixon	7.06	2.39	320 × 288	1	4.4	−2.2	36	12
2D SGE	125	Minimum	256 × 192	1	8	2	36	80

Pulse Sequence	Bandwidth	Fat-suppressed	Plane	Notes	Time (s)
SSFSE	62.5	No	C	—	15
T1 3D	83.3	No	A	—	21
T2 SSFSE	62.5	Yes	A	—	14
DWI	62.5	Yes	A	B50 b800	30
Gadolinium Injection					
3D FSPGR Dixon	—	—	Ax2	Dixon	22
	83.3	Dixon	C S	Water	—
2D SGE	31.25	Yes	A	—	22

Table shows imaging parameters for complete prostate MR examination.
Parallel imaging is used on all sequences.
Abbreviation: FOV, field of view.

with hydronephrosis, and direct tumor extension through the diaphragm with pleural metastases.

Finally, determining tumor resectability based on these findings on preoperative imaging can prevent unnecessary laparotomy in patients whose excessive tumor burden or involvement of critical structures would preclude successful cytoreduction.

TUMOR DETECTION AND DETERMINATION OF PERITONEAL CANCER INDEX SCORE
Preoperative Computed Tomography

Although CT is routinely used at almost all medical centers for peritoneal cancer assessment, its shortcomings in accurately detecting peritoneal tumors is well documented (**Fig. 3**). Chua and colleagues[7] found that the accuracy in depicting peritoneal lesions using CT, regardless of size, ranged from 51% to 88% in the 9 abdominal-pelvic regions and 21% to 25% in the 4 small intestinal regions in pseudomyxoma peritonei. In comparing the radiologic CT PCI with the operative PCI in this study, the radiologic PCI consistently underestimated the volume of peritoneal disease.

Peritoneal tumor depiction is directly related to the size of the metastases. Koh and colleagues[5] reported that CT identified the presence of disease and portrayed true lesion size in only 60% of the cases of colorectal carcinoma. Small nodules, less than 0.5 cm, were visualized on CT with a sensitivity of only 11%, whereas for lesions 0.5 to 5 cm, sensitivity was 37%, and for tumors greater than 5 cm, CT sensitivity was 94%. Jacquet and colleagues,[2] in a similar analysis of lesions seen on preoperative CT compared with findings at abdominal exploration, reported that CT sensitivity for

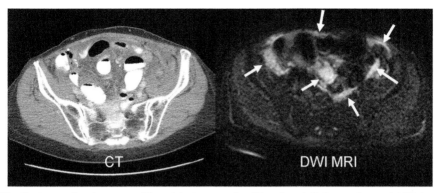

Fig. 3. Appendiceal cancer with pelvic tumors: On CT and gadolinium-enhanced MRI (not shown), it can be difficult to distinguish collapsed bowel from ascites, and tumors. CT shows (*left*) collapsed bowel and ascites which is difficult to distinguish from peritoneal and serosal tumors. DWI MRI, B-value 500 (*right*), images only the peritoneal and serosal tumors (*arrows*) and shows restricted diffusion, facilitating tumor depiction.

lesions less than 0.5 cm was 28%. Tumors 0.5 to 5 cm were depicted with a sensitivity of 72% and large tumors greater than 5 cm were depicted with a 90% sensitivity.

Accurate assessment of PCI based on preoperative imaging could provide valuable information useful in patient selection and surgical planning. In this calculation, radiologic PCI location of the peritoneal metastases in the 13 abdominal and pelvic regions clearly affects sensitivity for tumor detection.

Koh and colleagues[5] reported that CT PCI scores significantly underestimated the intraoperative PCI, with the operative score almost double the CT PCI score. CT detection of peritoneal nodules was 67% in the epigastrium, 54% in the right upper quadrant, and 60% in the pelvis. Small bowel involvement had the least sensitivity, 8% to 17%, of all the regions.

A recent review of multidetector CT for preoperative determination of PCI in subjects with primary and recurrent ovarian cancer found a regional sensitivity of 66% and accuracy of 77% for peritoneal tumor compared with histologic findings.[6] In a subject-level analysis, the sensitivity for small bowel or mesenteric tumor (regions 9–12) was 58%. All of these studies confirm the limitations of CT in identifying peritoneal metastases and its gross underestimation of PCI compared with surgical findings (see **Fig. 1**).

Preoperative MRI

MRI provides a much more accurate imaging examination for preoperative evaluation of patients being assessed for cytoreduction and HIPEC. In a direct comparison of MRI, CT, and operative findings, the site sensitivity of delayed gadolinium-enhanced MRI for peritoneal tumors less than 1 cm was 85% to 90% compared with 22% to 33% for CT. The mean sensitivity of MRI for depicting tumors of all sizes was 84% compared with 54% for CT.[17] The addition of diffusion-weighted MRI to the MR peritoneal examination improves tumor detection, particularly in the small bowel and mesentery. A study comparing preoperative CT and MRI with surgical findings at CRS and HIPEC surgery confirmed 222 sites of tumor. MRI demonstrated a per-site sensitivity of 95%, specificity of 70%, and accuracy of 88%. CT showed a corresponding per-site sensitivity of 55%, specificity of 85%, and accuracy of 63%.[10]

Preoperative MRI can estimate the PCI with good accuracy compared with surgical findings. In 33 subjects being considered for CRS and HIPEC, there was no significant difference between the preoperative MRI PCI and surgical PCI.[9] MRI correctly categorized the tumor volume found at surgery in 29 (88%) of 33 subjects. MRI accurately categorized the tumor volume as small-volume (PCI 0–9) in 89% of subjects, moderate volume (PCI 10–20) in 75% of subjects, and large-volume (PCI >20) in 90% of subjects. Klumpp and colleagues[13,14] confirmed these findings, reporting that the preoperative MRI findings correlated with the surgical PCI.

In a comparison of preoperative CT with MRI in 22 subjects being considered for CRS and HIPEC, the operative PCI was 33 compared with 36 for MRI and 15 for CT. The CT PCI underestimated the surgical PCI in 19 of 22 subjects.[10] The median percentage difference between the surgical PCI and the CT PCI was 50% compared with 6% for the MRI PCI. Compared with the surgical PCI, MRI PCI correctly categorized tumor volume as small, moderate, or large in 91% of the subjects as opposed to only 50% with CT scanning. Notably, in the small bowel areas (sites 9–12), MRI had an accuracy of 92% versus 48% for CT (see **Fig. 2**; **Fig. 4**).

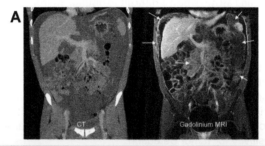

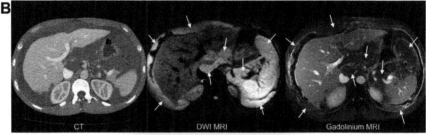

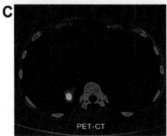

Fig. 4. Appendiceal cancer: (*A*) On CT (*left*) ascites, mucin, and tumors are difficult to distinguish due the limited soft tissue contrast of CT. On the gadolinium-enhanced MR (*right*) the ascites and mucin do not enhance, whereas the tumors (*arrows*) show moderate enhancement. (*B*) CT (*left*) does not distinguish tumors from ascites and mucin. DWI MRI (*middle*) shows bulky tumors (*arrows*) with high signal around the liver, spleen, and in the epigastrium. Gadolinium-enhanced MRI (*right*) shows the enhancing tumors (*arrows*) in the same locations. (*C*) PET-CT grossly underestimates the volume of peritoneal tumors, showing minimal metabolic activity in the ascites.

Preoperative PET–Computed Tomography

Pasqual and colleagues[28] compared the accuracy of CT and PET-CT for the quantification of peritoneal carcinomatosis in subjects before and after undergoing CRC and HIPEC for gastrointestinal malignancies. They concluded that, although there was a significant correlation between the preoperative PCI and the intraoperative PCI, both techniques significantly underestimated the intraoperative PCI volume and failed to adequately assess all the cases with a PCI greater than 20 (see **Fig. 4**). No significant difference was found between CT and FDG-PET-CT for preoperative staging, and both techniques were lacking in disease quantification and thus insufficient for adequate surgical staging.

Dromain and colleagues[29] reported results from a prospective study performed at a large HIPEC center in France (Institut Gustave Roussy), comparing CT with PET-CT preoperative findings and intraoperative findings in subjects scheduled for CRS and HIPEC. They concluded that neither CT nor PET-CT examination was a reliable imaging method in the preoperative assessment of the extent of peritoneal involvement; in particular, to predict small bowel involvement.

Wang and colleagues[30] reported their results of PET-CT in the perioperative assessments of subjects with peritoneal disease before CRS and HIPEC. In 64% of the study group, PET-CT provided no additional information compared with CT alone. They concluded that PET-CT is best as adjuvant to CT and/or MRI scans, when lesions in these studies were indeterminate and in subjects with nonmucinous tumors.

DeVos and colleauges[31] found that PET-CT underestimated extent of disease in subjects with carcinomatosis from colorectal cancer by 67% in nonmucinous tumors and 90% in mucinous tumors. PET-CT was best for detection of upper abdominal disease but poor for pelvic and mesenteric carcinomatosis and lesions less than 5 mm.[32]

PET-CT has had significant impact on preoperative evaluations of subjects with colorectal metastases.[33] Most of these subjects were found to be inoperable due to extrahepatic lymph node involvement in the periportal area and retroperitoneum. Extrahepatic disease to lung, mediastinal nodes, and bone was found in 6% to 17% of the subjects.[34–36]

In summary, PET-CT is most beneficial for evaluating gastrointestinal carcinomas if a CT or MRI is inconclusive or negative and tumor markers are increased but a recurrence is suspected. PET-CT should be used selectively in preoperative assessment in patients with large tumor volumes with poor prognostic histologies being considered for CRS and HIPEC to rule out extraabdominal metastases.

PET–computed tomography ovarian carcinomatosis

Studies comparing CT, MRI, and 18F FDG PET-CT have demonstrated greater accuracy of PET-CT in the detection of peritoneal implants in ovarian carcinoma.[37] However, this advantage was challenged in that whole-body diffusion-weighted and gadolinium-enhanced MRI demonstrate higher accuracy in detecting peritoneal disease compared with CT and PET-CT.[38] Several other studies have shown the inferiority of PET-CT compared with enhanced CT,[39,40] as well as inferior sensitivity and specificity based on subsequent surgical findings.[41] PET-CT, however, can diagnose extraabdominal lymph node metastases to mediastinal nodes, supraclavicular nodes, and other organ sites, such as bone and brain. It also can detect nodal involvement in normal-sized lymph nodes seen on conventional MRI or CT imaging.[42,43]

Elevation of serum cancer antigen (CA)-125 above normal range is the best predictor of recurrent ovarian carcinoma.[44] Although PET-CT has been reported to be superior to other imaging modalities for the detection of recurrent ovarian cancer,[45,46] diffusion-weighted and gadolinium-enhanced MRI abdomen-pelvis and CT chest are preferred as the initial imaging studies before proceeding to PET-CT.[9,10,17]

In summary, FDG PET-CT, when used for staging and pretreatment evaluation of ovarian cancer, demonstrates a higher accuracy than CT for node and metastasis staging but has limited sensitivity to detect peritoneal carcinomatosis, especially when there is small-volume disease.[47] For surveillance after treatment, FDG PET-CT is an accurate imaging technique for detecting tumor recurrence in patients with inconclusive, equivocal, or negative conventional imaging but suspected of having a recurrence due to an increase in CA-125 level. PET-CT is especially useful to identify possible extraabdominal metastases.

DETERMINING RESECTABILITY OF PERITONEAL METASTASES

Preoperative MRI, CT, and PET-CT of the abdomen and pelvis play an integral role in determining the extent of peritoneal and visceral disease in patients being considered for CRS.[1–3,9,10,27] Preoperative imaging can assist in patient selection by avoiding surgery in patients whose tumors are too extensive for adequate surgical cytoreduction.

As described by Sugarbaker,[3] the features that indicate an increased risk for incomplete tumor resection include

- Bowel obstruction or partial obstruction at more than one site
- Nonmucinous ascites
- Mesentery drawn together by tumor
- Tumor infiltrating leaves of small bowel mesentery
- Mesenteric or paraaortic lymphadenopathy
- Porta hepatis involvement
- Hydroureter
- Psoas muscle invasion
- Gastric outlet obstruction
- Pelvic sidewall invasion
- Tumor greater than or equal to 5 cm in jejunal areas
- CT PCI greater than 20 (excluding pseudomyxoma peritonei)
- Retroperitoneal lymphadenopathy
- Pleural effusion in the absence of extensive ascites.

Rivard and colleagues[1] noted that no single concerning feature was associated with unresectability. However, subjects with 2 or more concerning features were more likely to have a suboptimal cytoreduction (87.5% vs 36.4%) than subjects with a single concerning feature. Notably the PCI estimated on CT was not higher in unresectable subjects ($P = .851$) and significantly underestimated intraoperative PCI measurement ($P = .003$). Jacquet and colleagues[2] similarly found that in subjects with preoperative CT showing tumor causing bowel obstruction, surgical cytoreduction was suboptimal in 88%. If the obstructing tumor involving the jejunum or upper ileum was greater than 5 cm in diameter, no subjects had complete CRS.

Despite the promise of preoperative assessment of peritoneal tumor respectability, 16% to 26% of subjects undergoing laparotomy for possible CRS and HIPEC are found to be nonoperable owing to excessive tumor and involvement of critical structures.[48–54] Unfortunately, current imaging techniques often fail to alert the surgeon to nonresectable peritoneal tumor, which results in open-close procedures.[48,50,52] van Oudheusden and colleagues[52] reported similar experiences with the open-close procedure in 23.4% of 350 subjects with peritoneal cancer from colorectal cancer who were undergoing explorative surgery for possible CRS and HIPEC. Widespread peritoneal disease was the most common reason for discontinuing surgery in 50% of subjects. In a recent study of 533 subjects with peritoneal carcinomatosis who underwent preoperative CT, FDG PET, and MRI, the incidence of open-close laparotomy was improved but still 16%.[48]

In the authors' experience, MR determination of the tumor involving the mesentery and bowel serosal is critical for both patient selection and preoperative planning. MRI using gadolinium contrast material and DWI routinely depicts sheets of tumor cells involving the small bowel serosa and mesentery that is typically not seen on CT or PET (**Fig. 5**).

In a study of 51 subjects, the authors found that the results of preoperative MRI could be used to stratify subjects into surgical and nonsurgical management. Subjects were deemed to be nonsurgical if the MR PCI was greater than or equal to 25 or there was diffuse tumor involving the small bowel and mesentery; 74% of these subjects died within 14 months of the MRI. The surgical group with PCI less than 25 and no diffuse small bowel or mesenteric tumor all had resection (R) R0 or R1, and a mean disease-free interval of 40 months. Ten surgical subjects with MR PCI greater than or equal to 25 had incomplete surgical resection; 4 subjects had grade III-IV complications and the mean disease-free interval was less than 8 months for the non-DPAM subjects. (Low RN and Barone RM: Use of preoperative MRI for selection of

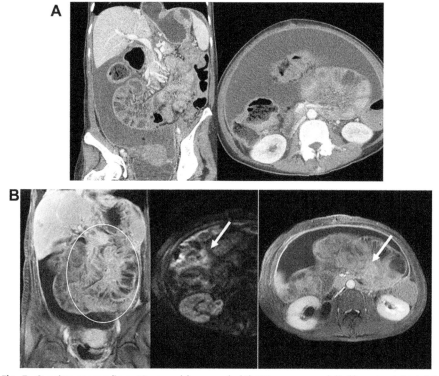

Fig. 5. Ovarian cancer (in a 48-year-old woman): (*A*) CT scan coronal (*left*) and axial (*right*) shows ascites but no mesenteric or small bowel tumors. (*B*) Coronal gadolinium-enhanced MRI (*left*); diffusion-weighted MRI, B-value 800 (*middle*); and delayed axial gadolinium-enhanced MRI (*right*) show bulky and diffuse mesenteric and small bowel serosal tumors (*arrows*). Patient was referred for chemotherapy and expired the same month.

subjects being considered for surgical cytoreduction and HIPEC. Submitted for publication.)

SURVEILLANCE IMAGING FOLLOWING CYTOREDUCTIVE SURGERY AND HEATED INTRAPERITONEAL CHEMOTHERAPY

Despite successful treatment, local intraperitoneal recurrence of tumor occurs in 28% to 44% of patients and remains a significant problem that reduces overall survival[7,55–57] (see **Fig. 5**). Second and third complete cytoreduction with repeated HIPEC for patients with recurrent tumor has been advocated as the best approach to achieve improved overall survival.[55] The early detection of recurrent tumor on serial laboratory tests and imaging studies plays a critical role in identifying patients who should be considered for repeat CRS and HIPEC.[7,49–58] (Low RN and Barone RM: Use of preoperative MRI for selection of patients being considered for surgical cytoreduction and HIPEC. Submitted for publication.)

Assessment of response following CRS and HIPEC using serial tumor markers alone is challenging.[58,59] In 1 study, preoperative Carcinoembryonic antigen (CEA) and CA-19.9 levels were increased in 75% and 58% of subjects' pseudomyxoma peritonei[57] and, during follow-up, a high CA-19.9 level was more predictive of recurrence. However, a progressive increase in serum tumor markers with disease recurrence is reliably seen in only some subjects and does not predict the volume of tumor recurrence or its location. Some subjects with large-volume recurrent tumor may not show an elevation in tumor markers. Tumor markers do not reliably monitor disease stabilization, partial response, or continued complete response.[60]

In a longitudinal study of 50 subjects with appendiceal neoplasm (DPAM 13, peritoneal mucinous carcinomatosis (PMCA) 37) MRI detected tumor recurrence earlier than serial tumor markers.[61,62] Following CRS and HIPEC, subjects entered follow-up surveillance with serial MRI every 6 months and serial laboratory studies, including CA-125, CEA, and CA-19-9. During surveillance, tumor recurrence was documented in 30 (60%) subjects with median time to recurrence of 13 months (range 5–56 months). MRI detected recurrent tumor in 28 subjects, including 11 subjects with normal laboratory values (sensitivity 0.93, specificity 0.95, accuracy 0.94, positive predictive value [PPV] 0.97, and negative predictive value [NPV] 0.90). Serial laboratory values showed tumor recurrence in 14 subjects (sensitivity 0.48, specificity 1.00, accuracy 0.69, PPV 1.0, and NPV 0.57). Median survival was 50 months for 11 subjects with earlier MRI detection of recurrence versus 33 months for the other 19 subjects with recurrence.[61]

Earlier intervention performed with smaller volume tumor should yield better surgical results with lower morbidity and mortality.[60] If the radiologist waits until the tumor burden is large enough to be detected on a CT scan, the delay in treatment could adversely affect outcome and survival. The importance of repeat CRS and HIPEC for treating recurrent appendiceal cancer has been described in prior reports.[55,56] Complete cytoreduction after repeat surgery was the only independent prognostic factor for improved survival resulting in a 70% 5-year survival rate for 402 subjects with appendiceal cancer.[55]

At the authors' institution, patients are routinely followed with serial serum laboratory values and a surveillance MRI every 6 months (**Fig. 6**).

Interpretation of Surveillance Magnetic Resonance Examinations

Following CRS and HIPEC, some peritoneal and bowel serosal thickening is present with enhancement on gadolinium-enhanced MRI and DWI. These changes reflect normal postoperative findings. Therefore, the initial MR examination following CRS and HIPEC establishes the patient's postoperative baseline appearance on MRI.

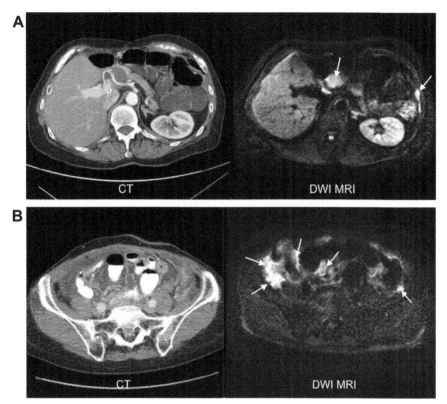

Fig. 6. Recurrent appendiceal cancer: (*A*) CT (*left*) shows fluid and air-filled bowel without definite tumors. DWI MRI (*right*) shows epigastric and left paracolic tumors (*arrows*). (*B*) CT (*left*) shows fluid and air-filled bowel without definite tumors. DWI MRI (*right*) shows epigastric and left paracolic tumors (*arrows*).

Assuming that the surgeon achieved an R0 tumor resection, at this initial surveillance examination all findings represent normal anatomy and postsurgical changes.

On subsequent MR examinations, we carefully assess for any interval changes that indicate disease progression or recurrence. Concerning findings include obvious tumor masses; however, more common findings include increasing peritoneal thickening, peritoneal nodules, and ascites. Identifying tumor on both gadolinium-enhanced MRI and DWI improves confidence and accuracy in detecting recurrent tumor.

An important point is that MR findings attributable to postsurgical changes do not progress on serial MR examinations. If progressively worsening bowel wall thickening and mesenteric infiltration on gadolinium-enhanced MRI and DWI is observed, this represents tumor recurrence. Postsurgical changes will gradually resolve on serial MR examinations and will not show progression. This assessment assumes that the patient is clinically stable and that there is no superimposed acute disease, such as a gastroenteritis or postoperative abscess.

SUMMARY

Compared with CT and PET, MRI of peritoneal tumor more accurately determines the location and extent of peritoneal tumor. The combination of DWI and gadolinium-enhanced MRI provides information that can estimate PCI and assist in patient selection for CRS and HIPEC. Following HIPEC surveillance, MRI can detect early tumor recurrence. Performing and interpreting the examination correctly requires careful attention to detail. A trained MR staff, an experienced MR radiologist, and close collaboration between the radiologist and oncologic surgeon are key elements in this team effort.

REFERENCES

1. Rivard JD, Temple WJ, McConnell YJ, et al. Preoperative computed tomography does not predict resectability in peritoneal carcinomatosis. Am J Surg 2014;207: 760–5.
2. Jacquet P, Jelinek JS, Chang D, et al. Abdominal computed tomographic scan in the selection of patients with mucinous peritoneal carcinomatosis for cytoreductive surgery. J Am Coll Surg 1995;181:530–8.
3. Sugarbaker PH. Preoperative assessment of cancer patients with peritoneal metastases for complete cytoreduction. Indian J Surg Oncol 2016;7(3):295–302.
4. Esquivel J, Chua TC, Stojadinovic A, et al. Accuracy and clinical relevance of computed tomography scan interpretation of peritoneal cancer index in colorectal cancer peritoneal carcinomatosis: a multi-institutional study. J Surg Oncol 2010;102:565–70.
5. Koh JL, Tan TD, Glenn D, et al. Evaluation of preoperative computed tomography in estimating peritoneal cancer index in colorectal peritoneal carcinomatosis. Ann Surg Oncol 2009;16:327–33.
6. Mazzei MA, Khader L, Cirigliano A. Accuracy of MDCT in the preoperative definition of Peritoneal Cancer Index (PCI) in patients with advanced ovarian cancer who underwent peritonectomy and hyperthermic intraperitoneal chemotherapy (HIPEC). Abdom Imaging 2013;38:1422–30.
7. Chua TC, AL-Zahrani A, Saxena A, et al. Determining the association between preoperative computed tomography findings and postoperative outcomes after cytoreductive surgery and perioperative intraperitoneal chemotherapy for pseudomyxoma peritonei. Ann Surg Oncol 2011;18:1582–9.
8. Torkzad M, Casta N, Bergman A, et al. Comparison between MRI and CT in prediction of peritoneal carcinomatosis index (PCI) in patients undergoing cytoreductive surgery in relation to the experience of the radiologist. J Surg Oncol 2015;111:746–51.
9. Low RN, Barone RM. Combined diffusion-weighted and gadolinium-enhanced MR imaging can accurately predict the peritoneal cancer index (PCI) preoperatively in patients being considered for cytoreductive surgical procedures. J Surg Oncol 2012;19:1394–401.
10. Low RN, Barone RM, Lucero J. Comparison of MRI and CT for predicting the peritoneal cancer index (PCI) preoperatively in patients being considered for cytoreductive surgical procedures. Ann Surg Oncol 2015;22:1708–15.
11. Ricke J, Sehouli J, Hach C, et al. Prospective evaluation of contrast-enhanced MRI in the depiction of peritoneal spread in primary or recurrent ovarian cancer. Eur Radiol 2003;13:943–9.
12. Low RN, Barone RM, Gurney JM. Mucinous appendiceal neoplasms: preoperative MR staging and classification compared with surgical and histopathologic findings. AJR Am J Roentgenol 2008;190:656–65.
13. Klumpp B, Aschoff P, Schwenzer N, et al. Correlation of preoperative magnetic resonance imaging of peritoneal carcinomatosis and clinical outcome after

peritonectomy and HIPEC after 3 years of follow-up: preliminary results. Cancer Imaging 2013;13:540–7.

14. Klumpp B, Aschoff P, Schwenzer N, et al. Peritoneal carcinomatosis: comparison of dynamic contrast-enhanced magnetic resonance imaging with surgical and histopathologic findings. Abdom Imaging 2012;37:834–42.

15. Klumpp B, Schwenzer N, Aschoff P, et al. Preoperative assessment of peritoneal carcinomatosis: intraindividual comparison of 18F-FSG PET/CT and MRI. Abdom Imaging 2012;38:64–71.

16. Elsayes KH, Staveteig PT, Narra VR, et al. MRI of the peritoneum: spectrum of abnormalities. AJR Am J Roentgenol 2006;186:1369–79.

17. Low RN, Barone RM, Lacey C, et al. Peritoneal tumor: MR imaging with dilute oral barium and intravenous gadolinium-containing contrast agents compared with unenhanced MR imaging and CT. Radiology 1997;204:513–20.

18. Koh DM, Collins DJ. Review. Diffusion-weighted MRI in the body: applications and challenges in oncology. AJR Am J Roentgenol 2007;188:1622–35.

19. Malayeri AA, El Khouli RH, Zaheer A, et al. Principles and applications of diffusion-weighted imaging in cancer detection, staging, and treatment follow-up. Radiographics 2011;31:1773–91.

20. Low RN, Sebrechts CP, Barone RM, et al. Diffusion-weighted MRI of peritoneal tumors: comparison with conventional MRI and surgical and histopathologic findings–a feasibility study. AJR Am J Roentgenol 2009;193:461–70.

21. Kyriazi S, Collins DJ, Messiou C, et al. Metastatic ovarian and primary peritoneal cancer: assessing chemotherapy response with diffusion-weighted mr imaging—value of histogram analysis of apparent diffusion coefficients. Radiology 2011; 261:182–92.

22. Kyriazi S, Collins DJ, Morgan VA, et al. Diffusion-weighted imaging of peritoneal disease for noninvasive staging of advanced ovarian cancer. Radiographics 2010;30:1269–85.

23. Bozkurt M, Doganay S, Kantacri M, et al. Comparison of peritoneal tumor imaging using conventional MR imaging and diffusion-weighted MR imaging with different b values. Eur J Radiol 2011;80:224–8.

24. Hanbridge A, Mester U. Mesentery, omentum, peritoneum: CT, ultrasound and MRI. Abdom Imaging 2013;1535–40.

25. Hanbidge A, Metser U. Mesentery, Omentum, Peritoneum: CT, Ultrasound and MRI. In: Hamm B, Ros PR, editors. Abdominal Imaging. Berlin, Heidelberg: Springer; 2013.

26. Espada M, Garcia-Flores JR, Jimenez M. Diffusion-weighted magnetic resonance imaging evaluation of intra-abdominal sites of implants to predict likelihood of suboptimal cytoreductive surgery in patients with ovarian carcinoma. Eur Radiol 2013;23:2636–42.

27. Pfannenberg C, Königsrainer I, Aschoff P. [18] F-FDG-PET/CT to select patients with peritoneal carcinomatosis for cytoreductive surgery and hyperthermic intraperitoneal chemotherapy. Ann Surg Oncol 2009;16:1295–303.

28. Pasqual EM, Bertozzi S, Bacchetti S, et al. Perioperative assessment of peritoneal carcinomatosis in patients undergoing hyperthermic chemotherapy following cytoreductive surgery. Anticancer Res 2014;34:2363–8.

29. Dromain C, Leboulleux S, Auperin A, et al. Staging of peritoneal carcinomatosis: enhanced CT vs. PET/CT. Abdom Imaging 2008;33:87–93.

30. Wang W, Tan G, Chia CS, et al. Are positron emission tomography-computed tomography (PET-CT) scans useful in preoperative assessment of patients with peritoneal disease before cytoreductive surgery (CRS) and hyperthermic

intraperitoneal chemotherapy (HIPEC)? Int J Hyperthermia 2017;1–8 [Epub ahead of print].

31. DeVos N, Goethols I, Ceelen W. Clinical value of 18F-FDG-PET/CT in the preoperative staging of peritoneal carcinomatosis from colorectal origin. Acta Chir Belg 2014;114:1–6.

32. Soussan M, Des Goetz G, Barrau V, et al. Comparison of FGD-18 FDG PET/CT and MR with diffusion weighted imaging for assessing peritoneal carcinomatosis from gastrointestinal malignancy. Eur Radiol 2012;22:1479–87.

33. Vegano Z, Lopci E, Costa G, et al. Positive emission tomography – computer tomography for patient's with recurrent colorectal metastases. Impact on restaging and treatment planning. Ann Surg Oncol 2017;24:1029–36.

34. Kong G, Jackson C, Koh M, et al. The use of 18F-FDG-PET/CT in Colorectal liver metastases comparison with CT and liver MRI. Eur J Nucl Med Mol Imaging 2008; 35:1323–9.

35. Briggs RH, Chowdhury FV, Lodge JPA, et al. Clinical impact of FDG PET/CT in patient's with potentially operable metastatic colorectal cancer. Clin Radiol 2011;66:1167–74.

36. Yip VS, Poston GJ, Fenwich SW, et al. FDG-PET-CT is effective in selecting patients with poor long term survival from colorectal liver metastases. Eur J Surg Oncol 2014;40:995–9.

37. Senli Y, Turkman C, Bakar B, et al. Diagnostic value of PET/CT is similar to that of conventional MRI and even better for detecting small peritoneal implants in recurrent ovarian cancer. Nucl Med Commun 2012;33:509–15.

38. Michielsen K, Vergeto I, Opde-Beeck K, et al. Whole body MRI with diffusion weighted sequence for staging of patient's with suspected ovarian cancer: a clinical feasibility study in comparison to CT and FDG-PET-CT. Eur J Radiol 2014;24: 809–911.

39. Hymminen J, Kemppainen M, Lavonius M, et al. A prospective comparison of integrated FDG-PET/contrast enhanced CT and contrast – enhanced CT for pretreatment imaging of advanced epithelial ovarian cancer. Gynecol Oncol 2013; 131:389–94.

40. Tsuyoshi H, Yoshida Y. Diagnostic imaging using positron emission tomography for gynecological malignancies. J Obstet Gynaecol Res 2017. https://doi.org/10.1111/jog.13436.

41. Rose P, Faulhaber P, Miraldi F, et al. Positron emission tomography for evaluating the complete response in patient's with ovarian and peritoneal carcinoma: correlation with second look laparotomy. Gynecol Oncol 2001;82:17–21.

42. Signorelli M, Guerra Z, Piravano C, et al. Detection of nodal metastases by 18F-FDG-PET/CT in apparent early stage ovarian cancer; a prospective study. Gynecol Oncol 2013;131:395–9.

43. Yuan Y, Gu ZX, Toa XF, et al. Computer tomography magnetic resonance and positron emission computer tomography or positive emission/computer tomography for detection of metastatic lymph nodes in patient's with ovarian cancer:a meta-analysis. Eur J Radiol 2012;81:1002–6.

44. Antunovic L, Cemitan M, Borsatti E, et al. Revealing the clinical value of 18F-FDG-PET/CT in detecting recurrent epithelial ovarian carcinomatosis: correlation with histology, serum CA 125 assay and conventional radiologic modalities. Clin Nucl Med 2012;37:184–8.

45. Gu P, Pan L, Wu S, et al. PET-CT, CT and MRI in diagnosing recurrent ovarian cancer; a systematic review and meta-analysis. Eur J Radiol 2009;71:164–74.

46. Risum S, Hogdall C, Markova E, et al. Influence of 2-(18F) fluoro-2-deoxy-D-glucose positron emission tomography in recurrent ovarian cancer diagnosis and in selection of patient's for secondary cytoreductive surgery. Int J Gynecol Cancer 2009;19:600–4.

47. Lopez-Lopez V, Cascales-Campos PA, Gil J, et al. Use of 18F-FDG PET/CT in pre-operative evaluation of patients diagnosed with peritoneal carcinomatosis of ovarian origin, candidates to cytoreduction HIPEC. A pending issue. Eur J Radiol 2016;85:1824–8.

48. Mohkam K, Passot G, Cotte E, et al. Resectability of peritoneal consecutive patients selected for cytoreductive surgery: learnings from a prospective cohort of 533 consecutive patients selected for cytoreductive surgery. Ann Surg Oncol 2016;23:1261–70.

49. Menassel B, Duclos A, Passot G, et al. Preoperative CT and MRI prediction of non-resectability for pseudomyxoma peritonei from mucinous appendiceal neoplasms. Eur J Surg Oncol 2016;42:558–66.

50. Spiliotis J, Halkia E, Rogdakis A, et al. Clinical history of patients with peritoneal carcinomatosis excluded from cytoreductive surgery & HIPEC. J BUON 2015;20: 244–7.

51. Marcotte E, Dube P, Drolet P, et al. Hyperthermic intraperitoneal chemotherapy with oxaliplatin as treatment for peritoneal carcinomatosis arising from the appendix and pseudomyxoma peritonei: a survival analysis. World J Surg Oncol 2014; 12:332.

52. van Oudheusden TR, Braam HJ, Luyer MDP, et al. Peritoneal cancer patients not suitable for cytoreductive surgery and HIPEC during explorative surger: risk factors, treatment options, and prognosis. Ann Surg Oncol 2015;22:1236–42.

53. Rodt AP, Svarrer RO, ZIversen LH. Clinical course for patients with peritoneal carcinomatosis excluded from cytoreductive surgery and hyperthermic intraperitoneal chemotherapy. World J Surg Oncol 2013;11:232.

54. Hompes D, Boot H, van Tinteren H, et al. Unresectable peritoneal carcinomatosis from colorectal cancer: a single center experience. J Surg Oncol 2011;104:269–73.

55. Yan TD, Bijelic L, Sugarbaker PH. Critical analysis of treatment failure after complete cytoreductive surgery and perioperative intraperitoneal chemotherapy for peritoneal dissemination from appendiceal mucinous neoplasms. Ann Surg Oncol 2007;14:2289–99.

56. Bijelic L, Tan TD, Sugarbaker PH. Treatment failure following complete cytoreductive surgery and perioperative intraperitoneal chemotherapy for peritoneal dissemination from colorectal or appendiceal mucinous neoplasms. J Surg Oncol 2008;15(98):295–9.

57. Smeenk RM, Verwaal VJ, Antonini N, et al. Survival analysis of pseudomyxoma peritonei patients treated by cytoreductive surgery and hyperthermic intraperitoneal chemotherapy. Ann Surg 2007;245:104–9.

58. van Ruth S, Hart AAM, Bonfrer JMG, et al. Prognostic value of baseline and serial carcinoembryonic antigen and carbohydrate antigen 19.1 measurements in patients with pseudomyxoma peritonei treated with cytoreduction and hyperthermic intraperitoneal chemotherapy. Ann Surg Oncol 2002;9:961–7.

59. Ross S, Sardi A, Nieroda C, et al. Clinical utility of elevated tumor markers in patients with disseminated appendiceal malignancies treated by cytoreductive surgery and HIPEC. Eur J Surg Oncol 2010;36:772–6.

60. Jacquet P, Sugarbaker PH. Clinical research methodologies in diagnosis and staging of patients with peritoneal carcinomatosis [Chapter 23]. In: Sugarbaker PH, editor. Peritoneal carcinomatosis. Springer; 1996.

Patient Selection for Cytoreductive Surgery

Travis E. Grotz, MD[a,b,]*, Keith F. Fournier, MD[a], Paul F. Mansfield, MD[a]

KEYWORDS

- Prognostic factors • Predicting • Patient selection • Outcomes • HIPEC
- Cytoreduction

KEY POINTS

- Clinical factors, such as age, comorbidities, smoking, and functional and nutritional status, are important to minimize morbidity from cytoreduction (CRS) and hyperthermic intraperitoneal chemotherapy (HIPEC).
- Simplified Preoperative Assessment for Appendix Tumor (SPAAT) score is helpful in determining expectations from CRS and HIPEC for well-differentiated mucinous appendiceal adenocarcinoma.
- Response to neoadjuvant chemotherapy and extent and volume of distribution of disease on laparoscopy are important for selecting patients with high-grade disease for CRS and HIPEC.
- Histology and various measures of proliferation (Ki-67, mitotic rate, and SUV-max on PET) are important in selecting patients with peritoneal mesothelioma for CRS and HIPEC.
- PCI of greater than 20 for high-grade appendiceal, greater than 17 to 20 for colorectal cancer, and greater than 7 for gastric cancer are relative contraindications for CRS and HIPEC.

CYTOREDUCTION FOR PERITONEAL MALIGNANCIES

"In the world of surgical oncology; biology is King; selection of cases is Queen, and the technical details of surgical procedures are princes and princesses of the realm who frequently try to overthrow the powerful forces of the King and Queen, usually to no long-term avail, although with some temporary apparent victories." This insight first shared by Blake Cady, MD more than 20 years ago remains just as true today. Nowhere is this more relevant than the group of cancers with a biologic predisposition

Disclosure: The authors have nothing to disclose.
[a] Division of Hepatobiliary and Pancreas Surgery, Mayo Clinic, 200 First Street Southwest, Rochester, MN 55905, USA; [b] Department of Surgical Oncology, MD Anderson Cancer Center, Houston, TX, USA
* Corresponding author. Division of Hepatobiliary and Pancreas Surgery, Mayo Clinic, 200 First Street Southwest, Rochester, MN 55905.
E-mail address: grotz.travis@mayo.edu

Surg Oncol Clin N Am 27 (2018) 443–462
https://doi.org/10.1016/j.soc.2018.02.012
1055-3207/18/© 2018 Elsevier Inc. All rights reserved.
surgonc.theclinics.com

for peritoneal dissemination collectively referred to as the peritoneal malignancies. The peritoneal malignancies span the biologic spectrum of aggressiveness from the indolent growth pattern and superficial nature of well-differentiated mucinous appendiceal adenocarcinoma to the rapidly growing and invasive nature of poorly differentiated signet ring cell adenocarcinomas of the appendix, colon, and stomach. Likewise, the peritoneum is a unique site of metastasis comprising 13 distinct abdominopelvic regions in the peritoneal carcinomatosis index (PCI) described by Sugarbaker. Each of these regions has its own associated challenges to evaluation and resection. The volume and distribution of disease within the peritoneal cavity are incorporated in the PCI and are consistently identified as an important prognostic factor for recurrence and survival. As the PCI increases the likelihood of complete cytoreduction and long-term survival decrease; however, there remains patients with extensive disease who are able to achieve a complete cytoreduction and improved survival. One of the limitations of the PCI is that it assigns points equally among the 13 abdominopelvic regions according to volume of disease and does not stratify points according to the difficulty of resection or presence of critical structures within each abdominopelvic region. This is a critical shortcoming because involvement of the upper and lower jejunum and the upper ileum are associated with a particularly worse outcome because of the inherent difficulties with removing all the disease in this location. In contrast, involvement of the left flank, left lower quadrant, and the right flank are associated with improved outcomes because of the relative lack of critical structures in these regions. An understanding of the biology, distribution, and volume of disease is critical to appropriately selecting patients for aggressive treatment with the goal of long-term survival.

Historically there has been little understanding of the tumor biology of peritoneal malignancies, which has until recently prevented a thoughtful approach to peritoneal metastasectomy. In 1998, the first randomized controlled trial for peritoneal carcinomatosis from colorectal and appendiceal adenocarcinoma began accrual. This trial randomized patients to the current standard of care at that time: systemic 5-FU chemotherapy alone or cytoreduction (cytoreductive surgery [CRS]) and hyperthermic intraperitoneal chemotherapy (HIPEC) followed by systemic 5-FU chemotherapy. Because of the uncommon nature of peritoneal carcinomatosis and the lack of any known selection factors there were few exclusion criteria. Both first presentation and recurrences were included. Abdominal computed tomography (CT) scan and chest radiograph were the only required staging imaging. The only clinical criteria were age less than 71 and normal hematologic, renal, and liver laboratory parameters. There were no stipulations regarding the volume and distribution of peritoneal disease. Despite the unselected nature of this study and the high perioperative mortality (8% in this study), which was a result of the steep learning curve associated with CRS and HIPEC and the advanced nature of the peritoneal disease studied, the trial demonstrated a doubling of survival compared with the control arm (22.3 months vs 12.6 months median overall survival [OS]). It was only in subset analysis of prognostic factors in the CRS and HIPEC arm that it was evident that patients with cancer deposits in six or seven of the seven possible regions in the Dutch Simplified Peritoneal Cancer Index do poorly, in respect to direct postoperative complications and long-term survival. In fact, the authors attributed 80% of all grade 4 toxicity and all treatment-related deaths to the patients with involvement of six or seven abdominal regions. Similarly, these are the same patients in whom a complete cytoreduction was unable to be obtained and the survival was similar for these patients whether they were treated with systemic chemotherapy alone or cytoreduction and HIPEC. These patients clearly did not benefit from cytoreduction. In contrast, the patients with 0 to 5 regions involved did significantly better with a median OS greater than 29 months. In fact, long-term follow-up demonstrates a median survival of 48 months and a 5-year survival of 45% for those patients for whom a complete cytoreduction could be achieved. Moreover, no treatment-related deaths occurred in these patients.[1,2] This randomized trial was not only critical in establishing cytoreduction and HIPEC as a potential standard of care in patients with peritoneal metastasis from colorectal cancer but it demonstrated that in carefully selected patients, perioperative morbidity and mortality can be reduced and long-term survival obtained. To maximize the benefits and minimize the risks of morbidity from CRS and HIPEC appropriate selection of patients is critical. Patient selection involves the thoughtful evaluation of clinical, biologic, and anatomic factors.

Clinical Factors

CRS and HIPEC is a major surgical undertaking that puts patients at risk for prolonged postoperative ileus, superficial and deep infections, anastomotic leakage, enteric fistula, sepsis, postoperative bleeding, respiratory distress, hematologic toxicity, and urinary disturbance. The most common causes of death include anastomotic leakage, sepsis, and postoperative bleeding. According to an analysis of the National Surgical Quality Improvement Program database, patients undergoing CRS and HIPEC have an average hospital stay of 13 days, an 11% readmission rate, an overall morbidity rate of 33%, and a mortality rate of 2%.[3] Single institutions with high case volumes have reported lower morbidity and mortality rates, suggesting that experience can mitigate some of the adverse events associated with surgeries for peritoneal malignancies. For example, at MD Anderson Cancer Center (MDACC) our 90-day major morbidity is less than 20% and the 90-day mortality rate is 0.8%. The individual and institutional learning curves are steep, and increased case volume has been associated with decreased morbidity and increased rates of complete cytoreduction suggesting that patient selection is likely improved with increased volume.[4,5] But what are these selection criteria? A study of 211 patients undergoing CRS and HIPEC in the Netherlands reported a 25% incidence of major complications. They identified previous surgery in more than one region of the abdomen (previous surgical score of >1), recent smoking history, poor functional status (Eastern Cooperative Oncology Group [ECOG] >1), and increasing number of visceral resections to be independently correlated with a higher risk of major morbidity. Severe morbidity, incidence of reoperation, readmission, and death were all stratified by the number of risk factors each patient had. For example, patients with no risk factors had a 5.3% risk of major morbidity compared with 14.7%, 29.3%, 66.7%, and 100% for patients with one, two, three, and four risk factors, respectively.[6] The authors constructed a decision-tree with the three preoperative factors such that patients who are current smokers, have a previous surgical score greater than 1, and ECOG functional status greater than 1 have a prohibitive, 70% risk of major morbidity. Baratti and colleagues[7] described similar findings in the largest single-institutional study of risk factors for complications. The authors reported a 28.2% incidence of major morbidity and 2.6% mortality in 426 consecutive CRS and HIPEC procedures. They were able to stratify these outcomes by the following independent risk factors: PCI greater than 30, more than five visceral resections, ECOG score greater than 0, such that patients with 2 risk factors had 65.7% incidence of major morbidity and a 16.6% risk of mortality. Patients with all three risk factors had a morbidity of 100% and mortality of 22.2%. Additional risk factors for morbidity and death in other reported series include longer operative times,[7] age greater than 70 years,[8] hypoalbuminemia,[9] diabetes,[9] gastrectomy, and intraoperative transfusion.[10] It is important to use the preoperative factors to guide patient selection, direct patient counseling, and instruct the preoperative optimization of patients before CRS and HIPEC.

Preoperative evaluation of the patient's candidacy for CRS and HIPEC includes a complete history and a physical examination detailing comorbidities and functional status. Obtaining a social history is also important, given the significance of smoking status on morbidity. Smoking cessation should be highly encouraged. Although improvements in oxygen-carrying capacity and oxygen consumption are seen in short-term abstinence, improvements in immune function, collagen production, lung capacity, mucous production, and ciliary function may take longer.[11] In fact, some studies suggest increased postoperative complications following short-term smoking cessation.[12] A Cochrane review found that smoking cessation 4 to 8 weeks before surgery had the largest impact on postoperative complications.[13] Therefore, smoking cessation strategies must be implemented early in the patient's evaluation. Other pertinent criteria include adequate renal, hepatic, and cardiac function to tolerate the effects of a long operation with significant fluid shifts. Medications must be reviewed to ensure cessation of any anticoagulants before surgery. Nutritional status is assessed with body mass index, recent weight changes, body habitus, and albumin and prealbumin levels. Nutritional prehabilitation for undernourished patients has been validated in a systematic review of clinical trials to be associated with reductions in morbidity, hospital and critical care length of stay, and infectious complications.[14] These trials consisted of 5 to 7 days of preoperative arginine-supplemented enteral nutritional support.[15] Therefore, careful attention to nutritional status is important and perioperative interventions warranted in those patients in whom oral intake is feasible. Unfortunately, we have found that feeding tube placement at the time of surgery fails to prevent postoperative weight loss and results in higher readmission rates and longer hospital stays; therefore we no longer routinely use feeding tubes.[16] In contrast, we have found parenteral nutrition to occasionally be necessary to supplement or maintain nutritional reserves in the perioperative period for patients with poor oral intake. At MDACC, the patients considered to be the best candidates for CRS and HIPEC are less than 70 years old, nonsmokers, have an ECOG functional status of 0 or 1, and have maintained their nutritional reserves (albumin >3.5 g/dL).

PATIENT SELECTION FOR WELL-DIFFERENTIATED MUCINOUS APPENDICEAL ADENOCARCINOMA

The abundance of mucin and the paucity of epithelial cells within well-differentiated mucinous appendiceal adenocarcinoma results in the superficial nature of these tumors. Exfoliated cells from the appendiceal primary are spread throughout the peritoneal cavity according to the redistribution phenomenon.[17] Briefly, cancer cells are exfoliated from the right lower quadrant and pool in the pelvis secondary to gravitational forces. The cancer-cell fluid is then distributed in a clockwise directional flow within the abdominal cavity. Subperitoneal lymphatic lacunae between muscle fibers of the diaphragm absorb the peritoneal fluid leading to layering of cancer cells along the diaphragm forming tumor plaques. Well-differentiated mucinous appendiceal cancer cells become attached to the visceral and parietal peritoneum but do not invade beyond the peritoneum and therefore are completely resected with the surgical technique of peritonectomy. Another common site of disease is the omentum, where milky spots serve as the major colonization and proliferation site for peritoneal cancer cells. Surrounding adipocytes in the omentum promote homing, migration, and invasion of cancer cells leading to the formation of characteristic "omental cake" deposits. This omental caking can be completely resected with a total omentectomy. Mucinous tumors spare mobile small bowel loops until late in the course of the disease. Therefore, the biology of well-differentiated mucinous appendiceal adenocarcinoma predicts that even patients with extensive peritoneal carcinomatosis can achieve complete cytoreduction.

In almost every analysis of clinical and pathologic factors, completeness of cytoreduction (CCR) is consistently an independent predictor of outcome. The CCR is characterized by the CCR score, which describes the amount of disease remaining after cytoreduction (**Fig. 1**). The scores are as follows: CCR-0, no visible tumor nodules remaining; CCR-1, persistence of tumor nodules less than 2.5 mm; CCR-2, tumor nodules greater than or equal to 2.5 mm but less than or equal to 2.5 cm; and CCR-3, tumor nodules greater than 2.5 cm.[18] Because HIPEC is thought to penetrate to a depth of at least 2.5 mm, scores of CCR-0 and CCR-1 have similar survival outcomes (**Fig. 2**) and therefore are considered a complete cytoreduction. In contrast, residual tumor of greater than 2.5 mm (CCR-2 and CCR-3) indicates incomplete cytoreduction and is associated with dismal survival not different from supportive management.[19] Therefore, CRS is only indicated for those in whom a CC0 or CC1 complete cytoreduction can be performed. The PCI is a scoring system that incorporates the volume and distribution of disease. Certain abdominopelvic regions are associated with poor outcomes compared with other regions. However, the PCI does not account for the difference in regions. All regions are weighted the same. Likely because of this the PCI is not a perfect indicator of resectability. Although the likelihood of complete cytoreduction decreases with increasing PCI score there is not a cutoff that sufficiently delineates resectability.[20] Furthermore, determining the PCI based on preoperative imaging is difficult and inaccurate because CT does not detect disease less than 5 mm, and underestimation of the PCI by imaging is likely. A small series from the Mayo Clinic comparing radiographic and clinical PCI at the time of CRS reported a

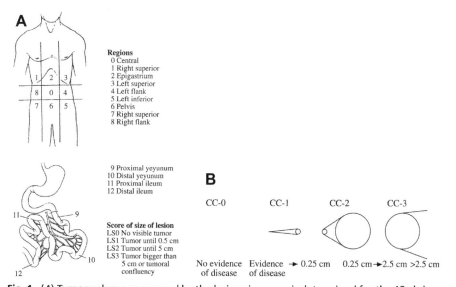

Fig. 1. (A) Tumor volume as assessed by the lesion size score is determined for the 13 abdominopelvic regions. The sum of these scores (0–39) is the peritoneal cancer index. (B) Completeness of cytoreduction after surgery. (*From* Carmignani P, Esquivel J, Sugarbaker PH. Cytoreductive surgery and intraperitoneal chemotherapy for the treatment of peritoneal surface malignancy. Clin Transl Oncol 2003;5(4):192–8; with permission.)

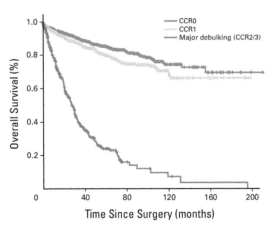

Fig. 2. Prognostic impact of CCR in surgery on overall survival (*P*<.001). (*From* Chua TC, Moran BJ, Sugarbaker PH, et al. Early- and long-term outcome data of patients with pseudomyxoma peritonei from appendiceal origin treated by a strategy of cytoreductive surgery and hyperthermic intraperitoneal chemotherapy. J Clin Oncol 2012;30(20):2449–56; with permission.)

poor correlation of 0.59 for appendiceal adenocarcinoma. Therefore, radiographic PCI alone is of limited value in determining the resectability of patients with well-differentiated mucinous appendiceal adenocarcinoma.

We reviewed the preoperative images of all patients with well-differentiated mucinous appendiceal adenocarcinoma and identified five anatomic regions that were indicative of resectability. The identification of scalloping, a radiographic finding where there is indentation of the solid organ by mucinous ascites, was assessed on the liver, spleen, pancreas, and portal vein and a single point awarded for its presence. Additionally, three points were awarded for the radiographic presence of mesenteric foreshortening where the small bowel appears tethered or retracted centrally, a term called "cauliflowering" of the small bowel. This compromised the Simplified Preoperative Assessment for Appendix Tumor (SPAAT) scoring system (**Fig. 3**).[21]

1. One point for the presence of scalloping on the liver.
2. One point for the presence of scalloping on the spleen.
3. One point for the presence of scalloping on the pancreas.
4. One point for the presence of scalloping on the portal vein.
5. Zero or three points for the absence or presence of mesenteric foreshortening of the small bowel.

A derivation cohort of 30 patients treated at MDACC demonstrated a SPAAT score of greater than or equal to three to have 100% sensitivity and specificity for the inability to achieve a complete cytoreduction. This was validated in a cohort of 70 patients from the National Cancer Institute. As a result, patients with a SPAAT greater than or equal to three are not offered CRS and HIPEC with curative intent, because the median OS for these patients was only 10 months.[21] A palliative debulking and HIPEC is still offered to the symptomatic patients with minimal comorbidities and preserved nutritional and functional status. In these patients, we offer an organ-sparing, incomplete debulking where the omentum is resected to improve the symptoms of ascites and we address potential sources of bowel obstruction. The patients also receive HIPEC, because it is effective in controlling ascites in greater than 90% of patients with

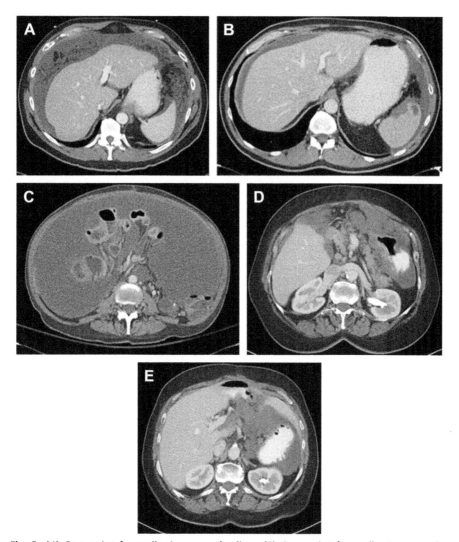

Fig. 3. (*A*) One point for scalloping over the liver. (*B*) One point for scalloping over the spleen. (*C*) Three points for mesenteric foreshortening. (*D*) One point for scalloping over the pancreas. (*E*) One point for scalloping around the portal vein.

malignant ascites, even in the absence of complete cytoreduction.[22] This approach is an attempt to maximize palliative benefit while minimizing potential morbidity. Several authors have demonstrated that palliative debulking is a safe procedure with an acceptable morbidity and mortality offering patients symptomatic benefits and immediate disease control.[22–24]

Tumor markers including CEA, CA19–9, and CA 125 are elevated in 56%, 67%, and 47% of patients with appendiceal adenocarcinoma, respectively.[25] Although the absolute value of the tumor markers does not correlate with survival a normal value is associated with improved survival.[25] The University of Pittsburgh reported an elevation of at least one tumor marker in 70% of patients and found absolute preoperative tumor marker values to correlate with the extent and distribution of peritoneal metastasis as measured by the PCI. Furthermore, an elevated CA19–9 was independently associated with poor progression-free survival (PFS) and an elevated CA-125 is associated with poor OS.[26] An elevated CA-125 was associated with a reduced likelihood of complete cytoreduction (70% vs 100%) in a study by Baratti and colleagues.[27] Similar to the Pittsburg group, Baratti and colleagues[27] reported an elevated CA19–9 to be independently associated with reduced PFS.[27] However, in clinical practice tumor markers are most useful in the evaluation treatment and recurrence but not in the initial evaluation.

Our algorithm for treating well-differentiated, mucinous appendiceal adenocarcinoma is shown in **Fig. 4**. We obtain laboratory studies, updated CT imaging with intravenous and oral contrast, colonoscopy, and review the previous operative report if any. All pathology is rereviewed by our pathologist. Patients with a previous

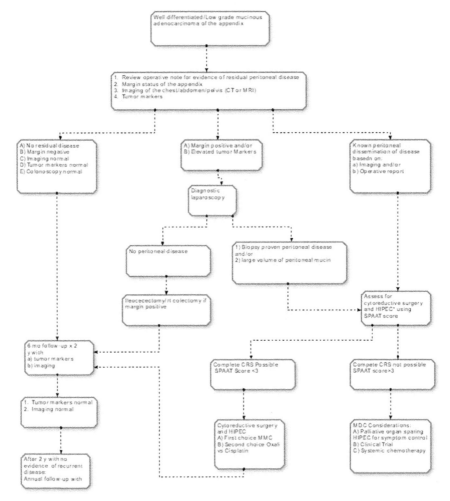

Fig. 4. Algorithm for treating well-differentiated, mucinous appendiceal adenocarcinoma. (*From* Grotz T. Patient selection in peritoneal malignancies. In: Feig B, editors. The MD Anderson surgical oncology handbook. 6th edition. Wolters Kluwer, in press. ISBN: 9781496358158; with permission.)

appendectomy with no suspicion of residual disease per the operative report and imaging with normal tumor markers and negative appendiceal margins are followed in surveillance. Completion colectomy is only offered to those with a positive appendiceal margin because there is no need for nodal staging, because the incidence of nodal metastasis for well-differentiated mucinous appendiceal adenocarcinoma is less than 5%. If a patient has a positive appendiceal margin or elevated tumor marker we recommend diagnostic laparoscopy with ileocectomy to obtain negative margins if no peritoneal disease is found at time of laparoscopy. If disease is identified on laparoscopy but not imaging then we recommend CRS and HIPEC. If a patient has residual disease on baseline imaging, we recommend determining the patient's SPAAT score to determine whether complete cytoreduction is possible. If a patient's medical comorbidities, nutritional status, and functional status permit, we then offer potentially curative CRS and HIPEC to a patient with a SPAAT score less than three. We typically wait 3 to 4 months from the last operation to allow inflammation to resolve. For patients with an SPAAT score greater than or equal to three who are symptomatic but have manageable comorbidities and preserved functional and nutritional status, we offer palliative, organ-preserving debulking and HIPEC. This approach attempts to balance morbidity and tumor debulking. For patients with unresectable well-differentiated mucinous appendiceal adenocarcinoma we do not recommend palliative chemotherapy because there has been no demonstrable benefit to systemic chemotherapy in these patients. These individuals are best managed with supportive care or a clinical trial.

PATIENT SELECTION FOR MODERATELY AND POORLY DIFFERENTIATED APPENDICEAL CANCER

Preoperative evaluation for patients with high-grade appendiceal cancer is similar to those with low-grade appendiceal cancer. High-quality imaging, tumor markers, and colonoscopy are routine. Patients should be fit to undergo a major abdominal operation and have no comorbid conditions that would prevent such. Our algorithm for high-grade appendiceal is outlined in **Fig. 5**. The additional consideration for high-grade appendiceal cancer is the nearly 40% incidence of lymph node metastasis. As such, in patients without peritoneal metastasis on imaging a formal right colectomy is indicated. At the time of the right colectomy we start with a diagnostic laparoscopy to formally assess the peritoneal cavity for evidence of peritoneal metastasis. If there is no evidence of peritoneal metastasis we proceed with laparoscopic right colectomy. In addition, we resect any omentum that was present in the area and we perform a right lower quadrant peritonectomy where the cecum and appendix previously contacted the peritoneum because these are the sites most likely to harbor occult disease. If at the time of laparoscopy there is evidence of peritoneal carcinomatosis we abort the right colectomy and initiate systemic chemotherapy, unless there is concern for obstruction or perforation of the primary tumor (discussed later). On completion of systemic chemotherapy, we obtain restaging studies and potentially repeat the diagnostic laparoscopy. If it seems that the patient is a good candidate for CRS and HIPEC, we proceed with formal right colectomy at the time of CRS/ HIPEC.

Chemotherapy

If after preoperative evaluation patients are considered a potential candidate for CRS and HIPEC then we initiate neoadjuvant systemic chemotherapy, generally with 5-FU/ oxaliplatin plus or minus bevacizumab for four to six cycles. Assuming patients are

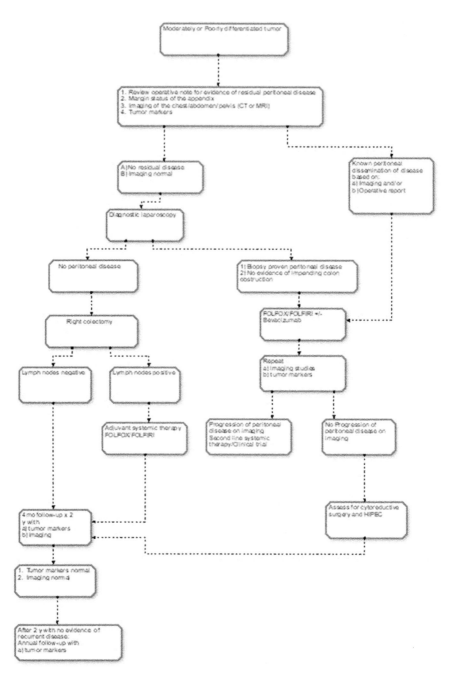

Fig. 5. Algorithm for high-grade appendiceal. (*From* Grotz T. Patient selection in peritoneal malignancies. In: Feig B, editors. The MD Anderson surgical oncology handbook. 6th edition. Wolters Kluwer, in press. ISBN: 9781496358158; with permission.)

able to tolerate chemotherapy, at the conclusion of their final cycle of chemotherapy, the patient undergoes restaging studies with CT imaging and serum tumor marker determination. The overall response rate to chemotherapy during a recent trial at MDACC was 44%. Stability disease occurred in 42% and progression of disease in only 14% of patients. The median PFS for this cohort of unresectable patients was 6.9 months with a median OS of 1.7 years.

Selection criteria for consideration of cytoreductive surgery and HIPEC are as follows:

1. Stability or response of tumor to neoadjuvant systemic chemotherapy seen on imaging.
2. The volume of disease on imaging must appear to be completely resectable.
3. No evidence of extraperitoneal metastasis.
4. No significant retroperitoneal or pericaval/periaortic lymphadenopathy.
5. Resectable liver metastasis are not a contraindication to CRS/HIPEC.

The response to systemic chemotherapy is an important predictor of biology because we found it to be independently associated with survival. Patients with high-grade appendiceal cancer with progression on systemic chemotherapy have a dismal prognosis with a median OS of 21 months compared with 44 months for those with stable or responsive disease. Therefore, we only offer CRS and HIPEC to those with stable or responsive disease. Patients with progression are treated with additional second- and third-line chemotherapy to achieve response before reconsideration for CRS and HIPEC.

Systemic chemotherapy, particularly with bevacizumab, has marked clinical activity and is associated with improvement in PFS and OS for unresectable high-grade appendiceal adenocarcinoma.[28] Extrapolating from the colorectal literature, Ceelen and coworkers[29] identified neoadjuvant systemic chemotherapy with bevacizumab to be an independent predictor of OS, reducing the risk of death by one-third. Unfortunately, there remains limited data for resectable moderately and poorly differentiated appendiceal adenocarcinoma and only a prospective randomized trial is able to definitively answer this question. Currently, there is a prospective phase II trial evaluating the use of adjuvant 5-FU-based chemotherapy with bevacizumab that is currently accruing and we look forward to the reporting of this trial (NCT02420509).

Diagnostic Laparoscopy

Nonmucinous and moderately and poorly differentiated appendiceal adenocarcinoma have outcomes following CRS and HIPEC that are remarkably similar to colon cancer.[30] Both are associated with increased desmoplasia and infiltration often leading to the necessity to resect underlying organs or structures of the overlying involved visceral and parietal peritoneum. This is in sharp contrast to the well-differentiated mucinous tumors that are removed easily with peritonectomy alone or with rough mechanical debridement. This difference in biology is important because it limits the extent and distribution of disease that can be resected. The PCI attributes points only based on the volume of disease in each of the 13 abdominopelvic regions and does not stratify points based on the ease or difficulty of resecting the organs/structures within the abdominopelvic region. Also, preoperative imaging consistently underestimates the extent of disease. Therefore, PCI based on preoperative imaging is not an adequate tool for patient selection for this population. Therefore, at MDACC diagnostic laparoscopy is used to evaluate the peritoneal cavity for PCI and distribution of disease.

The technique for diagnostic laparoscopy has been previously described. We typically perform a complete evaluation of the abdominal cavity using a video port and one instrument port, generally kept in the midline if possible so that these are resected with a midline incision. Loose adhesions are taken down and adhesiolysis is performed only to the extent needed to provide adequate visualization. During laparoscopy typically 80% of the abdominal cavity is visualized. Particular attention is paid to the small bowel serosal and mesenteric involvement and disease along the portal triad because these areas are particularly difficult to obtain complete cytoreduction. An assessment of the ability to obtain a complete cytoreduction is then made at time of laparoscopy. Tabrizian, and colleagues[32] in a multi-institutional study reported a successful completion of diagnostic laparoscopy in 92.6% of patients with minimal morbidity and no reported port site recurrence at short-term follow-up. Laparoscopy identified 31% of patients to have too extensive of disease burden for complete cytoreduction and were able to spare them an unnecessary laparotomy. These patients are given further systemic chemotherapy and a small proportion of them may have sufficient response to warrant repeat laparoscopy and reconsideration for CRS and HIPEC.[31,32] Patients considered amenable to CRS and HIPEC at laparoscopy are more likely to obtain complete cytoreduction.[32,33] The PCI can be calculated at the time of diagnostic laparoscopy and is an important independent prognostic factor. We use a PCI greater than 20 as a relative contraindication for proceeding to cytoreduction and HIPEC because we have found the median OS for a PCI of greater than 20 to be only 28 months compared with 65 months for those with PCI less than 20.[34] This is similar to the PCI cutoffs reported in the colorectal peritoneal carcinomatosis literature because they have similarly poor biology.[35–39] In addition, peritoneal cytology is obtained at the time of diagnostic laparoscopy. In our experience 45% of patients with gross peritoneal disease have positive cytology. All patients with positive peritoneal cytology were deceased by 49 months, whereas the median OS for those with negative cytology was 55 months. After controlling for other factors peritoneal cytology was an independent predictor of outcome. However, its use for selection of patients remains undefined and further investigation is warranted. Exclusionary findings at the time of diagnostic laparoscopy include the following:

1. Large-volume peritoneal carcinomatosis with a PCI greater than 20
2. Extensive involvement of the small bowel serosa or mesentery necessitating resection of greater than one-third of the small bowel
3. Extensive porta hepatis involvement
4. Extensive pelvic floor disease that would require an exenterative procedure

In addition to the previously stated important selection factors of response to neoadjuvant therapy and findings at diagnostic laparoscopy, pathologic factors, such as nonmucinous histology and presence of signet ring cells, are important independent predictors of outcome. However, long-term survival is achieved in these patients with poor biology if complete cytoreduction is achieved and therefore these are not absolute contraindications to CRS and HIPEC.[34,40]

PATIENT SELECTION FOR COLORECTAL PERITONEAL METASTASIS

Selection of patients with colorectal peritoneal carcinomatosis for CRS and HIPEC is similar to that for high-grade appendiceal in terms of our use of preoperative systemic chemotherapy and diagnostic laparoscopy. However, the Peritoneal Surface Malignancy Group has developed an additional consensus guideline for the appropriate patient selection for peritoneal carcinomatosis of colonic origin in which they defined eight clinical and radiologic variables that increase the probability of a complete cytoreduction and therefore improved survival[37]:

1. ECOG performance status ≤ 2
2. No evidence of extra-abdominal disease
3. Up to three small, resectable parenchymal hepatic metastases
4. No evidence of biliary obstruction
5. No evidence of ureteral obstruction
6. No evidence of intestinal obstruction at more than one site
7. Small bowel involvement: no evidence of gross disease in the mesentery with several segmental sites of partial obstruction
8. Small volume disease in gastrohepatic ligament

The PCI has been identified in several large cohort studies to be a major prognostic factor. Recently, Goéré and colleagues[35] even concluded that CRS and HIPEC does not offer any survival benefit in patients with a PCI score of 17 or higher. Others have also demonstrated this, reporting less than 10% 5-year OS for those with a PCI greater than or equal to 17,[36] although others have used higher cutoff points, such as PCI greater than 20.[39,41] The ambiguity of the PCI threshold is a limitation of the PCI because it does not account for the difference in resectability between tumors of the small bowel mesentery compared with the peritoneal lining. Therefore, we use these cutoffs as relative contraindications but reserve final decision of resectability until after visual inspection of the abdomen at diagnostic laparoscopy.

Similar to our experience with moderately and poorly differentiated appendiceal adenocarcinoma, the presence of signet ring cells is a marker of poor biology for colorectal cancer. A multi-institutional study from the Netherlands reported a median survival barely exceeding 1 year after CRS and HIPEC for patients with signet ring cell histology.[42] These results were mirrored at the University of Pittsburgh, which concluded that CRS and HIPEC does not confer a survival benefit in colorectal signet ring cell carcinomatosis unless complete cytoreduction is obtained.[40]

Prognostic scoring systems, which incorporate histology and PCI, have been developed to facilitate strict patient selection for CRS and HIPEC. The Peritoneal Surface Disease Severity Score (PSDSS) stratifies patients according to the severity of their peritoneal disease scored on a three-point scale that includes (1) symptoms, (2) extent of peritoneal dissemination (Peritoneal Cancer Index determined on a CT scan), and (3) primary tumor histology.

Multiple publications have validated the PSDSS as an independent positive predictive factor associated with survival for patients who are either treated with systemic chemotherapy alone or CRS and HIPEC.[43–46] However, even patients with a PSDSS III-IV have a median survival of 28 to 29 months and some long-term survivors. This still compares favorably with the stage IV patients treated with systemic chemotherapy alone (median survival, 8 and 6 months, respectively).[44] Similarly, the COMPAS nomogram has been developed, which takes into account, age, PCI, N2 lymph node status, and signet ring cell histology and predicts 1-, 2-, and 3-year OS based on the composite score. This model stratifies outcomes well with a median OS of only 16.5 months in patients with 82 or more points.[6] Therefore we use the PSDSS and COMPASS for patient education, prognostication, and to exclude patients with the highest scores from CRS and HIPEC.

A new and promising selection factor that needs further evaluation is peritoneal cytology. As more patients undergo laparoscopy to assess resectability, peritoneal cytology can be easily obtained and potentially providing additional prognostic information for determining appropriateness of CRS and HIPEC. A French study reviewed

162 patients with peritoneal disease from colon cancer who had undergone a complete cytoreduction. They obtained peritoneal lavage with 200-mL saline immediately at laparotomy and identified free-intraperitoneal cells using conventional cytology in 23.5% of patients. Positive cytology was also independently associated with worse PFS (median OS of 19 months compared with 44 months with negative cytology) in a retrospective review of 205 patients undergoing complete CRS and HIPEC by Yonemura and colleagues.[47] However, further evidence is lacking and additional studies are warranted before using peritoneal cytology clinically.

PATIENT SELECTION FOR PERITONEAL MESOTHELIOMA

Histologic subtype has become the most important determinant of survival for patients with peritoneal mesothelioma treated with CRS and HIPEC. Epithelioid is the most common histologic variant comprising 75% to 90% and is associated with a favorable outcome following complete CRS and HIPEC. Therefore, after previously described preoperative evaluation including high-quality imaging, tumor markers (CA-125 and CEA), and review of pathology, patients with epithelioid peritoneal mesothelioma that are considered amenable to complete cytoreduction based on imaging are offered CRS and HIPEC (**Fig. 6**).

In contrast, patients with sarcomatoid peritoneal mesothelioma have a different clinical course characterized by rapid progression and death. CRS and HIPEC is rarely of benefit in this histology and therefore palliative chemotherapy or enrollment in a clinical trial is best for this aggressive variant.

Biphasic peritoneal mesothelioma has histologic and clinical characteristics that are intermediate to epithelioid and sarcomatoid. Therefore, to better elicit the biology of this intermediate pathology we recommend neoadjuvant systemic chemotherapy with cisplatin and pemetrexed for four to six cycles. After completion of the last cycle patients are re-evaluated with imaging and tumor markers and those with a radiographic and/or biochemical response are considered for CRS and HIPEC.

Although straightforward, this algorithm fails to account for the complexity and heterogeneous biology exhibited within each histologic subtype. Therefore, there is great interest in improving the sophistication of understanding of tumor biology by replacing this crude histology-based stratification with more complex evaluation of tumor biology using Ki-67 proliferative index, mitotic rate, and PET avidity as surrogate markers of aggressiveness. An Australian group stratified 42 patients with malignant peritoneal mesothelioma into a low-proliferative group (Ki-67 <25%) and a high-proliferative group (Ki-67 ≥25%). This distinction was independently associated with survival with all low Ki-67 patients alive at 5 years compared with none of the high Ki67 patients.[48] Similarly, Kusamura and colleagues[49] evaluated the relationship of Ki-67 and PCI and identified a subgroup of patients with a Ki-67 greater than 9% and a PCI greater than 17 who had a median survival of only 10.3 months following CRS and HIPEC, suggesting these patients should be considered for other treatment protocols or clinical trials rather than CRS and HIPEC. Mitotic rate greater than 5/50 hpf is another dichotomized marker of proliferative capacity that has been demonstrated to hold prognostic significance with a median OS of 51 months compared with 23 months for those with a low and high mitotic rate, respectively.[50] Other studies have investigated the intensity of standardize uptake value (SUV)-max as a surrogate for proliferative capacity, and similarly have demonstrated an SUV-max of 3.63 best dichotomizes PFS, with a mean PFS of 29.2 months for SUV-max less than or equal to 3.63 and a mean PFS of 11.3 months for an SUV-max greater than 3.63.[51] In the

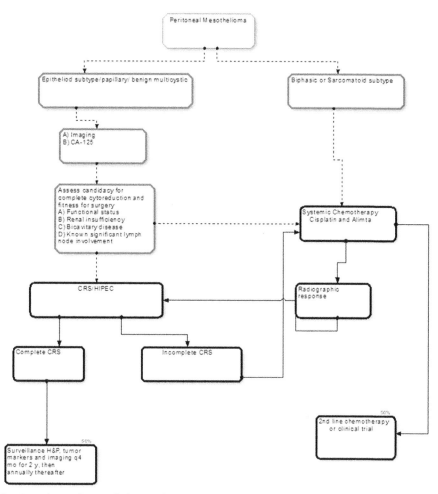

Fig. 6. Peritoneal mesothelioma algorithm. (*From* Grotz T. Patient selection in peritoneal malignancies. In: Feig B, editors. The MD Anderson surgical oncology handbook. 6th edition. Wolters Kluwer, in press. ISBN: 9781496358158; with permission.)

future, it is hoped that clinicians can incorporate more of these biochemical markers into the treatment decisions for patients with peritoneal mesothelioma.

PATIENT SELECTION FOR GASTRIC CANCER

There are two randomized controlled trials comparing CRS and HIPEC with systemic chemotherapy alone in patients with peritoneal carcinomatosis from gastric cancer. Both demonstrate a significant improvement in OS with CRS and HIPEC; however, the survival even after such an aggressive approach is dismal at 12 months.[52,53] This modest improvement in survival hardly seems worth it given what is known about the detrimental effects of CRS and HIPEC on quality of life, which last for up to 6 months following surgery. As a result, patient selection is likely even more critical for gastric cancer than the previously mentioned malignancies. The CCR is critical for gastric peritoneal carcinomatosis because only patients with a CCR of 0 have long-term survival.[54,55] To predict which patients are amenable to complete cytoreduction, several authors have used the PCI to demonstrate that only patients with a PCI less than seven have a long-term survival of 11%.[55,56] Importantly, there are no reported long-term survivors within the cohort of patients with a PCI greater than or equal to seven. Similarly, Fujimoto and colleagues[57] and Glehen and colleagues[58] reported all 5-year survivors having only Gilly stage I disease or less than 5-mm nodules confined to one region. Therefore, limited peritoneal disease that is amenable to complete cytoreduction is the most important preoperative selection factor. Because this low-volume disease is most likely to be missed on imaging, diagnostic laparoscopy is important for determining the extent of disease and likelihood of a complete CCR = 0 cytoreduction. We perform diagnostic laparoscopy and peritoneal cytology in patients with limited peritoneal disease from gastric cancer. We treat these patients with neoadjuvant systemic chemotherapy to convert patients to negative peritoneal cytology and at least show evidence of regression of peritoneal disease. Following this we have previously enrolled patients into a clinical trial (NCT02092298) in which patients were treated with laparoscopic HIPEC with mitomycin-C (30 mg) and cisplatin (200 mg) for 60 minutes every 2 to 8 weeks for up to five cycles. At each laparoscopy biopsies and repeat peritoneal cytology were obtained. For patients in whom staging imaging demonstrated no extraperitoneal metastasis and their peritoneal cytology and biopsies no longer demonstrated viable tumor we offered them curative-intent gastrectomy. We were able to complete conversion gastrectomy in 26% of patients with a median OS of 30.2 months, which compares favorably with the median OS of 24 and 35 months reported in the MAGIC and Intergroup trials, respectively, which both treated patients with gastric cancer without peritoneal metastasis with multimodality therapy.[59] We are currently enrolling patients into a phase II trial (NCT02891447) that includes CRS and HIPEC following induction chemotherapy for patients with peritoneal metastasis. It is hoped this study will bear further evidence for which patients will benefit most from CRS and HIPEC. We are in the infancy of experience with patient selection for CRS and HIPEC for gastric peritoneal carcinomatosis and further refinements to patient selection are needed and anticipated.

REFERENCES

1. Verwaal VJ, van Ruth S, de Bree E, et al. Randomized trial of cytoreduction and hyperthermic intraperitoneal chemotherapy versus systemic chemotherapy and palliative surgery in patients with peritoneal carcinomatosis of colorectal cancer. J Clin Oncol 2003;21(20):3737–43.
2. Verwaal VJ, Bruin S, Boot H, et al. 8-year follow-up of randomized trial: cytoreduction and hyperthermic intraperitoneal chemotherapy versus systemic chemotherapy in patients with peritoneal carcinomatosis of colorectal cancer. Ann Surg Oncol 2008;15(9):2426–32.
3. Jafari MD, Halabi WJ, Stamos MJ, et al. Surgical outcomes of hyperthermic intraperitoneal chemotherapy: analysis of the american college of surgeons national surgical quality improvement program. JAMA Surg 2014;149(2):170–5.
4. Smeenk RM, Verwaal VJ, Zoetmulder FA. Learning curve of combined modality treatment in peritoneal surface disease. Br J Surg 2007;94(11):1408–14.
5. Polanco PM, Ding Y, Knox JM, et al. Institutional learning curve of cytoreductive surgery and hyperthermic intraperitoneal chemoperfusion for peritoneal malignancies. Ann Surg Oncol 2015;22(5):1673–9.
6. Simkens GA, van Oudheusden TR, Luyer MD, et al. Predictors of severe morbidity after cytoreductive surgery and hyperthermic intraperitoneal

chemotherapy for patients with colorectal peritoneal carcinomatosis. Ann Surg Oncol 2016;23(3):833–41.

7. Baratti D, Kusamura S, Iusco D, et al. Postoperative complications after cytoreductive surgery and hyperthermic intraperitoneal chemotherapy affect long-term outcome of patients with peritoneal metastases from colorectal cancer: a two-center study of 101 patients. Dis Colon Rectum 2014;57(7):858–68.

8. Votanopoulos KI, Newman NA, Russell G, et al. Outcomes of cytoreductive surgery (CRS) with hyperthermic intraperitoneal chemotherapy (HIPEC) in patients older than 70 years; survival benefit at considerable morbidity and mortality. Ann Surg Oncol 2013;20(11):3497–503.

9. Ihemelandu CU, McQuellon R, Shen P, et al. Predicting postoperative morbidity following cytoreductive surgery with hyperthermic intraperitoneal chemotherapy (CS+HIPEC) with preoperative FACT-C (Functional Assessment of Cancer Therapy) and patient-rated performance status. Ann Surg Oncol 2013;20(11):3519–26.

10. Bartlett EK, Meise C, Roses RE, et al. Morbidity and mortality of cytoreduction with intraperitoneal chemotherapy: outcomes from the ACS NSQIP database. Ann Surg Oncol 2014;21(5):1494–500.

11. Tonnesen H, Nielsen PR, Lauritzen JB, et al. Smoking and alcohol intervention before surgery: evidence for best practice. Br J Anaesth 2009;102(3):297–306.

12. Wong J, Lam DP, Abrishami A, et al. Short-term preoperative smoking cessation and postoperative complications: a systematic review and meta-analysis. Can J Anaesth 2012;59(3):268–79.

13. Thomsen T, Villebro N, Moller AM. Interventions for preoperative smoking cessation. Cochrane Database Syst Rev 2014;(3):CD002294.

14. Drover JW, Dhaliwal R, Weitzel L, et al. Perioperative use of arginine-supplemented diets: a systematic review of the evidence. J Am Coll Surg 2011;212(3):385–99, 399.e1.

15. Jie B, Jiang ZM, Nolan MT, et al. Impact of preoperative nutritional support on clinical outcome in abdominal surgical patients at nutritional risk. Nutrition 2012;28(10):1022–7.

16. Dineen SP, Robinson KA, Roland CL, et al. Feeding tube placement during cytoreductive surgery and heated intraperitoneal chemotherapy does not improve postoperative nutrition and is associated with longer length of stay and higher readmission rates. J Surg Res 2016;200(1):158–63.

17. Sugarbaker PH. Pseudomyxoma peritonei. A cancer whose biology is characterized by a redistribution phenomenon. Ann Surg 1994;219(2):109–11.

18. Jacquet P, Sugarbaker PH. Clinical research methodologies in diagnosis and staging of patients with peritoneal carcinomatosis. Cancer Treat Res 1996;82:359–74.

19. Chua TC, Moran BJ, Sugarbaker PH, et al. Early- and long-term outcome data of patients with pseudomyxoma peritonei from appendiceal origin treated by a strategy of cytoreductive surgery and hyperthermic intraperitoneal chemotherapy. J Clin Oncol 2012;30(20):2449–56.

20. Lampe B, Kroll N, Piso P, et al. Prognostic significance of Sugarbaker's peritoneal cancer index for the operability of ovarian carcinoma. Int J Gynecol Cancer 2015;25(1):135–44.

21. Dineen SP, Royal RE, Hughes MS, et al. A simplified preoperative assessment predicts complete cytoreduction and outcomes in patients with low-grade mucinous adenocarcinoma of the appendix. Ann Surg Oncol 2015;22(11):3640–6.

22. Randle RW, Swett KR, Swords DS, et al. Efficacy of cytoreductive surgery with hyperthermic intraperitoneal chemotherapy in the management of malignant ascites. Ann Surg Oncol 2014;21(5):1474–9.

23. Funder JA, Jepsen KV, Stribolt K, et al. Palliative surgery for pseudomyxoma peritonei. Scand J Surg 2016;105(2):84–9.

24. Dayal S, Taflampas P, Riss S, et al. Complete cytoreduction for pseudomyxoma peritonei is optimal but maximal tumor debulking may be beneficial in patients in whom complete tumor removal cannot be achieved. Dis Colon Rectum 2013; 56(12):1366–72.

25. Carmignani CP, Hampton R, Sugarbaker CE, et al. Utility of CEA and CA 19-9 tumor markers in diagnosis and prognostic assessment of mucinous epithelial cancers of the appendix. J Surg Oncol 2004;87(4):162–6.

26. Wagner PL, Austin F, Sathaiah M, et al. Significance of serum tumor marker levels in peritoneal carcinomatosis of appendiceal origin. Ann Surg Oncol 2013;20(2): 506–14.

27. Baratti D, Kusamura S, Martinetti A, et al. Prognostic value of circulating tumor markers in patients with pseudomyxoma peritonei treated with cytoreductive surgery and hyperthermic intraperitoneal chemotherapy. Ann Surg Oncol 2007; 14(8):2300–8.

28. Choe JH, Overman MJ, Fournier KF, et al. Improved survival with anti-VEGF therapy in the treatment of unresectable appendiceal epithelial neoplasms. Ann Surg Oncol 2015;22(8):2578–84.

29. Ceelen W, Van Nieuwenhove Y, Putte DV, et al. Neoadjuvant chemotherapy with bevacizumab may improve outcome after cytoreduction and hyperthermic intraperitoneal chemoperfusion (HIPEC) for colorectal carcinomatosis. Ann Surg Oncol 2014;21(9):3023–8.

30. Cummins KA, Russell GB, Votanopoulos KI, et al. Peritoneal dissemination from high-grade appendiceal cancer treated with cytoreductive surgery (CRS) and hyperthermic intraperitoneal chemotherapy (HIPEC). J Gastrointest Oncol 2016; 7(1):3–9.

31. Jayakrishnan TT, Zacharias AJ, Sharma A, et al. Role of laparoscopy in patients with peritoneal metastases considered for cytoreductive surgery and hyperthermic intraperitoneal chemotherapy (HIPEC). World J Surg Oncol 2014;12:270.

32. Tabrizian P, Jayakrishnan TT, Zacharias A, et al. Incorporation of diagnostic laparoscopy in the management algorithm for patients with peritoneal metastases: a multi-institutional analysis. J Surg Oncol 2015;111(8):1035–40.

33. Marmor RA, Kelly KJ, Lowy AM, et al. Laparoscopy is safe and accurate to evaluate peritoneal surface metastasis prior to cytoreductive surgery. Ann Surg Oncol 2016;23(5):1461–7.

34. Grotz TE, Overman MJ, Eng C, et al. Cytoreductive surgery and hyperthermic intraperitoneal chemotherapy for moderately and poorly differentiated appendiceal adenocarcinoma: survival outcomes and patient selection. Ann Surg Oncol 2017;24(9):2646–54.

35. Goéré D, Souadka A, Faron M, et al. Extent of colorectal peritoneal carcinomatosis: attempt to define a threshold above which HIPEC does not offer survival benefit: a comparative study. Ann Surg Oncol 2015;22(9):2958–64.

36. Elias D, Faron M, Goéré D, et al. A simple tumor load-based nomogram for surgery in patients with colorectal liver and peritoneal metastases. Ann Surg Oncol 2014;21(6):2052–8.

37. Esquivel J, Sticca R, Sugarbaker P, et al. Cytoreductive surgery and hyperthermic intraperitoneal chemotherapy in the management of peritoneal surface

malignancies of colonic origin: a consensus statement. Society of Surgical Oncology. Ann Surg Oncol 2007;14(1):128–33.

38. Cashin PH, Graf W, Nygren P, et al. Cytoreductive surgery and intraperitoneal chemotherapy for colorectal peritoneal carcinomatosis: prognosis and treatment of recurrences in a cohort study. Eur J Surg Oncol 2012;38(6):509–15.

39. Maggiori L, Elias D. Curative treatment of colorectal peritoneal carcinomatosis: current status and future trends. Eur J Surg Oncol 2010;36(7):599–603.

40. Winer J, Zenati M, Ramalingam L, et al. Impact of aggressive histology and location of primary tumor on the efficacy of surgical therapy for peritoneal carcinomatosis of colorectal origin. Ann Surg Oncol 2014;21(5):1456–62.

41. Cashin PH, Dranichnikov F, Mahteme H. Cytoreductive surgery and hyperthermic intra-peritoneal chemotherapy treatment of colorectal peritoneal metastases: cohort analysis of high volume disease and cure rate. J Surg Oncol 2014; 110(2):203–6.

42. van Oudheusden TR, Braam HJ, Nienhuijs SW, et al. Poor outcome after cytoreductive surgery and HIPEC for colorectal peritoneal carcinomatosis with signet ring cell histology. J Surg Oncol 2015;111(2):237–42.

43. Pelz JO, Stojadinovic A, Nissan A, et al. Evaluation of a peritoneal surface disease severity score in patients with colon cancer with peritoneal carcinomatosis. J Surg Oncol 2009;99(1):9–15.

44. Pelz JO, Chua TC, Esquivel J, et al. Evaluation of best supportive care and systemic chemotherapy as treatment stratified according to the retrospective peritoneal surface disease severity score (PSDSS) for peritoneal carcinomatosis of colorectal origin. BMC Cancer 2010;10:689.

45. Esquivel J, Lowy AM, Markman M, et al. The American Society of Peritoneal Surface Malignancies (ASPSM) Multiinstitution Evaluation of the Peritoneal Surface Disease Severity Score (PSDSS) in 1,013 patients with colorectal cancer with peritoneal carcinomatosis. Ann Surg Oncol 2014;21(13):4195–201.

46. Chua TC, Morris DL, Esquivel J. Impact of the peritoneal surface disease severity score on survival in patients with colorectal cancer peritoneal carcinomatosis undergoing complete cytoreduction and hyperthermic intraperitoneal chemotherapy. Ann Surg Oncol 2010;17(5):1330–6.

47. Trilling B, Cotte E, Vaudoyer D, et al. Intraperitoneal-free cancer cells represent a major prognostic factor in colorectal peritoneal carcinomatosis. Dis Colon Rectum 2016;59(7):615–22.

48. Pillai K, Pourgholami MH, Chua TC, et al. Prognostic significance of Ki67 expression in malignant peritoneal mesothelioma. Am J Clin Oncol 2015;38(4):388–94.

49. Kusamura S, Torres Mesa PA, Cabras A, et al. The role of Ki-67 and pre-cytoreduction parameters in selecting diffuse malignant peritoneal mesothelioma (DMPM) patients for cytoreductive surgery (CRS) and hyperthermic intraperitoneal chemotherapy (HIPEC). Ann Surg Oncol 2016;23(5):1468–73.

50. Krasinskas AM, Borczuk AC, Hartman DJ, et al. Prognostic significance of morphological growth patterns and mitotic index of epithelioid malignant peritoneal mesothelioma. Histopathology 2016;68(5):729–37.

51. Dubreuil J, Giammarile F, Rousset P, et al. The role of 18F-FDG-PET/ceCT in peritoneal mesothelioma. Nucl Med Commun 2017;38(4):312–8.

52. Yang XJ, Huang CQ, Suo T, et al. Cytoreductive surgery and hyperthermic intraperitoneal chemotherapy improves survival of patients with peritoneal carcinomatosis from gastric cancer: final results of a phase III randomized clinical trial. Ann Surg Oncol 2011;18(6):1575–81.

53. Rudloff U, Langan RC, Mullinax JE, et al. Impact of maximal cytoreductive surgery plus regional heated intraperitoneal chemotherapy (HIPEC) on outcome of patients with peritoneal carcinomatosis of gastric origin: results of the GYMSSA trial. J Surg Oncol 2014;110(3):275–84.

54. Yang XJ, Li Y, Yonemura Y. Cytoreductive surgery plus hyperthermic intraperitoneal chemotherapy to treat gastric cancer with ascites and/or peritoneal carcinomatosis: results from a Chinese center. J Surg Oncol 2010;101(6):457–64.

55. Chia CS, You B, Decullier E, et al. Patients with peritoneal carcinomatosis from gastric cancer treated with cytoreductive surgery and hyperthermic intraperitoneal chemotherapy: is cure a possibility? Ann Surg Oncol 2016;23(6):1971–9.

56. Yonemura Y, Elnemr A, Endou Y, et al. Multidisciplinary therapy for treatment of patients with peritoneal carcinomatosis from gastric cancer. World J Gastrointest Oncol 2010;2(2):85–97.

57. Fujimoto S, Takahashi M, Mutou T, et al. Improved mortality rate of gastric carcinoma patients with peritoneal carcinomatosis treated with intraperitoneal hyperthermic chemoperfusion combined with surgery. Cancer 1997;79(5):884–91.

58. Glehen O, Gilly FN, Arvieux C, et al. Peritoneal carcinomatosis from gastric cancer: a multi-institutional study of 159 patients treated by cytoreductive surgery combined with perioperative intraperitoneal chemotherapy. Ann Surg Oncol 2010;17(9):2370–7.

59. Macdonald JS, Smalley SR, Benedetti J, et al. Chemoradiotherapy after surgery compared with surgery alone for adenocarcinoma of the stomach or gastroesophageal junction. N Engl J Med 2001;345(10):725–30.

Genomics of Peritoneal Malignancies

Enusha Karunasena, PhD[a], Jonathan Sham, MD[b], Kevin Wyatt McMahon, PhD[b],
Nita Ahuja, MD, MBA[b,c,d,*]

KEYWORDS

- Colorectal • Ovarian • Pancreatic • Microarray • Sequencing • Mutations
- Epigenetics • Genomics

KEY POINTS

- Inherited and somatic genetic mutations, epigenetic alterations, and other genomic aberrations contribute to peritoneal metastasis in select gastrointestinal, gynecologic, and orphan cancers.
- Classifications systems for disease subtypes based on genomic variants for colorectal, pancreatic, and epithelial ovarian cancers linked to peritoneal metastasis are highlighted.
- Genomic markers with associations to immunologic and cellular pathways important to cancer metastasis, and future significance to precision medicine, are emphasized.

GENOMICS OF GASTROINTESTINAL CANCERS AND PERITONEAL METASTASIS
Colorectal Cancer

Colorectal cancer (CRC) is the second leading cause of cancer mortality in the United States and third globally.[1] Patient morbidity is due to metastases, which develop in up to 50% of patients.[1] The majority of metastatic CRC are initially responsive to chemotherapy; however, resistance develops rapidly, such that the median survival for metastatic CRC has plateaued at 23 to 27 months despite the development of multiple targeted therapies.[1] Prognosis for early stage disease with localized tumor have improved with 5-year survival reaching upwards of 70% and up to 90%.[1] However, approximately 10% metastasize only into peritoneal tissues, although peritoneal

Disclosure: The authors have nothing to disclose.
[a] Department of Oncology, GI Clinical Cancer Research and Cancer Immunology, Sidney Kimmel Comprehensive Cancer Center, Johns Hopkins Medical Institute, 600 North Wolfe Street, Baltimore, MD 21287, USA; [b] Department of Surgery, Johns Hopkins Medical Institute, 600 North Wolfe Street, Baltimore, MD 21287, USA; [c] Cancer Biology, Department of Oncology, Sidney Kimmel Comprehensive Cancer, Johns Hopkins Medical Institute, 600 North Wolfe Street, Baltimore, MD 21287, USA; [d] Department of Surgery, Yale School of Medicine, PO Box 208062, New Haven, CT 06520-8062, USA
* Corresponding author. Department of Surgery, Yale School of Medicine, PO Box 208062, New Haven, CT 06520-8062.
E-mail address: nita.ahuja@yale.edu

metastases can often be a late stage finding of disease along with multifocal metastases at other sites. Moreover, synchronous peritoneal carcinomatosis occur in 5% to 6% of colon cancers and 1% to 2% of rectal cancers.[2] These patients with isolated peritoneal metastases are treated with systemic chemotherapy but increasingly with extensive surgery termed cytoreductive surgery, along with intraoperative delivery of chemotherapy or hyperthermic intraperitoneal chemotherapy, a combined approach to chemotherapy administration applied at the site of tumor resection; the median survival with this procedure is 30 months with a 5-year survival of 26%.[2,3] (See Paul H. Sugarbakers' article, "Peritoneal Metastases, A Frontier for Progress," and Travis E. Grotz colleagues' article, "Patient Selection for Cytoreductive Surgery," in this issue.)

Somatic mutations in genes known as driver mutations are associated with peritoneal metastases and are also predicative markers for treatment and survival prognostics. With peritoneal dissemination, TP53 gene mutations are observed in 35% to 75% of cases as compared with primary adenocarcinomas, and are the most common mutations observed with peritoneal metastasis.[4,5] Mutations occurring in KRAS occur in approximately 40% to 50% of patients with CRC, and are also associated with metastases. Reports of KRAS mutations in primary tumors resulting in metastases has a correlation of 95%.[6,7] A third common driver mutation is BRAF, occurring in approximately 10% of patients as a missense mutation resulting in V600E and is associated with peritoneal disease and poor overall survival, in addition to propagation via the lymphatic system.[2] Detection of PIK3CA mutations occur in 15% of metastatic diseases, and within peritoneal carcinomatosis anti-epidermal growth factor receptor therapy combined with an oxaliplatin regimen (ie, FOLFOX) has resulted in some benefit, although PIK3CA status and therapy benefits from antiangiogenic and MAPK pathway inhibitors remain uncertain.[2,8]

Additional new biomarkers arising from next-generation sequencing technologies include epigenetic markers. Tumor suppressor genes are notably silenced through hypermethylation and hypomethylation at tandem repeat loci known as CpG islands, and modification at promoter regions typically results in gene silencing; several of these genes are correlated with metastasis, including peritoneal disease. Better screening for familial CRCs, through mutation or epigenetic silencing, of mismatch repair genes (*MLH1*, *MSH2*, *MSH6*, *PMS2*, *STK11*, and *SMAD/DPC4*) and mutation of adenomatous polyposis coli[9–12] provide earlier disease detection capabilities and insight in metastatic potential. Typically, microsatellite instable cancers are more responsive to immune-therapies owing to mutational burden resulting in better antigenicity.[13] Other epigenetic marks are discussed in **Table 1**. Although microsatellite instable cancers account for less than 15% of CRCs, the prognostics for metastatic peritoneal disease remain better than microsatellite stable phenotypes.[1] Downstream transcriptional elements, including RNAs resulting from epigenetic modifications and driver gene mutations, has produced a new cohort of metastatic and recurrence-associated markers. Within these, changes in microRNA expression are associated specifically with peritoneal metastasis, such as miR-139-5p, others are linked to metastasis in additional sites, including miR-121.[25–27] The role of these and other macromolecular and micromolecular genetic elements are nascent, and our knowledge of their role in cancer is developing with several promising studies revealing prognostic markers and targets for future therapy.

Appendiceal Cancer

Distinct from CRC, appendiceal malignancies are rare, accounting for approximately 0.4% of gastrointestinal tumors.[28] Patients most commonly present with right lower quadrant pain and acute appendicitis, with tumors found incidentally on pathologic

Table 1
Epigenetic changes

	Function
Genes	
APC[a]	Tumor suppressor[14]
MGMT[a]	DNA damage repair[15]
CDKN2A/p16[a]	Tumor suppressor[16]
hMLH1, hMLH2[a]	DNA damage repair[9]
COX2[b]	Metastasis[17]
RASSF1A[a]	Tumor suppressor[18]
SOCS1[b]	Signal transduction[19]
CHFR[a]	Tumor suppressor/check point inhibitor[20]
ADAM23[b]	Metalloprotease[21,22]
miRNAs	
miR-21[b]	Invasion/metastasis[23]
miR-34a[a]	Tumor suppressor[24]

[a] Epigenetic changes associated with colorectal cancers and metastasis gene expression is inhibited by hypermethylation.
[b] Genes are overexpressed after hypermethylation.

review in approximately 1% of appendectomies.[29] Adenocarcinomas and mucinous neoplasms account for less than 10% of all appendiceal cancers, but are the predominate histologic subtypes accounting for peritoneal spread.[30] Appendiceal malignancies are of particular interest to surgeons, because they are among the few neoplasm with robust data demonstrating benefit with cytoreductive surgery and hyperthermic intraperitoneal chemotherapy in the setting of carcinomatosis.[31]

When disseminated disease is present, profound differences have been observed in clinical outcomes[32] and genetic features[33,34] of appendiceal neoplasms compared with CRCs. Whole-exome sequencing demonstrated KRAS mutations in 90% of metastatic mucinous neoplasms of the appendix compared with less than 50% of CRCs.[33] In contrast, mutations in TP53 and adenomatous polyposis coli, which are common in CRC, were virtually absent (<5%) in mucinous neoplasms of the appendix. These variations may have clinical significance. In at least one study of patients with pseudomyxoma peritonei undergoing cytoreductive surgery and hyperthermic intraperitoneal chemotherapy, multivariate analysis demonstrated poorer progression-free survival with KRAS-mutant tumors (hazard ratio, 14.96; 95% confidence interval, 1.95–114.77), whereas mutations in GNAS were associated with incomplete cytoreduction.[35]

Several studies have explored the molecular profiles of various appendiceal neoplasms – mucoceles, low-grade appendiceal mucinous neoplasms, low-grade appendiceal mucinous neoplasms with pseudomyxoma peritonei, and appendiceal adenocarcinoma—and finding striking molecular heterogeneity among these tumors.[35,36] KRAS and GNAS predominate in low-grade appendiceal mucinous neoplasms and low-grade appendiceal mucinous neoplasms with pseudomyxoma peritonei, whereas SMAD4 and TP53 are most commonly found in appendiceal adenocarcinoma. Activating GNAS mutations, which have been implicated in the Ras-PI3K-Akt and cAMP-PKA signaling pathways, were also found in high frequency in low-grade appendiceal mucinous neoplasms (24%) and low-grade appendiceal mucinous neoplasms with pseudomyxoma peritonei (22%). GNAS-mutant cells are predicted to be more invasive through increased exocytosis of vascular endothelial growth factor, matrix metalloproteases, and mucins.[37–39] However, it is unclear whether these genetic mutations or mucin secretion within the unique anatomic structure of the appendix (ie, blind pouch predisposed to obstruction and perforation) play a greater role in increased rates of peritoneal spread observed in mucin-secreting tumors.

Gastric Cancer

The incidence of gastric cancer has been steadily decreasing since the early 1970s when it was estimated to be most common global malignancy.[40] Despite this trend, it remains the third leading cause of cancer death worldwide, with 55% to 60% of patients presenting with metastatic peritoneal disease.[41]

Although some authors have suggested hematogenous spread as a potential mechanism for peritoneal dissemination, most believe that carcinomatosis occurs in a dynamic yet stepwise fashion stemming from direct extension of the primary tumor.[41] Once a primary invades to breach the gastric serosa, intracellular adhesion molecules such as E-cadherin can become downregulated, allowing cellular detachment and access to the peritoneal cavity.[42] These free malignant cells can then adhere to distant peritoneal sites through adhesion molecules such as selectins and CD44, with subsequent local invasion via matrix metalloproteinases and other motility factors.[43] The genomic alterations that enable this invasive transformation have only recently been explored.

While comparing matched pairs of whole-exome sequences between primary tumors and malignant ascites of patients with gastric cancer, Lim and colleagues[41] demonstrated an unusually high rate of C-to-A transversions in the exomes of metastatic cells (59.4%) when compared with their primary tumors (39.3%). Patients who received systemic chemotherapy (5-fluoracil, leucovorin) for their peritoneal disease exhibited a higher proportion of C-to-T transitions (43%) when compared with their nontreated counterparts (22.2%). As a control, cirrhosis-derived benign ascites was analyzed and also demonstrated high rates of C-to-A transversions, leading to between 10 and 21 somatic mutations per patient. The authors suggest the presence of a yet-to-be-defined process within ascitic fluid that may promote C-to-A transversions and thereby mutagenesis.

Whole genome sequencing of primary and metastatic gastric cancer have identified several somatic variations associated with carcinomatosis.[44] Mutations in retinitis pigmentosa 1-like 1 gene (RP1L1), PRB1 (BstNI subfamily), dynactin (DCTN1), and HS6ST3 were all observed in both primary lesions and metastatic tumor deposits. Although RP1L1, PRB1, and DCTN1 have no known oncologic association, HS6ST3 is implicated in proliferation, differentiation, adhesion, migration, and is highly expressed in chondrosarcomas.[45] In another study, more than 50% of patients with gastric cancer carcinomatosis had mutations in Rho-ROCK pathway components (RHOA, ROCK1, ROCK2, FYN, and MYO9B), which are involved in actin cytoskeleton formation, focal adhesion, and the Rho-protein signaling, suggesting that these mutations could play a role in peritoneal spread.[41]

Pancreatic Cancer

Pancreatic cancer metastases most often spread to the liver and peritoneum.[46] Improvements in morbidity and therapy efficacy in pancreatic ductal adenocarcinomas (PDAC) remain limited, with the overall median survival between 6 and 10 months for metastatic disease and 12 and 19 months for resectable tumors followed with chemotherapy.[1] Among cancers, PDAC (accounting for approximately 95% of pancreatic cancers) continues to rank among the worst for 1- or 5-year survival and is predicted to become the second most common cancer in the United States within 2 decades.[1,47] Identifying disease-associated mutations, including those important to metastasis, has been challenging owing to low neoplastic cellularity of pancreatic tumors (5%–20%) and the heterogeneous stromal environment that propagates metastasis through signaling and communication with tumor cells.[48]

Genomic sequencing of PDAC creates for a landscape of genetic aberrations and of these, several driver gene mutations important to metastasis, including KRAS, TP53, CDKN2A, and SMAD4—the most commonly identified somatic mutations in PDAC; additional oncogenic mutations include those observed in RNF43, ARID1A, TFGβR2, GNAS, RREB1, PBRM1, and BRAF and CTNNB1 in KRAS-wild type cancers.[49] Several classification systems to stratify PDAC into molecular subclassifications based on mutation profiles has resulted in 3 clinically informative cohorts and most recently a compendium of these profiles combined with The Cancer Genome Atlas (TCGA) data, further delineating subtypes with a propensity for metastasis.[48]

One classification system was based on gene transcription and described by Collison and colleagues[50] in 2011: the 3 groups consisted of a classical subtype with increased expression of epithelial and adhesion specific genes; the second subtype, quasimesenchymal, showed high expression of mesenchymal genes; and the third group showed higher expression for tumor-associated genes important to digestive enzymes; select groups of these genes are noted in **Table 2**.

A second classification system was described by Moffitt and colleagues[51] in 2015, consisting of microarray analysis of gene expression, in this stratification system stromal cells and neoplastic tissues were analyzed, creating 4 groups: basal-like tumor with normal stroma, basal-like tumor and activated stroma, classical tumor and normal stroma, and classical tumor and activated stroma. Basal-like tumors were described as similar in gene expression to breast and bladder cancers versus classical, which typically demonstrate lower expression of these markers.[51] Stroma described as normal exhibits gene expression associated with pancreatic stellate cells, whereas activated populations have greater Wnt family gene expression, and immunogenic genes linked to tumor promoting macrophage (chemokine and integrin expression).[51] Typically, patients with classical normal stroma have better prognostics compared with basal-like tumors; however,

Table 2
Compendia of genomic analyses resulting in PDAC subtype classifications

PDAC Genomic Analysis	Select Genes with Aberrations Important to PDAC Classification
Collison et al,[50] 2011: Analysis of gene expression (microarray analysis). 3 subtypes	*TMEM45B, TTF1, MUC13, AIM2, GPM6B, NT5E, CFTR, PNLIPRP2, REG1B*
Moffitt et al,[51] 2015: Gene expression (microarray analysis). 4 subtypes	*ACTA2, VIM, DES, WNT2, WNT5A, MMP9, MMP11, VGLL1, BTNL8, FAM3D*
Bailey et al,[52] 2016: Gene expression (RNAseq analysis). 4 subtypes	*GATA6, KRAS, TP53, KDM6A,TP63,NR5A2, RBPJL, NEUROD1, NKX2-2*
Waddell et al,[53] 2015: chromosomal structural variants (whole genome sequencing) 4 subtypes	*TP53, SMAD4, CDKN2A, ARID1A, ROBO2, KRAS, SOC9, GATA6, ERBB2, MET, CDK6, PIK3CA, PIK3R3*

Described above are 4 studies resulting in pancreatic ductal adenocarcinoma (PDAC) classification that were described based on microarray, RNAseq, and whole-genome sequencing studies of PDAC tumor and germline samples. Listed are those genes important to subtype classifications and characteristic of metastatic disease phenotypes.

basal-like tumors with normal stroma respond well to adjuvant therapies.[51] Genes associated with the Moffitt classification system are described in **Table 2**.[51]

With the advent of RNA sequencing platforms, quantification and better depth of sequencing coverage provides for more informative and accurate analysis; Bailey and colleagues[52] in 2016 combined these data with genomic sequencing data from mutations to describe disease-specific PDAC cohorts. From these results immunogenic characteristics, exocrine- and endocrine-associated differentiation and subtypes associated with disease-specific pathways were characterized; a subset of these classes and mutations are described in **Table 2**.[52]

Structural changes in genetic sequences, and most often near driver mutations, have created a signature in PDAC genomics; whole-genome sequencing by Waddell and colleagues[53] shows structural variants to be important in PDAC carcinogenesis. Specifically, they describe copy number variations and rearrangements in genes that cluster into subtypes. Subtype 1 is associated most often with classical disease and occurs in 20% with 50 or fewer variants; subtype 2 (30% of samples) demonstrates copy number variation gains near oncogenes; subtype 3 shows fewer than 200 variants but greater than 50 with chromosomal damage; and subtype 4 is seen in 14% of samples and is considered unstable, with more than 200 variants with structural rearrangements resulting in DNA damage.[53]

These classification systems and genetic variants were further analyzed and compared with tumor and germline samples by TCGA.[48] The TCGA produced a compendia of driver mutations, also described by other groups, and a loss-of-function mutation in RREB1, which has previously been reported as downregulated in PDAC and is important to PDAC carcinogenesis.[48] Notably, from the TCGA analysis heterogeneity in KRAS mutations within clonal populations were identified with biallelic mutation in subclones (G12R/G12V) and multiple KRAS mutations in subsets of clones (G12R, G12V, and Q12V); KRAS mutations are observed in approximately 93% of PDAC and G12R mutations may be indicative of tumors with a propensity for biallelic subclones or heterogeneous clonal populations which can be advantageous to tumor progression including, potentially to, metastasis.[48,54]

In addition to these compendia of collective drive mutations promoting PDAC and metastases, earlier studies by Yachida and colleagues[55] in 2010 described progressor mutations present in primary PDAC tumors and associated with peritoneal, liver, or lung metastasis; these mutations (including those described herein) comprised peritoneal specific cohorts (C20orf2 and FAT4) in clonal populations that consisted of millions of cells, consequently readying primary tumors with tissue specific metastatic potential as observed when later compared with patient-matched metastatic lesions.

Most recently, Feinberg and colleagues[56] in 2017 described epigenomic modifications in metastatic PDAC in large sequences (approximately 1000 bp) that were hypomethylated and in heterochromatin regions, and these metastasis were especially dependent on the oxidative branch of the pentose-phosphate pathway for glucose metabolism, demonstrating alternative metabolic pathways that are activated in conjunction with uniquely hypomethylated genomic sequences in metastatic PDAC; although peritoneal disease-specific variants remain to be identified, these epigenetic changes may be additive to metastatic growth, including in the peritoneum.

GYNECOLOGIC CANCERS WITH METASTASIS TO PERITONEAL TISSUES
Ovarian Cancer

Epithelial ovarian cancer (EOC) is the most common form of this disease and accounts for 90% of ovarian cancer cases (22,000 new cases and 15,500 reported deaths in the United States per year); it also remains the fifth leading cause of cancer death in women in the United States.[1] EOC has traditionally been divided into 4 phenotypes based on molecular and histopathologic traits: serous, endometrioid, clear cell, and mucinous.[57] Serous ovarian cancer will be the focus of this discussion because associated metastatic disease into the peritoneal cavity is common (70%, respectively) and several genomic studies have produced genetic aberrations with insight into peritoneal metastasis.[58] Similar to breast cancer, the risk for ovarian cancer owing to familial inheritance of mutated BRCA1 and/or BRCA2 accounts for 5% to 10% of EOC cases.[59,60] Surgical resection of tumors at stage 1 results in a more than 90% survival at 5 years.[57] However, EOCs are most often detected at higher stages (II–IV; 70%-80% of EOCs), with resulting metastasis commonly into the peritoneal tissues followed by other organs within the gastrointestinal tract.[58,59] EOC at higher stages typically have less than 30% survival rate at 5 years.[59,60] Metastatic disease is currently treated with surgery followed with chemotherapy (platinum-taxane regimen), in which 25% of patients progressed within 6 months after treatment.[61]

Whole exome sequencing, tumor and bloodline methylome analyses, and proteomic efforts have further validated previously identified genetic markers and introduced novel disease-specific aberrations. TCGA analyses of 316 serous ovarian cancer samples identified 6 genes with somatic mutations in addition to BRCA1/BRCA2 germline (8%–9%) and somatic (3%) mutations: RB1, NF1, FAT3, CSMD3, GABRA6, and CDK12; of these RB1 and NF1 were the most significantly mutated and 2% of tumors having homozygous deletions in PTEN, RB1, and NF1.[61] Additional somatic gene mutations previously identified (although rarer in EOC) included variants in BRAF, PIK3CA, KRAS, and NRAS—all of which demonstrate transforming activity.[61] Somatic copy number variants were located as focal amplifications in CCNE1, MYC, and MECOM (and were identified in ≥20% of tumors).[60] Most recently, notable efforts to describe genome-wide variants was conducted by Phelan and colleagues,[62] which included genomic sequences from multiple ovarian cancers and from several consortia (>25,000 EOC samples), this effort resulted in the identification of 12 distinct chromosomal loci, with genotypes unique to ovarian cancer subtypes: 6 loci were unique to serous EOC (3q28, 4q32.3, 8q21.11, 10q24.33, 18q11.2 and 22q12.1), three from BRCA1 and BRCA2 mutated ovarian cancers, and 3 disease susceptibility markers were newly identified (2q13, 8q24.1, and 12q24.31).

Given the permeability of the peritoneum, what is normally a protective asset is exploited by tumor-promoting inflammatory cells.[57] With peritoneal metastasis, physiologic changes result in thickening and increased vascularization; associated with these events are increased macrophage infiltration, specifically M2 CD68+ cells (M2 cells are commonly associated with increased Tregs in the tumor microenvironment and decreased CD8+, CD4+, and M1 macrophages; these cells typically produce an immune response associated with tumor inhibition).[63] Expression of TIE2 by M2 macrophages have been identified in EOC among other cancers, including hepatocellular carcinoma. TIE2 is a receptor for Ang2 that promotes angiogenesis and promotes the Erk 1/2 and Akt pathways.[63] TIE2 expression and the increased occurrence of TIE2 by M2 macrophages may be a diagnostic marker for metastasis.[63] Previously described and established immunologic markers also include macrophage specific induction of nuclear factor-κB and c-Jun kinase signaling pathways resulting in increased interleukin-6, interleukin-8, and vascular endothelial growth factor-C, which promote metastasis.[64,65] As immunotherapy and targeted therapies improve disease management, such expression markers may be essential to controlling metastatic peritoneal disease.[66]

Studies propose that ovarian cancer cells shed from tumors with high expression of human growth factor are contributive to the implantation of cancerous cells into the peritoneum, and that these cells attach to mesothelial cells resulting in their embedment.[67] Human growth factor overexpression is also implicated in hepatic metastasis and is overexpressed in hepatocellular carcinoma.[67] In addition to the seed and soil hypothesis, others suggest peritoneal metastasis, as observed often in the omentum of the peritoneum with serous ovarian cancers, may be due to inherent genetic aberrations that are yet to be identified.[57,68]

ORPHAN CANCERS WITH PERITONEAL METASTASIS
Cholangiocarcinoma

Intrahepatic cholangiocarcinoma arises in epithelial cells lining the bile duct system and is the fifth most common cancer worldwide with 600,000 new cases reported annually.[69] Disease burden is higher in Asiatic nations but incidence is increasing in the United States and is expected to be a major cause of cancer death by 2050.[69] The 5-year survival is 12% for localized intrahepatic cholangiocarcinoma and 2% for metastatic disease (including peritoneal malignancies).[70,71] Diagnosis is typically made at advanced stages, at which point palliative chemotherapy is the common course of treatment.[69,70,72] At present, there is only 1 standard line of therapy for these patients, indicating a substantial unmet need for this cancer with an increasing prevalence. Companion diagnostics and therapeutics for intrahepatic cholangiocarcinoma have been restricted by a lack of targetable molecular markers, limiting precision-based treatment and continued overall poor prognosis.[71] With the advent of high-throughput genomic sequencing technologies and a collective international effort toward characterizing genomic variations in ICC has yielded, multiple driver mutations (including *KRAS* and *ARID1A*) and targetable oncogenic mutants — in particular isocitrate dehydrogenase 1 (*IDH1*).[69,71,73] IDH mutations have been reported in multiple cancers including myeloid cancers (15%), gliomas (80% low grade), chondrosarcomas (50%), and intrahepatic cholangiocarcinoma (20%).[73–75] IDH1 is an oncogene with a gain-of-function mutation, producing the oncometabolite 2-hydroxyglutarate (2-HG).[73,76] High 2-HG levels inhibit multiple normal cellular processes such as differentiation as well as epigenetic regulators of DNA including DNA methyltransferases and chromatin remodeling proteins such as histone demethylases.[72,76,77] As with many orphan cancers, and peritoneum specific malignancies, genetic markers remain unknown.

Leiomyosarcoma

Uterine leiomyosarcomas are rare but deadly cancers of the smooth muscle around the uterus, with a reported 1 in 100,000 cases in the United States. The 5-year survival is typically between 44% and 27% for stages II through IV disease.[78] This tissue is also the origin of uterine leiomyomas (also known as fibroids), which are a major source of female infertility.[78] Uterine leiomyosarcomas typically metastasize to peritoneal tissues. Somatic mutations in MED12, a member of the large multiprotein complex called "the mediator" that regulates RNA polymerase II transcription, are found in 70% of leiomyosarcomas, and the mediator interacts with epigenetic modifiers as part of its regulation of transcription.[79–81] Additional driver mutations identified from Uterine leiomyosarcomas tumors included TP53, RB1, and ATRX1; ATRX is also notably mutated in diffusive glioblastoma.[82–84]

SUMMARY

With advancements in cost-effective sequencing and collaborative international and national efforts, sequencing studies on common and orphan cancers will continue to catalyze precision oncology, resulting in better therapy decisions based on genetic and genomic aberrations, as demonstrated with immunotherapy and other target-specific small molecule inhibitors. Pan-cancer sequencing profiles will also contribute to our understanding of which genetic and genomic aberrations contribute to selective pressures that result in metastasis including tissue-specific metastasis.

REFERENCES

1. Siegel RL, Miller KD, Fedewa SA, et al. Colorectal cancer statistics, 2017. CA Cancer J Clin 2017;67(3):177–93.
2. Massalou D, Benizri E, Chevallier A, et al. Peritoneal carcinomatosis of colorectal cancer: novel clinical and molecular outcomes. Am J Surg 2017;213(2):377–87.
3. Glehen O, Gilly FN, Boutitie F, et al. Toward curative treatment of peritoneal carcinomatosis from nonovarian origin by cytoreductive surgery combined with perioperative intraperitoneal chemotherapy: a multi-institutional study of 1,290 patients. Cancer 2010;116(24):5608–18.
4. Sclafani F, Gonzalez D, Cunningham D, et al. TP53 mutational status and cetuximab benefit in rectal cancer: 5-year results of the EXPERT-C trial. J Natl Cancer Inst 2014;106(7) [pii:dju121].
5. Pino MS, Chung DC. The chromosomal instability pathway in colon cancer. Gastroenterology 2010;138(6):2059–72.
6. Karapetis CS, Khambata-Ford S, Jonker DJ, et al. K-ras mutations and benefit from cetuximab in advanced colorectal cancer. N Engl J Med 2008;359(17): 1757–65.
7. De Roock W, Claes B, Bernasconi D, et al. Effects of KRAS, BRAF, NRAS, and PIK3CA mutations on the efficacy of cetuximab plus chemotherapy in chemotherapy-refractory metastatic colorectal cancer: a retrospective consortium analysis. Lancet Oncol 2010;11(8):753–62.
8. Tian S, Simon I, Moreno V, et al. A combined oncogenic pathway signature of BRAF, KRAS and PI3KCA mutation improves colorectal cancer classification and cetuximab treatment prediction. Gut 2013;62(4):540–9.
9. Herman JG, Umar A, Polyak K, et al. Incidence and functional consequences of hMLH1 promoter hypermethylation in colorectal carcinoma. Proc Natl Acad Sci U S A 1998;95(12):6870–5.
10. Fu T, Liu Y, Li K, et al. Tumors with unmethylated MLH1 and the CpG island methylator phenotype are associated with a poor prognosis in stage II colorectal cancer patients. Oncotarget 2016;7(52):86480–9.
11. Curtin K, Samowitz WS, Wolff RK, et al. MSH6 G39E polymorphism and CpG island methylator phenotype in colon cancer. Mol Carcinog 2009;48(11):989–94.
12. Fu T, Pappou EP, Guzzetta AA, et al. CpG island methylator phenotype-positive tumors in the absence of MLH1 methylation constitute a distinct subset of duodenal adenocarcinomas and are associated with poor prognosis. Clin Cancer Res 2012;18(17):4743–52.
13. Le DT, Durham JN, Smith KN, et al. Mismatch-repair deficiency predicts response of solid tumors to PD-1 blockade. Science 2017;357(6349):409–13.
14. Powell SM, Zilz N, Beazer-Barclay Y, et al. APC mutations occur early during colorectal tumorigenesis. Nature 1992;359(6392):235–7.
15. Esteller M, Garcia-Foncillas J, Andion E, et al. Inactivation of the DNA-repair gene MGMT and the clinical response of gliomas to alkylating agents. N Engl J Med 2000;343(19):1350–4.

16. Xiong Y, Zhang H, Beach D. Subunit rearrangement of the cyclin-dependent kinases is associated with cellular transformation. Genes Dev 1993;7(8):1572–83.
17. Nakae D, Kotake Y, Kishida H, et al. Inhibition by phenyl N-tert-butyl nitrone of early phase carcinogenesis in the livers of rats fed a choline-deficient, L-amino acid-defined diet. Cancer Res 1998;58(20):4548–51.
18. van Engeland M, Roemen GM, Brink M, et al. K-ras mutations and RASSF1A promoter methylation in colorectal cancer. Oncogene 2002;21(23):3792.
19. Kishimoto T, Kikutani H. Knocking the SOCS off a tumor suppressor. Nat Genet 2001;28(1):4–5.
20. Brandes JC, van Engeland M, Wouters KA, et al. CHFR promoter hypermethylation in colon cancer correlates with the microsatellite instability phenotype. Carcinogenesis 2005;26(6):1152–6.
21. Costa FF, Verbisck NV, Salim AC, et al. Epigenetic silencing of the adhesion molecule ADAM23 is highly frequent in breast tumors. Oncogene 2004;23(7):1481–8.
22. Takada H, Imoto I, Tsuda H, et al. ADAM23, a possible tumor suppressor gene, is frequently silenced in gastric cancers by homozygous deletion or aberrant promoter hypermethylation. Oncogene 2005;24(54):8051–60.
23. Chan JA, Krichevsky AM, Kosik KS. MicroRNA-21 is an antiapoptotic factor in human glioblastoma cells. Cancer Res 2005;65(14):6029–33.
24. Tazawa H, Tsuchiya N, Izumiya M, et al. Tumor-suppressive miR-34a induces senescence-like growth arrest through modulation of the E2F pathway in human colon cancer cells. Proc Natl Acad Sci U S A 2007;104(39):15472–7.
25. Miyoshi J, Toden S, Yoshida K, et al. MiR-139-5p as a novel serum biomarker for recurrence and metastasis in colorectal cancer. Sci Rep 2017;7:43393.
26. Dalmay T, Edwards DR. MicroRNAs and the hallmarks of cancer. Oncogene 2006;25(46):6170–5.
27. Hur K. MicroRNAs: promising biomarkers for diagnosis and therapeutic targets in human colorectal cancer metastasis. BMB Rep 2015;48(4):217–22.
28. Connor SJ, Hanna GB, Frizelle FA. Appendiceal tumors: retrospective clinicopathologic analysis of appendiceal tumors from 7,970 appendectomies. Dis Colon Rectum 1998;41(1):75–80.
29. McCusker ME, Coté TR, Clegg LX, et al. Primary malignant neoplasms of the appendix: a population-based study from the surveillance, epidemiology and end-results program, 1973-1998. Cancer 2002;94(12):3307–12.
30. Sugarbaker PH, Kern K, Lack E. Malignant pseudomyxoma peritonei of colonic origin. Natural history and presentation of a curative approach to treatment. Dis Colon Rectum 1987;30(10):772–9.
31. Bryant J, Clegg AJ, Sidhu MK, et al. Systematic review of the Sugarbaker procedure for pseudomyxoma peritonei. Br J Surg 2005;92(2):153–8.
32. Sugarbaker PH, Jablonski KA. Prognostic features of 51 colorectal and 130 appendiceal cancer patients with peritoneal carcinomatosis treated by cytoreductive surgery and intraperitoneal chemotherapy. Ann Surg 1995;221(2):124–32.
33. Alakus H, Babicky ML, Ghosh P, et al. Genome-wide mutational landscape of mucinous carcinomatosis peritonei of appendiceal origin. Genome Med 2014; 6(5):43.
34. Green DE, Jayakrishnan TT, Hwang M, et al. Immunohistochemistry - microarray analysis of patients with peritoneal metastases of appendiceal or colorectal origin. Front Surg 2014;1:50.
35. Pietrantonio F, Perrone F, Mennitto A, et al. Toward the molecular dissection of peritoneal pseudomyxoma. Ann Oncol 2016;27(11):2097–103.

36. Liu X, Mody K, de Abreu FB, et al. Molecular profiling of appendiceal epithelial tumors using massively parallel sequencing to identify somatic mutations. Clin Chem 2014;60(7):1004–11.
37. Bradbury NA. Protein kinase-A-mediated secretion of mucin from human colonic epithelial cells. J Cell Physiol 2000;185(3):408–15.
38. Jarry A, Merlin D, Hopfer U, et al. Cyclic AMP-induced mucin exocytosis is independent of Cl- movements in human colonic epithelial cells (HT29-Cl.16E). Biochem J 1994;304(Pt 3):675–8.
39. Ernens I, Rouy D, Velot E, et al. Adenosine inhibits matrix metalloproteinase-9 secretion by neutrophils: implication of A2a receptor and cAMP/PKA/Ca2+ pathway. Circ Res 2006;99(6):590–7.
40. Ferlay J, Soerjomataram I, Dikshit R, et al. Cancer incidence and mortality worldwide: sources, methods and major patterns in GLOBOCAN 2012. Int J Cancer 2015;136(5):E359–86.
41. Lim B, Kim C, Kim JH, et al. Genetic alterations and their clinical implications in gastric cancer peritoneal carcinomatosis revealed by whole-exome sequencing of malignant ascites. Oncotarget 2016;7(7):8055–66.
42. Kusamura S, Baratti D, Zaffaroni N, et al. Pathophysiology and biology of peritoneal carcinomatosis. World J Gastrointest Oncol 2010;2(1):12–8.
43. Jayne D. Molecular biology of peritoneal carcinomatosis. Cancer Treat Res 2007; 134:21–33.
44. Zhang J, Huang JY, Chen YN, et al. Whole genome and transcriptome sequencing of matched primary and peritoneal metastatic gastric carcinoma. Sci Rep 2015;5:13750.
45. Waaijer CJ, de Andrea CE, Hamilton A, et al. Cartilage tumour progression is characterized by an increased expression of heparan sulphate 6O-sulphation-modifying enzymes. Virchows Arch 2012;461(4):475–81.
46. Yamada H, Hirano S, Tanaka E, et al. Surgical treatment of liver metastases from pancreatic cancer. HPB (Oxford) 2006;8(2):85–8.
47. Rahib L, Smith BD, Aizenberg R, et al. Projecting cancer incidence and deaths to 2030: the unexpected burden of thyroid, liver, and pancreas cancers in the United States. Cancer Res 2014;74(11):2913–21.
48. Cancer Genome Atlas Research Network. Integrated genomic characterization of pancreatic ductal adenocarcinoma. Cancer Cell 2017;32(2):185–203.e13.
49. Jones S, Zhang X, Parsons DW, et al. Core signaling pathways in human pancreatic cancers revealed by global genomic analyses. Science 2008;321(5897): 1801–6.
50. Collisson EA, Sadanandam A, Olson P, et al. Subtypes of pancreatic ductal adenocarcinoma and their differing responses to therapy. Nat Med 2011;17(4): 500–3.
51. Moffitt RA, Marayati R, Flate EL, et al. Virtual microdissection identifies distinct tumor- and stroma-specific subtypes of pancreatic ductal adenocarcinoma. Nat Genet 2015;47(10):1168–78.
52. Bailey P, Chang DK, Nones K, et al. Genomic analyses identify molecular subtypes of pancreatic cancer. Nature 2016;531(7592):47–52.
53. Waddell N, Pajic M, Patch AM, et al. Whole genomes redefine the mutational landscape of pancreatic cancer. Nature 2015;518(7540):495–501.
54. Maddipati R, Stanger BZ. Pancreatic cancer metastases harbor evidence of polyclonality. Cancer Discov 2015;5(10):1086–97.
55. Yachida S, Jones S, Bozic I, et al. Distant metastasis occurs late during the genetic evolution of pancreatic cancer. Nature 2010;467(7319):1114–7.

56. McDonald OG, Li X, Saunders T, et al. Epigenomic reprogramming during pancreatic cancer progression links anabolic glucose metabolism to distant metastasis. Nat Genet 2017;49(3):367–76.

57. Yeung TL, Leung CS, Yip KP, et al. Cellular and molecular processes in ovarian cancer metastasis. A review in the theme: cell and molecular processes in cancer metastasis. Am J Physiol Cell Physiol 2015;309(7):C444–56.

58. Seidman JD, Horkayne-Szakaly I, Haiba M, et al. The histologic type and stage distribution of ovarian carcinomas of surface epithelial origin. Int J Gynecol Pathol 2004;23(1):41–4.

59. Pal T, Permuth-Wey J, Betts JA, et al. BRCA1 and BRCA2 mutations account for a large proportion of ovarian carcinoma cases. Cancer 2005;104(12):2807–16.

60. Ramus SJ, Harrington PA, Pye C, et al. Contribution of BRCA1 and BRCA2 mutations to inherited ovarian cancer. Hum Mutat 2007;28(12):1207–15.

61. Cancer Genome Atlas Research Network. Integrated genomic analyses of ovarian carcinoma. Nature 2011;474(7353):609–15.

62. Phelan CM, Kuchenbaecker KB, Tyrer JP, et al. Identification of 12 new susceptibility loci for different histotypes of epithelial ovarian cancer. Nat Genet 2017; 49(5):680–91.

63. Wang X, Zhu Q, Lin Y, et al. Crosstalk between TEMs and endothelial cells modulates angiogenesis and metastasis via IGF1-IGF1R signalling in epithelial ovarian cancer. Br J Cancer 2017;117(9):1371–82.

64. Hagemann T, Wilson J, Kulbe H, et al. Macrophages induce invasiveness of epithelial cancer cells via NF-κB and JNK. J Immunol 2005;175(2):1197–205.

65. Wang X, Deavers M, Patenia R, et al. Monocyte/macrophage and T-cell infiltrates in peritoneum of patients with ovarian cancer or benign pelvic disease. J Transl Med 2006;4(1):30.

66. Hardwick N, Frankel PH, Cristea M. New approaches for immune directed treatment for ovarian cancer. Curr Treat Options Oncol 2016;17(3):14.

67. Nakamura M, Ono YJ, Kanemura M, et al. Hepatocyte growth factor secreted by ovarian cancer cells stimulates peritoneal implantation via the mesothelial-mesenchymal transition of the peritoneum. Gynecol Oncol 2015;139(2):345–54.

68. Lengyel E. Ovarian cancer development and metastasis. Am J Pathol 2010; 177(3):1053–64.

69. Putra J, de Abreu FB, Peterson JD, et al. Molecular profiling of intrahepatic and extrahepatic cholangiocarcinoma using next generation sequencing. Exp Mol Pathol 2015;99(2):240–4.

70. Goyal L, Govindan A, Sheth RA, et al. Prognosis and clinicopathologic features of patients with advanced stage isocitrate dehydrogenase (IDH) mutant and IDH wild-type intrahepatic cholangiocarcinoma. Oncologist 2015;20(9):1019–27.

71. Zou S, Li J, Zhou H, et al. Mutational landscape of intrahepatic cholangiocarcinoma. Nat Commun 2014;5:5696.

72. Saha SK, Gordan JD, Kleinstiver BP, et al. Isocitrate dehydrogenase mutations confer dasatinib hypersensitivity and SRC dependence in intrahepatic cholangiocarcinoma. Cancer Discov 2016;6(7):727–39.

73. Fujii T, Khawaja MR, DiNardo CD, et al. Targeting isocitrate dehydrogenase (IDH) in cancer. Discov Med 2016;21(117):373–80.

74. Wang P, Dong Q, Zhang C, et al. Mutations in isocitrate dehydrogenase 1 and 2 occur frequently in intrahepatic cholangiocarcinomas and share hypermethylation targets with glioblastomas. Oncogene 2013;32(25):3091–100.

75. Yan H, Parsons DW, Jin G, et al. IDH1 and IDH2 mutations in gliomas. N Engl J Med 2009;360(8):765–73.

76. Borodovsky A, Salmasi V, Turcan S, et al. 5-azacytidine reduces methylation, promotes differentiation and induces tumor regression in a patient-derived IDH1 mutant glioma xenograft. Oncotarget 2013;4(10):1737–47.
77. Emadi A, Faramand R, Carter-Cooper B, et al. Presence of isocitrate dehydrogenase mutations may predict clinical response to hypomethylating agents in patients with acute myeloid leukemia. Am J Hematol 2015;90(5):E77–9.
78. Stewart EA. Clinical practice. Uterine fibroids. N Engl J Med 2015;372(17): 1646–55.
79. Malik S, Roeder RG. The metazoan Mediator co-activator complex as an integrative hub for transcriptional regulation. Nat Rev Genet 2010;11(11):761–72.
80. Makinen N, Mehine M, Tolvanen J, et al. MED12, the mediator complex subunit 12 gene, is mutated at high frequency in uterine leiomyomas. Science 2011; 334(6053):252–5.
81. Tsutsui T, Fukasawa R, Shinmyouzu K, et al. Mediator complex recruits epigenetic regulators via its two cyclin-dependent kinase subunits to repress transcription of immune response genes. J Biol Chem 2013;288(29):20955–65.
82. Conconi D, Chiappa V, Perego P, et al. Potential role of BCL2 in the recurrence of uterine smooth muscle tumors of uncertain malignant potential. Oncol Rep 2017; 37(1):41–7.
83. Bodner-Adler B, Bodner K, Czerwenka K, et al. Expression of p16 protein in patients with uterine smooth muscle tumors: an immunohistochemical analysis. Gynecol Oncol 2005;96(1):62–6.
84. Yang C-Y, Liau J-Y, Huang W-J, et al. Targeted next-generation sequencing of cancer genes identified frequent TP53 and ATRX mutations in leiomyosarcoma. Am J Transl Res 2015;7(10):2072–81.

Pharmacokinetics and Tissue Transport of Intraperitoneal Chemotherapy

Nick Lagast, MSE, Charlotte Carlier, MS, Wim P. Ceelen, MD, PhD*

KEYWORDS

- Pharmacokinetics • Chemotherapy • HIPEC • Carcinomatosis

KEY POINTS

- During intraperitoneal (IP) chemotherapy delivery, the peritoneal barrier results in a pharmacokinetic advantage, which can be characterized using a 2-compartment model.
- The anticancer efficacy of IP chemotherapy depends on the extent of tumor tissue penetration.
- Tissue transport of IP chemotherapy is governed by diffusion and convection; their relative contribution can be expressed using the Péclet number, which is higher for macromolecular drugs.
- Results from mathematical models, in vitro experiments, animal research, and clinical studies demonstrate that tissue penetration of IP chemotherapy is very limited (0.5–3 mm at most).
- Several physical and pharmacologic approaches are currently being studied in order to improve tissue penetration of small molecular and macromolecular anticancer drugs after IP instillation.

INTRODUCTION

Anticancer drugs are usually administered systemically, resulting in exposure of healthy tissue, which limits their therapeutic index. Locoregional drug delivery, targeted at the tissue or organ of interest, may allow an increase in treatment intensity while at the same time limiting systemic toxicity. Over the past decades, several methods of locoregional anticancer therapy have been clinically implemented. These therapies include instillation in an anatomic cavity (intraperitoneal [IP], intravesical, intrathecal, intrapleural) or selective infusion into a feeding artery with or without vascular isolation of the target organ.

Disclosure Statement: The authors have nothing to disclose.
Department of Surgery, Ghent University, Cancer Research Institute Ghent (CRIG), Ghent B-9000, Belgium
* Corresponding author. Department of GI Surgery, Ghent University Hospital, Route 1275, Corneel Heymanslaan 10, Ghent B-9000, Belgium.
E-mail address: Wim.ceelen@ugent.be

Surg Oncol Clin N Am 27 (2018) 477–494
https://doi.org/10.1016/j.soc.2018.02.003
1055-3207/18/© 2018 Elsevier Inc. All rights reserved.
surgonc.theclinics.com

In parallel, innovative pharmaceutical platforms, such as targeted agents, nano-sized medicine, and drug-eluting beads, have the potential to further increase the appeal of locoregional drug delivery.

The peritoneal cavity, with its serosal exchange surface of approximately 1.5 to 2 m^2, is a well-established route of drug delivery. Examples include renal replacement using peritoneal dialysis and IP instillation of analgesic compounds following laparoscopic surgery. Recently, there has been an increased interested from clinicians in IP instillation of anticancer drugs for abdominal malignancy. The concept of IP therapy is not entirely new. The earliest IP "drug therapy" was reported in 1744 by the English surgeon Christopher Warrick, who, apparently with great success, injected a mixture of "Bristol water" and "claret" (a Bordeaux wine) in the peritoneal cavity of a woman suffering from intractable ascites.[1] In the 1940s, interest arose in IP administration of radionuclides. IP colloidal radioactive gold (Au-198) was used as adjuvant treatment or as palliation of ascites and pleural effusions in patients with ovarian cancer. Although some success was reported, serious complications and deaths were also observed.[2] Similarly, adjuvant IP instillation of radioactive chromic phosphate (^{32}P) was associated in early stage ovarian cancer with inadequate distribution and small bowel perforation.[3] In 1958, Economou and coworkers[4] reported the use of intraoperative IP delivery of nitrogen mustard (HN2, bis(2-chloroethyl)methylamine, mustine) in 36 patients undergoing laparotomy for cancer.[4] The product was administered IP in 500 mL of saline "as the last peritoneal stitch was taken." They concluded that IP instillation of nitrogen mustard "is a safe procedure." The interest in IP chemotherapy was encouraged by the work of Robert Dedrick and colleagues[5] in the 1970s, who proposed a theoretic framework for IP therapy based on the assumption that, because peritoneal clearance is much lower than plasma clearance, a regional pharmacokinetic (PK) advantage results in much higher IP drug concentrations with limited systemic exposure and toxicity.[5] The same investigators, however, were also some of the first to highlight the fact that, despite the PK advantage of IP-instilled chemotherapy, tissue penetration depth remains very limited.[6]

Here, the authors provide an overview of the pharmacologic aspects of IP drug treatment, as they pertain to intraoperative chemoperfusion as an adjuvant therapy following cytoreductive surgery for peritoneal metastases.

STRUCTURE AND TRANSPORT BARRIER FUNCTION OF THE PERITONEUM

Both the interior aspect of the abdominal wall and the viscera are covered by a peritoneal layer consisting of mesothelial cells, which are flat, squamouslike cells approximately 25 μm in diameter, and by an underlying extracellular matrix (ECM).[7] Recent cadaveric research showed that the mean peritoneal surface area in the adult female is approximately 1.43 m^2, with the small bowel and its mesentery accounting for 39% of the total surface.[8] The mesothelial cells provide a protective, nonadhesive surface by production of surfactant, proteoglycans, and glycosaminoglycans. Also, they have a role in transporting fluid and cells across the peritoneal cavity, presenting antigens to T cells, and participating in inflammation and tissue repair by the secretion of chemokines (monocyte chemoattractant protein-1 and interleukin-8 [IL-8]), cytokines (IL-6 and IL-1), growth factors (transforming growth factor-β, fibroblast growth factor , platelet-derived growth factor), ECM components, and other biological mediators.[9]

The peritoneal cavity contains a small amount of free fluid, the movement of which is in a cephalad direction due to the movement of the diaphragm, which creates a relatively low pressure zone in the upper abdomen. The peritoneum that covers the diaphragmatic surfaces is characterized by "stomata," cavities with a diameter of 3 to 12 μm between the mesothelial cells. These stomata provide direct access to an underlying network of lymphatic vessels, lacunae, and cisternae, which allow clearance of particulate matter, bacteria, and cells from the peritoneal cavity into the circulation.[10,11]

Functionally, the mesothelial lining does not represent a significant barrier to drug transport, as demonstrated by preclinical and clinical studies showing that peritonectomy does not affect transport characteristics of IP chemotherapy.[12] The transport barrier consists of the submesothelial stroma and, importantly, the endothelial glycocalyx lining the submesothelial capillaries.[13]

COMPARTMENTAL KINETIC MODELING OF PERITONEAL DRUG TRANSPORT

For PK modeling of drug transport, the anatomy and physiology of the peritoneal cavity and its surrounding tissue are usually represented by "compartments." In pharmacokinetics, compartments are mathematical constructs representing a space that a drug occupies after it has been absorbed and may or may not correspond to actual anatomic structures. Although numerous such compartments are relevant for IP drug delivery (liver, abdominal wall, visceral surface, diaphragm, and so forth), a simple linear 2-compartment approach is sufficient to describe the PK of IP drug transport (**Fig. 1**). These compartments are the following:

- A systemic compartment, characterized by a certain drug concentration and distribution volume, and from which the drug is cleared by a first-order elimination process;
- A peritoneal compartment, characterized by perfusate concentration and volume, and from which bidirectional transport occurs toward and from the systemic compartment.

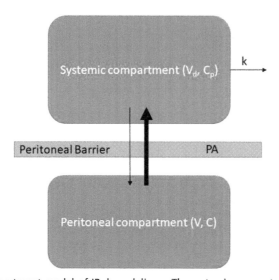

Fig. 1. Two-compartment model of IP drug delivery. The systemic compartment is characterized by the drug distribution volume (V_d) and the systemic concentration (C_p), whereas drug is cleared from the body at a rate defined by the elimination constant (k). The peritoneal compartment corresponds to the perfusate-filled abdominal cavity and is characterized by an instilled volume (V) and drug concentration (C). Mass transport occurs over the peritoneal barrier, which is characterized by a PA product.

Both compartments are separated by the peritoneal barrier, characterized by a permeability-area (PA) product. The PA product of the peritoneal barrier cannot be directly measured. However, from correlations of drug clearance with molecular properties, it was estimated that the PA decreases approximately with the square root of the molecular weight.[6]

The change in systemic and peritoneal drug concentrations over time can be derived from the mass balance equations:

$$V_d \frac{dC_p}{dt} = PA(C - C_p) - kC_p$$

$$V \frac{dC}{dt} = PA(C_p - C)$$

Both equations can be solved simultaneously to yield:

$$C_p = \frac{PA(e^{-\alpha t} - e^{-\beta t})}{V_d(\beta - \alpha)}$$

$$C = \frac{e^{-\alpha t}}{\beta - \alpha}\left[\frac{PA+k}{V_d} - \alpha\right] - \frac{e^{-\beta t}}{\beta - \alpha}\left[\frac{PA+k}{V_d} - \beta\right]$$

where α and β are the solutions to the following pair of simultaneous equations:

$$\alpha + \beta = \frac{PA}{V} + \frac{PA}{V_d} + \frac{k}{V_d}$$

$$\alpha\beta = \frac{(PA)k}{VV_d}$$

Fig. 2 illustrates the simulated time course of systemic and perfusate concentrations of cisplatin and paclitaxel. The regional advantage of IP drug delivery is usually expressed as the ratio of the area under the concentration-time curve (AUC) in the perfusate divided by the AUC in the systemic compartment (represented by the blood plasma). In steady-state conditions (constant perfusate concentration), the ratio of perfusate over systemic drug concentration can be expressed as (P denotes plasma):

$$\frac{C}{C_p} = 1 + \frac{k}{PA}$$

From the above equation, it is immediately clear that the PK advantage is proportional to systemic drug clearance (k) and inversely proportional to the PA product of the peritoneal barrier.

The concentrations predicted in the peritoneal cavity by the 2-compartment model are only experienced by free floating cancer cells. In order to take into account the importance of drug penetration into tissue, more advanced ("distributed") models were developed that incorporate capillary and lymphatic vessels, assumed to be uniformly distributed within the tissue.[14]

PHARMACOKINETIC PROPERTIES OF CHEMOTHERAPY USED FOR INTRAPERITONEAL DRUG DELIVERY

A rational choice of chemotherapy for intraperitoneal drug delivery (IPDD) should be based on the following considerations:

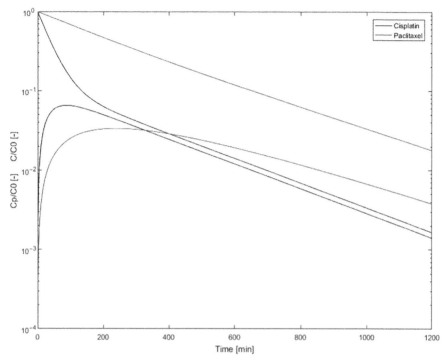

Fig. 2. Simulation of peritoneal and plasma concentration over time of cisplatin and pacli-taxel based on a linear 2-compartment model and using the following parameters: cisplatin: k = 160 mL/min, PA = 95.7 mL/min, Alpha = 26.7 e^{-3}, Beta = 3.58 e^{-3}; paclitaxel: k = 174 mL/min, PA = 15.6 mL/min, Alpha = 5.62 e^{-3}, Beta = 3.02 e^{-3}.

- It should have (continued) demonstrated activity against the cancer type of origin;
- Because exposure time is a critical parameter for cancer cell kill and intraoperative IPDD administration time is typically limited (30–120 minutes), the drug should ideally be non-cell-cycle specific;
- When used under hyperthermic conditions (hyperthermic intraperitoneal chemoperfusion [HIPEC]), there should be demonstrated thermal enhancement of cytotoxicity (eg, alkylating agents);
- Its physicochemical properties (molecular weight, charge, size, water solubility) and PK behavior (metabolism, first pass effect, peritoneal clearance, excretion) should result in a favorable (high) peritoneal/plasma AUC ratio;
- It should not cause locoregional (peritoneal) toxicity, such as inflammation or fibrosis. Vesicant agents (mitomycin C, doxorubicin, mitoxantrone, oxaliplatin) are, in theory, more likely to cause peritoneal inflammation;
- It should be safe for the health care staff and environment. Specifically, drugs that are volatile at 20°C to 43°C (ifosfamide, carmustin, nitrogen mustard) should not be used.

Table 1 summarizes the PK properties of the most commonly used chemotherapy drugs for HIPEC. Unfortunately, there is significant heterogeneity in treatment methods and protocols, and virtually no formal dose finding studies were performed. As a consequence of this heterogeneity, makes comparison between drugs difficult.

Table 1
Pharmacokinetic and pharmacodynamic properties of cytotoxic agents used during intraoperative or early postoperative intraperitoneal chemotherapy

Drug	MW (Da)	IP Dose (mg/m²)	AUC Ratio[a]	Drug Penetration Distance	TE
Alkylating agents					
Mitomycin C	334.3	35	10–23.5	2 mm	+
Platinum compounds					
Cisplatin	300.1	90–250	13–21	1–3 mm	+
Carboplatin	371.3	350–800	1.9–5.3	0.5 mm	+
Oxaliplatin	397.3	200–460	3.5	1–2 mm	+
Antimicrotubule agents					
Paclitaxel	853.9	20–175	1000	0.5 mm	?
Docetaxel	861.9	40–156	207	NA	+
Topoisomerase Interactive Agents					
Topotecan	457.9	NA	NA	NA	?
Irinotecan	677.2	NA	NA	NA	±
Mitoxantrone	517.4	28	15.2	5–6 cell layers	±
Doxorubicin	543.5	60–75	162	4–6 cell layers	+
Antimetabolites					
5-Fluorouracil	130.1	650	NA	0.2 mm	...
Gemcitabine	300	120–1000	847	...	...

Abbreviations: MW, molecular weight (Dalton); NA, not available; TE, thermal enhancement.
[a] Only data referring to clinical studies with hyperthermic chemoperfusion (HIPEC).

TISSUE TRANSPORT OF INTRAPERITONEALLY ADMINISTERED CHEMOTHERAPY

The presence of the peritoneal barrier allows the escalation of the IP drug dose and concentration. Because most chemotherapy displays an exponential dose-cell kill response, significant activity is assumed against peritoneal metastases. However, preclinical and clinical experiments that incorporated direct measurement of chemotherapy distribution in the tumor following IPDD suggest that, despite a high drug dose, the ability to penetrate normal as well as tumor tissue is extremely limited, averaging less than 1 mm. Poor tissue penetration represents a major obstacle for the efficacy of the IP, compared with the systemic route of chemotherapy administration. In the next part, the authors describe the basic mechanisms of tissue transport and the relevant findings from published literature and their own data and provide an overview of methods that have the potential to improve tissue penetration.

BASIC MECHANISMS OF TISSUE DRUG TRANSPORT

The physiology of drug transport usually considers tumor tissue an isotropic (homogeneous) porous medium (**Fig. 3**). Interstitial mass transport is driven by 2 main mechanisms: convection or bulk fluid flow, driven by a pressure gradient, and diffusion, which results from a concentration gradient. The ratio of convective versus diffusive transport is defined as the dimensionless Péclet number. The Péclet number is low for small molecules and higher for larger substances, such as antibodies or nucleic acids.

Convection describes the interstitial fluid flow resulting from a pressure gradient. Because tumor tissue is characterized by an elevated interstitial fluid pressure (IFP), which decreases sharply at the tumor periphery, a net outward convective flow results in "oozing" from the tumor surface.[15] IFP ranges from 4 to 100 mm Hg, and this has to

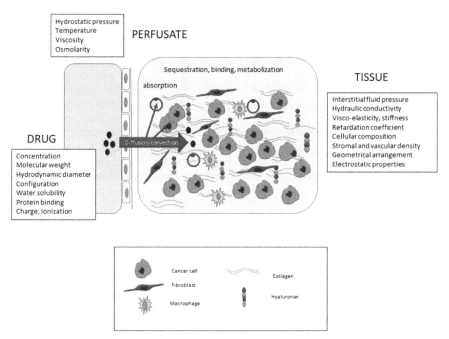

Fig. 3. Overview of physical and pharmacologic parameters that affect tissue transport after IP drug delivery.

be balanced against the pressure exerted by the IP fluid column (average of 10–20 cm H_2O or 7.4–14.8 mm Hg). The degree of convective transport depends on the hydraulic conductivity of the tissue, which is determined by the viscosity of the interstitial fluid and by the stromal architecture or mechanical "stiffness".[16] Because chemotherapy will interact with cellular and stromal structures, solute transport velocity is always slower than fluid velocity. The ratio of both velocities is termed the retardation or hindrance coefficient.

The rate of drug diffusion is proportional to a concentration gradient, according to Fick's first law of diffusion. The rate of diffusion depends on temperature, the physicochemical drug properties, and the stromal architecture.[17] The temperature dependence is explained by the Einstein-Stokes equation, which states that diffusion is proportional to temperature and inversely proportional to the viscosity of the medium. The extent of diffusive transport depends on properties of the drug (molecular weight, size, charge, configuration) and the ECM (cellular composition, density, viscoelasticity, geometric arrangement, electrostatic properties).[18] Because the shape of a molecule will affect its diffusive behavior more than its molecular weight, the Stokes-Einstein radius of a molecule is often used as a measure of its size. Tumor stroma mainly consists of adipose tissue, smooth muscle, and epithelial cells, but also includes pericytes, endothelial cells, leukocytes, and activated fibroblasts (cancer-associated fibroblasts).[19,20] Interestingly, because of intense reciprocal interaction with the tumor microenvironment, stromal cells develop a modified phenotype and altered function.[19] Tumor tissue is characterized by increased deposition of collagen I, the most abundant ECM protein. As a result, tumor stroma is characterized by increased stiffness or rigidity compared with normal tissue. Rigidity (or stiffness) is measured using Young's modulus of elasticity, which is the ratio of stress to strain along an axis. Tissue elasticity can be measured using a mechanical device that directly applies a mechanical load and measures the resulting deformation. Alternatively, noninvasive elastography techniques can be used with ultrasound or MRI.[21,22] In addition to increased collagen deposition, tumors were shown to further exacerbate matrix stiffness by increased expression of the collagen cross-linking enzyme LOX (lysyl oxidase).[23] Paszek and coworkers[24] found that tissue stiffness of mouse mammary tumors far exceeded that of normal breast tissue (elastic modulus 4049 ± 938 Pa vs 167 ± 31 Pa), whereas mechanical disturbances were shown to enhance the malignant phenotype through "mechanoregulatory" circuits.[25] In addition to the density of the collagen fibers that are deposited in the ECM, their geometric arrangement may affect drug diffusion. Fibers that are oriented tangentially from the tumor surface may direct drug diffusion away from the tumor, whereas the opposite may result from fibers that are radially aligned.[26] In addition to stromal components, the tumor cell population in itself represents a barrier to diffusive drug transport. Using advanced imaging techniques, Chauhan and coworkers[27] demonstrated a significant improvement of macromolecular diffusion when colorectal xenografts were treated with diphtheria toxin, which causes apoptosis of tumor cells but leaves the mouse stroma intact. Other cell types include fibroblasts, myofibroblasts, mesenchymal cells such as pericytes, endothelial cells, and immune cells, all of which contribute to a high cellular density and solid stress, compressing the interstitial matrix.

TISSUE PENETRATION FOLLOWING INTRAPERITONEAL DRUG DELIVERY: MEASUREMENT METHODS AND CLINICAL DATA

Chemotherapy drug penetration in tissue has been extensively studied using in vitro 3-dimensional organoids, mathematical models, and animal studies.[28] On the contrary, clinical data on tissue penetration after IPDD with or without HIPEC are scarce. First, it complicates surgical treatment by the requirement that tumor tissue is left in situ during chemoperfusion. Second, measurement of chemotherapy distribution and penetration distance necessitates advanced sample preparation and analytical techniques. Several investigators have measured drug concentrations on tumor tissue *homogenates* using standard analytical techniques such as high-performance liquid chromatography or mass spectrometry, but this method does not allow gaining insight into the parameters of interest. Methods that do allow analysis of tissue distribution include autoradiography, nuclear imaging, fluorescence imaging, and mass spectrometry–based imaging. Autoradiography and nuclear imaging methods, such as PET, require radiolabeling of the drug, thereby altering its behavior, are very difficult to use clinically because of regulatory issues with the use of radioactive tracers. Fluorescence imaging requires labeling of the compound or the use of fluorescent antibodies; some chemotherapeutic agents (doxorubicin) possess autofluorescent properties and therefore do not require labeling. Recently, mass spectrometry imaging (MSI) techniques were introduced in the study of drug distribution in biological tissues. The principal MSI techniques are matrix-assisted laser desorption ionization-mass spectrometry imaging (MALDI-MSI), laser ablation-inductively coupled plasma mass spectrometry imaging (LA-ICP-MSI), and secondary ion mass spectrometry (SIMS) techniques, including nanoscale ion microprobe SIMS (NanoSIMS), and time-of-flight SIMS.[29] Inductively coupled plasma-mass spectrometry (ICP-MS) is ideally suited to study fate of metallodrugs (platinum compounds: cisplatin, carboplatin, oxaliplatin) in biological systems due to low limits of detection (parts-per-trillion to parts-per-quadrillion range). However, the method is destructive (samples are either digested or homogenized). MSI combined with MALDI or desorption electrospray ionization is a nondestructive method and measures molecules instead of atoms.[30] Quantification of drugs using MSI remains a challenge, but methods achieving this are underway.[31] Finally, laser ablation-inductively coupled plasma mass spectrometry (LA-ICP-MS) offers the capability not only to visualize and measure tissue distribution but also to quantify drug concentration.[32] However, the method is destructive and time consuming. In a recent study comparing MALDI and LA-ICP-MS to study platinum distribution following HIPEC in human tumor samples, MALDI imaging was found to suffer in some cases from signal suppression by the matrix, leading to false negatives.[33]

Only very limited clinical data are available on spatial tissue distribution of chemotherapy after IPDD. Ansaloni and coworkers[34] studied tissue penetration using MALDI imaging of paclitaxel after HIPEC in patients with ovarian cancer (175 mg/m², 41°C–43°C, 90 minutes) and found that drug penetration in normal peritoneum was limited to ~0.5 mm (**Fig. 4**). Bianga and colleagues[33] used both LA-ICP-MS and MALDI to study drug penetration in tumor tissue after HIPEC with oxaliplatin (460 mg/m², 30 minutes, 42°C) or cisplatin (75 mg/m², 60 minutes, 42°C). They found a poor tissue penetration of oxaliplatin (approximately 2–3 mm) compared with cisplatin. The authors have studied cisplatin penetration using LA-ICP-MS in tumor tissue from patients

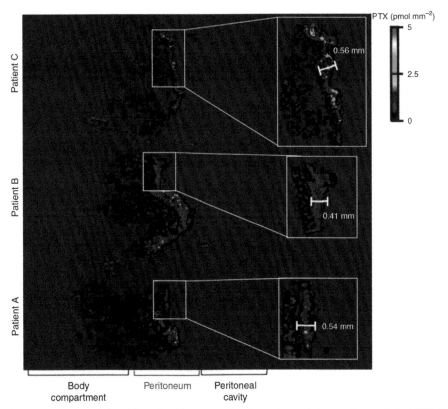

Fig. 4. MALDI imagining of paclitaxel penetration in peritoneal tissue after a clinical HIPEC procedure. (*From* Ansaloni L, Coccolini F, Morosi L, et al. Pharmacokinetics of concomitant cisplatin and paclitaxel administered by hyperthermic intraperitoneal chemotherapy to patients with peritoneal carcinomatosis from epithelial ovarian cancer. Br J Cancer 2015;112(2):310; with permission.)

with ovarian cancer after normothermic or hyperthermic chemoperfusion and found an average penetration distance of approximately 0.5 to 1 mm (**Fig. 5**).

APPROACHES TO IMPROVE TISSUE PENETRATION

Numerous physical and pharmacologic interventions have been described aiming to improve drug transport and tissue penetration after IPDD (**Table 2**).[34] Given its widespread clinical use, this article only discusses the potential benefit of hyperthermia for drug penetration. In theory, the Einstein-Stokes equation, which states that diffusion is proportional to temperature and inversely proportional to the viscosity of the medium, predicts increased drug diffusion with increasing temperature. Also, the hydraulic conductivity, the primary determinant of convective transport, is increased due to enhanced matrix permeability and reduced fluid viscosity at higher temperature. Nevertheless, the potential of hyperthermia to enhance IP drug delivery remains uncertain. Preclinical studies using murine colon, melanoma, and mammary tumors showed that whole body hyperthermia (39.5°C during 6 hours) lowers IFP, improves blood flow, and enhances the efficacy of radiotherapy.[35] Others, however, were unable to observe IFP lowering upon locoregional heating (41.8°C during 2 hours) in a glioma xenograft model.[36] Several investigators have studied chemotherapy concentrations in tumor tissue after hyperthermic IP delivery. Los and colleagues[37] found that, compared with normothermic administration, locoregional heating (41.5°C for 60 minutes) resulted in a 4-fold increase in cisplatin tumor concentration in a rat CC531 colon carcinomatosis model. Of note, plasma cisplatin levels were also significantly elevated after hyperthermic treatment, which raises the question whether the difference in tumor tissue drug concentration resulted from increased peritoneal to tumor transport, or from increased systemic exposure. Later work by Zeamari and coworkers[38] was unable to confirm the benefit of hyperthermia: mild hyperthermic perfusion with cisplatin (40°C for 90 minutes) did not improve drug uptake in small IP tumors in a rat model. Similarly, Facy and colleagues[39] did not find a significant difference in cisplatin concentration of ovarian peritoneal tumors in a rat model after normothermic or hyperthermic (42°C for 60 minutes) chemoperfusion. These investigators hypothesized that increased peritoneal drug clearance due to vasodilation and increased blood flow may explain the lack of benefit associated with

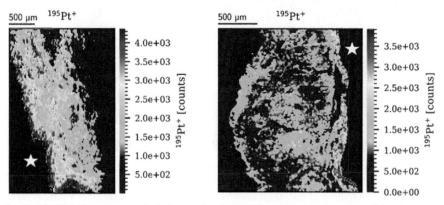

Fig. 5. LA-ICP-MS mappings of platinum distribution in peritoneal tumor nodules from patients with ovarian cancer after intraoperative IP chemoperfusion with cisplatin (120 mg/m^2) for 90 minutes at 37°C (*left*) or 41°C (*right*). Color scale bars indicate the amount of ^{195}Pt in counts. Star denotes peritoneal (exposed) surface.

Table 2
Physical and pharmacologic interventions to improve drug transport and tissue penetration

Physical Interventions	Compound(s)	Species	Tumor Model	Route of Administration	Ref.
Increased intra-abdominal pressure	Cisplatin	Rat	IP	IAP	40
	Doxorubicin	Rat	NA	IAP	41
	Oxaliplatin	Pig	NA	IAP	42
	Doxorubicin + Cisplatin	Human	NA	PIPAC	43–46
Increased exposure time	Doxorubicin	In vitro	Colorectal spheroids	In vitro	47
Hyperthermia	NA	Mouse	SC	NA	35
	NA	Mouse	SC	NA	36
	Cisplatin	Rat	IP	IP	37
	Cisplatin	Rat	IP	IP	38
	Cisplatin	Rat	IP	IP	39
Hyperbaric oxygen	5-FU	Rat	Orally induced mammary tumors	IP	48
Photodynamic therapy	Photofrin	Hamster	SC	IV	49
	Liporubicin	Rat	SPL	IV	50
Radiation therapy	Cisplatin	Human	NA	HIPEC	51
	NA	Mouse	SC	NA	52
	Liposomal doxorubicin	Mouse	OT or SC	IV	53
	Doxorubicin	Ex vivo: pig	NA	PIPAC	54
Ultrasound	Doxorubicin and Gemcitabine	Mouse	SC	IV	55
	MAb B3	Mouse	SC	IV	56

Pharmacologic Interventions	Compound(s)	Species	Tumor Model	Route of Administration	Ref.
Targeting tumor vasculature	[Bevacizumab or Pazopanib] + Oxaliplatin	Mouse	SP	Bevacizumab: IV; Pazopanib: Oral; Oxaliplatin: IP	57
	ZD6126	Mouse	ID	IP	58
Vasoactive drugs	[Vasopressin] + Carboplatin, Etoposide, and 5-FU	Pig	NA	Vasopressin: IV; Carboplatin, Etoposide, and 5-FU: IP	59
	[Norbormide or Epinephrine] + 5-FU	Rat	SP	IP	60
	[Epinephrine] + Cisplatin	Rat	IP and SC	Epinephrine: IP; Cisplatin: IV or IP	61
	[Epinephrine] + Cisplatin	Human	NA	IP	62,63
	[Vasopressin] + 5-FU	Human	NA	Vasopressin: IV; 5-FU: IP	64
	Hydralazine	Mouse	SC	IV	65

(continued on next page)

Table 2
(continued)

Pharmacologic Interventions	Compound(s)	Species	Tumor Model	Route of Administration	Ref.
Targeting stromal components	[PEGPH20] + Gemcitabine	Mouse	KPC	IV	66
	[PEGPH20] + Gemcitabine	Human	NA	IV	67
	Collagenase-1	Mouse	SC	IV	68
	[Collagenase] + MAb TP-3	Mouse	SC	IV	69
	[Relaxin] + IgG or Dextran	Mouse	DSC	Relaxin: Implanted relaxin-loaded osmotic pumps; IgG or Dextran: IP	70,71
	[Losartan] + 5-Fu or Doxil	Mouse	OT	Losartan: IP; 5-FU or Doxil: IV	72–74
	[IPI-926] + Gemcitabine	Mouse	KPC, SC, and OT	IPI-926: Oral; Gemcitabine: IV	75
	[IPI-926] + FOLFIRINOX	Human	NA	IPI-926: Oral; FOLFIRINOX: IV	76
	[GDC-0449] ± Gemcitabine	Human	NA	GDC-0449: Oral; Gemcitabine: IV	77
	[Calcipotriol] + and/or Gemcitabine	Mouse	KPC, and OT	IP	78
Targeting tumor cell density	[F8-IL2] + Paclitaxel	Mouse	SC	IV	79
	Paclitaxel + Doxorubicin	Human	NA	IV	80
	[Cyclophosphamide] + MM-302	Mouse	SC	Cyclophosphamide: IP; MM-302: IV	81
	Diphtheria toxin	Mouse	DSC	NA	27
	Apo2L/TRAIL	Mouse	SC	IP	82
	Tumor priming microparticles loaded with Paclitaxel	Mouse	IP	IP	83
	[iRGD] + Doxorubicin, Abraxane, Doxorubicin liposomes, or Trastuzumab	Mouse	OT	IV	84
	[FAM-iRGD]	Mouse	OT	IV	85
	[iRGD] ± Gemcitabine	Mouse	OT	iRGD: IV; Gemcitabine: IP	86
	[iRGD] ± Doxorubicin or Dextran	Mouse	IP	IP	87
	iRGD loaded with Paclitaxel	Mouse	IP	IP	88
Altering stromal pH	[Pantoprazole] ± Doxorubicin	Mouse	SC	Pantoprazole: IP; Doxorubicine: IV	89
	[Lansoprazole] ± Doxorubicin	Mouse	SC	Lansoprazole: IP; Doxorubicine: IV	90

Abbreviations: ±, with or without; 5-FU, 5-Fluorouracil; DSC, dorsal skinfold chambers; IAP, intra-abdominal pressure; ID, intradermal; IV, intravenous; KPC, *K-rasLSL.G12D/+; p53R172H/+; PdxCre*; NA, not applicable; OT, orthotopic; PIPAC, pressurized intraperitoneal aerosol chemotherapy; SC, subcutaneous; SP, subperitoneal; SPL, subpleural; [X], pharmacological intervention.

hyperthermia. Results from an ongoing trial (clinicaltrials.gov identifier NCT02567253) comparing normothermic with hyperthermic chemoperfusion using cisplatin in ovarian cancer will provide important answers on the potential risk versus benefit of hyperthermic drug delivery.

SUMMARY AND FUTURE PERSPECTIVES

IP chemotherapy delivery is associated with a PK advantage, resulting in higher locoregional drug concentrations. However, this PK advantage does not necessarily result in enhanced anticancer efficacy, as evidenced by very limited tissue penetration in preclinical as well as clinical studies. Several physical or pharmaceutical approaches hold promise to enhance drug penetration in preclinical models.

REFERENCES

1. Warrick C. An improvement on the practice of tapping; whereby that operation, instead of a relief for symptoms, becomes an absolute cure for an ascites, exemplified in the case of Jane Roman; and recommended to the consideration of the Royal Society, by Christopher Warrick, of Truro, Surgeon. Phil Trans 1744;43(473):12-19.
2. Saxena A, Yan TD, Morris DL. A critical evaluation of risk factors for complications after cytoreductive surgery and perioperative intraperitoneal chemotherapy for colorectal peritoneal carcinomatosis. World J Surg 2010;34(1):70–8.
3. Chua TC, Yan TD, Zhao J, et al. Peritoneal carcinomatosis and liver metastases from colorectal cancer treated with cytoreductive surgery perioperative intraperitoneal chemotherapy and liver resection. Eur J Surg Oncol 2009;35(12):1299–305.
4. Economou SG, Mrazek R, Mc DG, et al. The intraperitoneal use of nitrogen mustard at the time of operation for cancer. Ann N Y Acad Sci 1958;68(3):1097–102.
5. Dedrick RL, Myers CE, Bungay PM, et al. Pharmacokinetic rationale for peritoneal drug administration in the treatment of ovarian cancer. Cancer Treat Rep 1978; 62(1):1–11.
6. Dedrick RL. Theoretical and experimental bases of intraperitoneal chemotherapy. Semin Oncol 1985;12(3 Suppl 4):1–6.
7. Mutsaers SE, Prele CM, Pengelly S, et al. Mesothelial cells and peritoneal homeostasis. Fertil Steril 2016;106(5):1018–24.
8. Albanese AM, Albanese EF, Mino JH, et al. Peritoneal surface area: measurements of 40 structures covered by peritoneum: correlation between total peritoneal surface area and the surface calculated by formulas. Surg Radiol Anat 2009;31(5):369–77.
9. Yung S, Chan TM. Mesothelial cells. Perit Dial Int 2007;27(Suppl 2):S110–5.
10. Michailova KN, Wassilev WA, Kuhnel W. Features of the peritoneal covering of the lesser pelvis with special reference to stomata regions. Ann Anat 2005;187(1): 23–33.
11. Ohtani O, Ohtani Y, Li RX. Phylogeny and ontogeny of the lymphatic stomata connecting the pleural and peritoneal cavities with the lymphatic system–a review. Ital J Anat Embryol 2001;106(2 Suppl 1):251–9.
12. de Lima Vazquez V, Stuart OA, Mohamed F, et al. Extent of parietal peritonectomy does not change intraperitoneal chemotherapy pharmacokinetics. Cancer Chemother Pharmacol 2003;52(2):108–12.
13. Flessner MF. Endothelial glycocalyx and the peritoneal barrier. Perit Dial Int 2008; 28(1):6–12.
14. Flessner MF, Dedrick RL, Schultz JS. A distributed model of peritoneal-plasma transport: theoretical considerations. Am J Physiol 1984;246(4 Pt 2):R597–607.

15. Butler TP, Grantham FH, Gullino PM. Bulk transfer of fluid in the interstitial compartment of mammary tumors. Cancer Res 1975;35(11 Pt 1):3084–8.
16. Netti PA, Berk DA, Swartz MA, et al. Role of extracellular matrix assembly in interstitial transport in solid tumors. Cancer Res 2000;60(9):2497–503.
17. Jain RK. Transport of molecules in the tumor interstitium: a review. Cancer Res 1987;47(12):3039–51.
18. Young EW. Cells, tissues, and organs on chips: challenges and opportunities for the cancer tumor microenvironment. Integr Biol (Camb) 2013;5(9):1096–109.
19. Li H, Fan X, Houghton J. Tumor microenvironment: the role of the tumor stroma in cancer. J Cell Biochem 2007;101(4):805–15.
20. De Wever O, Mareel M. Role of tissue stroma in cancer cell invasion. J Pathol 2003;200(4):429–47.
21. Jamin Y, Boult JK, Li J, et al. Exploring the biomechanical properties of brain malignancies and their pathologic determinants in vivo with magnetic resonance elastography. Cancer Res 2015;75(7):1216–24.
22. Zaleska-Dorobisz U, Kaczorowski K, Pawlus A, et al. Ultrasound elastography - review of techniques and its clinical applications. Adv Clin Exp Med 2014; 23(4):645–55.
23. Baker AM, Bird D, Lang G, et al. Lysyl oxidase enzymatic function increases stiffness to drive colorectal cancer progression through FAK. Oncogene 2013; 32(14):1863–8.
24. Paszek MJ, Zahir N, Johnson KR, et al. Tensional homeostasis and the malignant phenotype. Cancer Cell 2005;8(3):241–54.
25. Sun Z, Guo SS, Fassler R. Integrin-mediated mechanotransduction. J Cell Biol 2016;215(4):445–56.
26. Butcher DT, Alliston T, Weaver VM. A tense situation: forcing tumour progression. Nat Rev Cancer 2009;9(2):108–22.
27. Chauhan VP, Lanning RM, Diop-Frimpong B, et al. Multiscale measurements distinguish cellular and interstitial hindrances to diffusion in vivo. Biophys J 2009;97(1):330–6.
28. Steuperaert M, Falvo D'Urso Labate G, Debbaut C, et al. Mathematical modeling of intraperitoneal drug delivery: simulation of drug distribution in a single tumor nodule. Drug Deliv 2017;24(1):491–501.
29. Lee RFS, Theiner S, Meibom A, et al. Application of imaging mass spectrometry approaches to facilitate metal-based anticancer drug research. Metallomics 2017;9(4):365–81.
30. Morosi L, Zucchetti M, D'Incalci M, et al. Imaging mass spectrometry: challenges in visualization of drug distribution in solid tumors. Curr Opin Pharmacol 2013; 13(5):807–12.
31. Giordano S, Morosi L, Veglianese P, et al. 3D mass spectrometry imaging reveals a very heterogeneous drug distribution in tumors. Sci Rep 2016;6:37027.
32. Becker JS, Matusch A, Wu B. Bioimaging mass spectrometry of trace elements - recent advance and applications of LA-ICP-MS: a review. Anal Chim Acta 2014; 835:1–18.
33. Bianga J, Bouslimani A, Bec N, et al. Complementarity of MALDI and LA ICP mass spectrometry for platinum anticancer imaging in human tumor. Metallomics 2014;6(8):1382–6.
34. Ansaloni L, Coccolini F, Morosi L, et al. Pharmacokinetics of concomitant cisplatin and paclitaxel administered by hyperthermic intraperitoneal chemotherapy to patients with peritoneal carcinomatosis from epithelial ovarian cancer. Br J Cancer 2015;112(2):306–12.

35. Sen A, Capitano ML, Spernyak JA, et al. Mild elevation of body temperature reduces tumor interstitial fluid pressure and hypoxia and enhances efficacy of radiotherapy in murine tumor models. Cancer Res 2011;71(11):3872–80.

36. Hauck ML, Coffin DO, Dodge RK, et al. A local hyperthermia treatment which enhances antibody uptake in a glioma xenograft model does not affect tumour interstitial fluid pressure. Int J Hyperthermia 1997;13(3):307–16.

37. Los G, Sminia P, Wondergem J, et al. Optimisation of intraperitoneal cisplatin therapy with regional hyperthermia in rats. Eur J Cancer 1991;27(4):472–7.

38. Zeamari S, Floot B, van der Vange N, et al. Pharmacokinetics and pharmacodynamics of cisplatin after intraoperative hyperthermic intraperitoneal chemoperfusion (HIPEC). Anticancer Res 2003;23(2B):1643–8.

39. Facy O, Radais F, Ladoire S, et al. Comparison of hyperthermia and adrenaline to enhance the intratumoral accumulation of cisplatin in a murine model of peritoneal carcinomatosis. J Exp Clin Cancer Res 2011;30:4.

40. Esquis P, Consolo D, Magnin G, et al. High intra-abdominal pressure enhances the penetration and antitumor effect of intraperitoneal cisplatin on experimental peritoneal carcinomatosis. Ann Surg 2006;244(1):106–12.

41. Jacquet P, Stuart OA, Chang D, et al. Effects of intra-abdominal pressure on pharmacokinetics and tissue distribution of doxorubicin after intraperitoneal administration. Anticancer Drugs 1996;7(5):596–603.

42. Facy O, Al Samman S, Magnin G, et al. High pressure enhances the effect of hyperthermia in intraperitoneal chemotherapy with oxaliplatin: an experimental study. Ann Surg 2012;256(6):1084–8.

43. Tempfer CB, Celik I, Solass W, et al. Activity of pressurized intraperitoneal aerosol chemotherapy (PIPAC) with cisplatin and doxorubicin in women with recurrent, platinum-resistant ovarian cancer: preliminary clinical experience. Gynecol Oncol 2014;132(2):307–11.

44. Solass W, Kerb R, Murdter T, et al. Intraperitoneal chemotherapy of peritoneal carcinomatosis using pressurized aerosol as an alternative to liquid solution: first evidence for efficacy. Ann Surg Oncol 2014;21(2):553–9.

45. Solass W, Giger-Pabst U, Zieren J, et al. Pressurized intraperitoneal aerosol chemotherapy (PIPAC): occupational health and safety aspects. Ann Surg Oncol 2013;20(11):3504–11.

46. Blanco A, Giger-Pabst U, Solass W, et al. Renal and hepatic toxicities after pressurized intraperitoneal aerosol chemotherapy (PIPAC). Ann Surg Oncol 2013; 20(7):2311–6.

47. Toley BJ, Tropeano Lovatt ZG, Harrington JL, et al. Microfluidic technique to measure intratumoral transport and calculate drug efficacy shows that binding is essential for doxorubicin and release hampers doxil. Integr Biol (Camb) 2013; 5(9):1184–96.

48. Moen I, Tronstad KJ, Kolmannskog O, et al. Hyperoxia increases the uptake of 5-fluorouracil in mammary tumors independently of changes in interstitial fluid pressure and tumor stroma. BMC Cancer 2009;9:446.

49. Leunig M, Goetz AE, Gamarra F, et al. Photodynamic therapy-induced alterations in interstitial fluid pressure, volume and water content of an amelanotic melanoma in the hamster. Br J Cancer 1994;69(1):101–3.

50. Perentes JY, Wang Y, Wang X, et al. Low-dose vascular photodynamic therapy decreases tumor interstitial fluid pressure, which promotes liposomal doxorubicin distribution in a murine sarcoma metastasis model. Transl Oncol 2014;7(3): 393–9.

51. Osborne EM, Briere TM, Hayes-Jordan A, et al. Survival and toxicity following sequential multimodality treatment including whole abdominopelvic radiotherapy for patients with desmoplastic small round cell tumor. Radiother Oncol 2016;119(1):40–4.
52. Znati CA, Rosenstein M, Boucher Y, et al. Effect of radiation on interstitial fluid pressure and oxygenation in a human tumor xenograft. Cancer Res 1996;56(5):964–8.
53. Davies Cde L, Lundstrom LM, Frengen J, et al. Radiation improves the distribution and uptake of liposomal doxorubicin (caelyx) in human osteosarcoma xenografts. Cancer Res 2004;64(2):547–53.
54. Khosrawipour V, Bellendorf A, Khosrawipour C, et al. Irradiation does not increase the penetration depth of doxorubicin in normal tissue after pressurized intra-peritoneal aerosol chemotherapy (PIPAC) in an ex vivo model. In Vivo 2016;30(5):593–7.
55. Li T, Wang YN, Khokhlova TD, et al. Pulsed high-intensity focused ultrasound enhances delivery of doxorubicin in a preclinical model of pancreatic cancer. Cancer Res 2015;75(18):3738–46.
56. Wang S, Shin IS, Hancock H, et al. Pulsed high intensity focused ultrasound increases penetration and therapeutic efficacy of monoclonal antibodies in murine xenograft tumors. J Control Release 2012;162(1):218–24.
57. Gremonprez F, Descamps B, Izmer A, et al. Pretreatment with VEGF(R)-inhibitors reduces interstitial fluid pressure, increases intraperitoneal chemotherapy drug penetration, and impedes tumor growth in a mouse colorectal carcinomatosis model. Oncotarget 2015;6(30):29889–900.
58. Skliarenko JV, Lunt SJ, Gordon ML, et al. Effects of the vascular disrupting agent ZD6126 on interstitial fluid pressure and cell survival in tumors. Cancer Res 2006;66(4):2074–80.
59. Lindner P, Heath D, Howell S, et al. Vasopressin modulation of peritoneal, lymphatic, and plasma drug exposure following intraperitoneal administration. Clin Cancer Res 1996;2(2):311–7.
60. Mahteme H, Sundin A, Larsson B, et al. 5-FU uptake in peritoneal metastases after pretreatment with radioimmunotherapy or vasoconstriction: an autoradiographic study in the rat. Anticancer Res 2005;25(2A):917–22.
61. Duvillard C, Benoit L, Moretto P, et al. Epinephrine enhances penetration and anticancer activity of local cisplatin on rat sub-cutaneous and peritoneal tumors. Int J Cancer 1999;81(5):779–84.
62. Guardiola E, Chauffert B, Delroeux D, et al. Intraoperative chemotherapy with cisplatin and epinephrine after cytoreductive surgery in patients with recurrent ovarian cancer: a phase I study. Anticancer Drugs 2010;21(3):320–5.
63. Royer B, Kalbacher E, Onteniente S, et al. Intraperitoneal clearance as a potential biomarker of cisplatin after intraperitoneal perioperative chemotherapy: a population pharmacokinetic study. Br J Cancer 2012;106(3):460–7.
64. Oman M, Lundqvist S, Gustavsson B, et al. Phase I/II trial of intraperitoneal 5-Fluorouracil with and without intravenous vasopressin in non-resectable pancreas cancer. Cancer Chemother Pharmacol 2005;56(6):603–9.
65. Podobnik B, Sersa G, Miklavcic D. Effect of hydralazine on interstitial fluid pressure in experimental tumours and in normal tissue. In Vivo 2001;15(5):417–24.
66. Provenzano PP, Cuevas C, Chang AE, et al. Enzymatic targeting of the stroma ablates physical barriers to treatment of pancreatic ductal adenocarcinoma. Cancer Cell 2012;21(3):418–29.
67. Hingorani SR, Harris WP, Beck JT, et al. Phase Ib study of PEGylated recombinant human hyaluronidase and gemcitabine in patients with advanced pancreatic cancer. Clin Cancer Res 2016;22(12):2848–54.

68. Kato M, Hattori Y, Kubo M, et al. Collagenase-1 injection improved tumor distribution and gene expression of cationic lipoplex. Int J Pharm 2012;423(2):428–34.

69. Eikenes L, Bruland OS, Brekken C, et al. Collagenase increases the transcapillary pressure gradient and improves the uptake and distribution of monoclonal antibodies in human osteosarcoma xenografts. Cancer Res 2004;64(14):4768–73.

70. Brown E, McKee T, diTomaso E, et al. Dynamic imaging of collagen and its modulation in tumors in vivo using second-harmonic generation. Nat Med 2003;9(6): 796–800.

71. Perentes JY, McKee TD, Ley CD, et al. In vivo imaging of extracellular matrix remodeling by tumor-associated fibroblasts. Nat Methods 2009;6(2):143–5.

72. Chauhan VP, Martin JD, Liu H, et al. Angiotensin inhibition enhances drug delivery and potentiates chemotherapy by decompressing tumour blood vessels. Nat Commun 2013;4:2516.

73. Kumar V, Boucher Y, Liu H, et al. Noninvasive assessment of losartan-induced increase in functional microvasculature and drug delivery in pancreatic ductal adenocarcinoma. Transl Oncol 2016;9(5):431–7.

74. Diop-Frimpong B, Chauhan VP, Krane S, et al. Losartan inhibits collagen I synthesis and improves the distribution and efficacy of nanotherapeutics in tumors. Proc Natl Acad Sci U S A 2011;108(7):2909–14.

75. Olive KP, Jacobetz MA, Davidson CJ, et al. Inhibition of Hedgehog signaling enhances delivery of chemotherapy in a mouse model of pancreatic cancer. Science 2009;324(5933):1457–61.

76. Ko AH, LoConte N, Tempero MA, et al. A phase I study of FOLFIRINOX plus IPI-926, a hedgehog pathway inhibitor, for advanced pancreatic adenocarcinoma. Pancreas 2016;45(3):370–5.

77. Kim EJ, Sahai V, Abel EV, et al. Pilot clinical trial of hedgehog pathway inhibitor GDC-0449 (vismodegib) in combination with gemcitabine in patients with metastatic pancreatic adenocarcinoma. Clin Cancer Res 2014;20(23):5937–45.

78. Sherman MH, Yu RT, Engle DD, et al. Vitamin D receptor-mediated stromal reprogramming suppresses pancreatitis and enhances pancreatic cancer therapy. Cell 2014;159(1):80–93.

79. Moschetta M, Pretto F, Berndt A, et al. Paclitaxel enhances therapeutic efficacy of the F8-IL2 immunocytokine to EDA-fibronectin-positive metastatic human melanoma xenografts. Cancer Res 2012;72(7):1814–24.

80. Taghian AG, Abi-Raad R, Assaad SI, et al. Paclitaxel decreases the interstitial fluid pressure and improves oxygenation in breast cancers in patients treated with neoadjuvant chemotherapy: clinical implications. J Clin Oncol 2005;23(9): 1951–61.

81. Geretti E, Leonard SC, Dumont N, et al. Cyclophosphamide-mediated tumor priming for enhanced delivery and antitumor activity of HER2-targeted liposomal doxorubicin (MM-302). Mol Cancer Ther 2015;14(9):2060–71.

82. Hylander BL, Sen A, Beachy SH, et al. Tumor priming by Apo2L/TRAIL reduces interstitial fluid pressure and enhances efficacy of liposomal gemcitabine in a patient derived xenograft tumor model. J Control Release 2015;217:160–9.

83. Lu Z, Tsai M, Lu D, et al. Tumor-penetrating microparticles for intraperitoneal therapy of ovarian cancer. J Pharmacol Exp Ther 2008;327(3):673–82.

84. Sugahara KN, Teesalu T, Karmali PP, et al. Coadministration of a tumor-penetrating peptide enhances the efficacy of cancer drugs. Science 2010; 328(5981):1031–5.

85. Sugahara KN, Teesalu T, Karmali PP, et al. Tissue-penetrating delivery of compounds and nanoparticles into tumors. Cancer Cell 2009;16(6):510–20.

86. Akashi Y, Oda T, Ohara Y, et al. Anticancer effects of gemcitabine are enhanced by co-administered iRGD peptide in murine pancreatic cancer models that over-expressed neuropilin-1. Br J Cancer 2014;110(6):1481–7.

87. Sugahara KN, Scodeller P, Braun GB, et al. A tumor-penetrating peptide enhances circulation-independent targeting of peritoneal carcinomatosis. J Control Release 2015;212:59–69.

88. Simon-Gracia L, Hunt H, Scodeller P, et al. iRGD peptide conjugation potentiates intraperitoneal tumor delivery of paclitaxel with polymersomes. Biomaterials 2016;104:247–57.

89. Patel KJ, Lee C, Tan Q, et al. Use of the proton pump inhibitor pantoprazole to modify the distribution and activity of doxorubicin: a potential strategy to improve the therapy of solid tumors. Clin Cancer Res 2013;19(24):6766–76.

90. Yu M, Lee C, Wang M, et al. Influence of the proton pump inhibitor lansoprazole on distribution and activity of doxorubicin in solid tumors. Cancer Sci 2015; 106(10):1438–47.

Techniques and Safety Issues for Intraperitoneal Chemotherapy

Santiago González-Moreno, MD, PhD[a],*, Gloria Ortega-Pérez, MD[a],
Oscar Alonso-Casado, MD, PhD[b], Javier Galipienzo-García, MD, PhD[c],
Manuel J. Linero-Noguera, MD[c], David Salvatierra-Díaz, MD[c]

KEYWORDS

- Hyperthermia • Safety • Intraperitoneal chemotherapy • Technique
- Peritoneal neoplasms • Occupational hazard

KEY POINTS

- Several methods of delivering hyperthermic intraperitoneal chemotherapy (HIPEC) have been described, but no significant differences in treatment outcomes, morbidity, or safety have been found among them, and the ultimate choice between them is left to individual preference or institutional criteria.
- Administration of HIPEC is safe for the personnel working in the operating room; chemotherapy exposure during the procedure is negligible provided universal precautions, individual protection measures, and environmental safety guidelines are followed.
- Proper education of operating room staff about the essentials of HIPEC and proper chemotherapy handling is the first safety requirement.

INTRODUCTION

The combination of complete cytoreductive surgery (CRS) and perioperative intraperitoneal chemotherapy (PIC) provides the best chance for long-term survival for selected patients diagnosed with a variety of peritoneal neoplasms, either primary or secondary to digestive or gynecologic malignancies.[1–4] Its clinical application is fully developed and well-established in specialized centers around the world.[5] New treatment centers are emerging on a yearly basis.

Hyperthermic intraperitoneal chemotherapy (HIPEC) delivered in the operating room once the cytoreductive surgical procedure is finalized constitutes the most common

Disclosure: The authors have nothing to disclose.
[a] Peritoneal Surface Oncology Program, Department of Surgical Oncology, MD Anderson Cancer Center, Calle Arturo Soria 270, Madrid 28033, Spain; [b] Hepatobiliary and Pancreatic Surgery, Department of Surgical Oncology, MD Anderson Cancer Center, Calle Arturo Soria 270, Madrid 28033, Spain; [c] Department of Anesthesiology, MD Anderson Cancer Center, Calle Arturo Soria 270, Madrid 28033, Spain
* Corresponding author.
E-mail address: sgonzalezm@mdanderson.es

form of administration of PIC. HIPEC combines the pharmacokinetic advantage inherent to the intracavitary delivery of certain cytotoxic drugs, which results in regional dose intensification, with the direct cytotoxic effect of hyperthermia. Hyperthermia exhibits a selective cell-killing effect in malignant cells by itself, potentiates the cytotoxic effect of certain chemotherapy agents, and enhances the tissue penetration of the administered drug.[6] HIPEC may be complemented in some instances with early postoperative intraperitoneal chemotherapy (EPIC), delivered for the first 5 postoperative days in normothermia, although EPIC may be used alone.

The specific contribution of PIC to the overall oncological outcomes observed for the combined procedure remains to be elucidated. This issue is addressed by the French randomized trial PRODIGE-7, whose final outcome results are still awaited.[7]

Randomized controlled studies have not been performed to formally assess which modality of PIC is more advantageous. A few retrospective comparative studies are available showing a trend for or even an advantage for HIPEC alone over HIPEC followed by EPIC or EPIC alone, in terms of morbidity (fistula formation), although not in terms of survival.[8,9] These conclusions, however, need to be interpreted with caution.

Although the use of HIPEC has gained wider acceptance, the specifics of its administration still lack uniformity. This article describes different techniques in use and the technology available for the administration of HIPEC, discussing its advantages and disadvantages. It also reviews the safety features that must be taken into consideration when performing this procedure to prevent occupational hazards.

HYPERTHERMIC INTRAPERITONEAL CHEMOTHERAPY TECHNIQUES

By principle, HIPEC is delivered in the operating room once a complete macroscopic cytoreduction has been achieved. There are 2 main methods for intraperitoneal administration of hyperthermic chemotherapy: open abdomen technique and closed abdomen technique. Mixed methods (semiopen or semiclosed) have been reported also.

Open Technique

The open technique is referred to as the coliseum technique, as described by Sugarbaker.[10] Once the cytoreductive phase has been finalized, 4 closed-suction drains are placed through the abdominal wall and made watertight with a purse-string suture at the skin. These drains will remain in place for the postoperative period. An inflow line is placed over the abdominal wall into the peritoneal cavity and may be secured by a silk tie at the retractor frame. A different number of temperature probes may be used for intraperitoneal temperature monitoring; at least one in the in-flow line or under the right diaphragm and another one at a distance from this point (pelvis) are employed, but a more intensive monitoring may be used. Probes' tips may be secured with a silk tie to the tip of the corresponding drains to prevent migration. The skin edges of the abdominal incision are suspended up to a self-retaining retractor whose frame has previously been elevated 15 to 20 cm over the patient, thus creating an open space in the abdominal cavity. This is done by a running monofilament number 1 suture. A silastic sheet is incorporated into this suture to prevent chemotherapy solution splashing from occurring. A cut in the plastic cover is made to allow the surgeon's double-gloved hand access to the abdomen and pelvis. Impervious gown, double gloving, and protection goggles are mandatory. A smoke evacuator is placed under the plastic sheet to clear chemotherapy vapors or small droplets that may be liberated during the procedure. During the 30 to 90 minutes of perfusion, all the anatomic structures within the peritoneal cavity and the laparotomy incision are uniformly exposed to heat and chemotherapy by continuous manual stirring of the perfusate performed by the surgeon. After completion of HIPEC, the chemotherapy solution is drained and applicable anastomoses performed. However, some teams do the anastomoses before HIPEC is administered.

A variation of the open technique described and mainly used in Japan uses a device called peritoneal cavity expander (PCE). The PCE is an acrylic cylinder containing inflow and outflow lines that is secured over the laparotomy wound. When filled with heated perfusate, the PCE can accommodate the small bowel, allowing it to float freely and be manipulated within the perfusate. After HIPEC is completed, the perfusate is drained, and the PCE is removed. Fujimura and colleagues[11] and Yonemura and colleagues[12] reported about HIPEC with a PCE in carcinomatosis from various malignancies. The use of the PCE is limited (if any) at the present time and has rarely been employed outside Japan. Its interest is somewhat historical.

Closed Technique

The closed technique has become a commonly used method to deliver HIPEC. After macroscopic cytoreduction, 1 inflow catheter and 2 outflow catheters are typically placed. The outflow catheters are placed in dependent positions, such as the pelvis and under the right hemidiaphragm. Temperature probes are placed in the abdomen attached to the catheter tips to monitor in-flow and out-flow temperatures. After temporary watertight closure of the abdominal skin, the heated chemotherapy solution is administered. The abdominal cavity is manually agitated externally during the perfusion period to promote uniform distribution of the heated chemotherapy perfusate. After completion of perfusion, the abdomen is reopened, and the perfusate is evacuated. Appropriate anastomoses are performed, and the patient is closed in the standard fashion. Some teams apply the HIPEC closed method after constructing the anastomoses and performing a definitive closure of the abdominal wall.

Mixed Methods

The mixed methods (semiopen or semiclosed) have been developed as an evolution of an open method, in an attempt to reduce the chance of operating room staff exposure to chemotherapy and prevent heat loss. The group from Dijon, France, led by Rat,[13] use a latex sheet (abdominal cavity expander) water-tight sutured to the skin edges and then secured to the retractor frame, allowing a controlled overflow of the perfusate and allowing its level to reach well above the skin edges with no spillage. A transparent methacrylate cover with a laparoscopy hand port in its center is placed over the retractor's frame and the latex piece, hermetically closing the abdominal cavity. Sugarbaker[14] also reported the use of a closed acrylic device with a lid, mounted on top of the coliseum to provide perfusate containment while allowing manual access to the peritoneal cavity for manipulation.

In a HIPEC procedure using any of these techniques, a roller pump forces the chemotherapy solution into the abdomen through the inflow line and pulls it out through the drains, with a flow rate around 1 L per minute. The instillate's temperature reaches up to 43°C to 45°C after passing through a heat exchanger, so that the intraperitoneal fluid is maintained at 41°C to 43°C. The perfusate may be first recirculated between a reservoir and the heat exchanger so that it can be heated to an adequate temperature. At this point, full closed-circuit circulation of the perfusate in and out of the peritoneal cavity is established until a minimum intraperitoneal temperature of 41.5°C is achieved and maintained. The drug is then added to the circuit, and the timer for the perfusion is started. In bidirectional chemotherapy protocols, the intravenous infusion of the appropriate drugs may be started at this time point as well, although some authors advocate doing it 1 hour before the initiation of HIPEC.

Comparative Analysis and Choice of Hyperthermic Intraperitoneal Chemotherapy Technique

Each HIPEC technique has its own advantages and disadvantages.

Advantages of the closed technique include

- Ability to rapidly achieve and maintain hyperthermia as there is minimal heat loss
- Minimal contact or aerosolized exposure of the operating room staff to the chemotherapy; the only way for exposure is leakage through the surgical wound or catheter wounds
- A higher abdominal pressure is achieved during the perfusion, which may facilitate drug tissue penetration[15]

Disadvantages of the closed technique include

- Lack of uniform distribution of the heat and chemotherapy, for which continuous external manual agitation of the abdominal wall is needed
- A larger volume of perfusate is generally needed to establish the circuit compared with the open technique

Advantages of the open technique include assurance that heated chemotherapy is adequately distributed throughout the abdominal cavity. Because of direct manipulation of the intra-abdominal viscera during perfusion, all peritoneal surfaces are equally exposed to the therapy (both heat and chemotherapy). This limits pooling of the heated perfusate and thereby theoretically reduces systemic absorption of chemotherapy, post-operative ileus, perforation or fistula formation.

Disadvantages of the open technique include

- The open abdomen naturally leads to heat dissipation, which can make it more difficult and time-consuming to achieve hyperthermia, particularly if higher temperatures are desired
- The abdominal wall is suspended, and thus may be inadequately exposed to the perfusate
- Theoretic increased exposure of operating room personnel to chemotherapy (because the surgeon's gloved hand is in direct contact with the cytotoxic solution, increased potential exists for contact exposure, and because the abdomen is open during perfusion, heated chemotherapy can aerosolize, creating inhalational exposure; these concerns have never been substantiated in the different ad hoc studies performed)

To the authors' knowledge, no formal large-scale prospective controlled comparison of HIPEC techniques has been carried out to date. Elias and colleagues[16] performed an early phase trial in which they successively tested 7 HIPEC procedures. The authors concluded that closed methods were not satisfactory and that the open technique with traction of the skin upwards was superior in terms of technical feasibility, thermal homogeneity, and perfusate distribution. Ortega-Deballon and colleagues[17] published a comparative experimental study in a small number of pigs, concluding that intraperitoneal hyperthermia can be achieved with both techniques and that the open technique had higher systemic absorption and abdominal tissue penetration of chemotherapy (oxaliplatin) than the closed technique.

The panel of experts assembled for the 2006 Consensus Conference in Milan concluded that there is no evidence to establish the superiority of one method over the others regarding patient outcomes, morbidity, or surgical staff safety.[18] A call for future studies to definitively answer this question has not been answered. Therefore, any of the methods listed may be used for the delivery of HIPEC.

The criteria that may be taken into consideration when choosing a HIPEC method by emerging treatment programs are completely subjective and have to do with perceptions, not facts. They have to do mainly with the perceived risk of environmental or staff chemotherapy exposure or concerns on possible differences in the uniform distribution of chemotherapy or heat throughout the peritoneal cavity that may result in visceral thermal injury. Possible differences in dosage and perfusate volume inherent to the closed method can play a role as well.

Each program should use the method that best fits its institutional needs or demands in terms of operational features, safety, and occupational hazard regulations, becoming used to deal with its own advantages and disadvantages. Some teams have changed their method of choice over time, even after extensive experience with one of them.

TECHNOLOGY FOR THE DELIVERY OF HYPERTHERMIC INTRAPERITONEAL CHEMOTHERAPY

Regardless of the method employed, an external device that heats the chemotherapy perfusate and continuously circulates it in and out of the patient in order to keep a target intraperitoneal temperature and volume within the peritoneal cavity is always needed. Key components of this apparatus are

- A single-use circuit tubing that incorporates in most cases a reservoir to withdraw the perfusate in case of an emergency or keep it before the perfusion starts.
- A heat source
- A heat exchanger, where the perfusate is actually heated
- A roller pump that forces the perfusate from the reservoir into the patient
- A return method from patient to reservoir, which could be a second roller pump or a vacuum source
- Several temperature monitors (heat source, heat exchanger, inflow line, various points in the peritoneal cavity)

All these components, except for the single-use circuit tubing that comes inside its own sterile box, are assembled together, creating a machine. Most of these devices also incorporate a computerized continuous recording of thermal data that may be displayed in situ for monitoring during the procedure and then exported or printed with different formats. This adds security and comfortability to the procedure, avoiding the need to create written records and also allowing efficient data recording for clinical research.

Commercially available compact HIPEC machines have been developed since the late 1990s, and the number of companies manufacturing them has gradually increased over the years; this may be regarded as an indirect sign of the acceptability and applicability of HIPEC in clinical practice. This was also a step forward in the regulatory field, since these machines must be approved specifically for HIPEC use by the appropriate regulatory agencies (eg, US Food and Drug Administration), which definitely addresses any institutional medico-legal concerns about the use of this technology in people.[19] On the other hand, availability of HIPEC machines for purchase may bring the opportunity to perform surgical treatment of peritoneal carcinomatosis in suboptimal conditions, without the appropriate training and knowledge, under the false assumption that the machine does the work. The peritoneal surface oncology community and these companies must work together to prevent against this opportunistic approach.

The choice of a specific HIPEC apparatus is certainly a subjective issue. Several factors may be taken into account in this decision: ability to achieve adequate hyperthermia in a short time period, adjustable flow rate, user friendliness, ease of assembly for the circuit by the surgical support staff, easy-reading and continuous registration of temperatures, availability of technical support, and of course, pricing of the machine itself and of the disposable circuit tubing kits. Testing different options in one's own operating room is advisable before making a final decision.

An original alternative to the use of a closed-circuit external apparatus to deliver HIPEC has been described by Ortega-Deballon and colleagues.[20] Their method uses a heat source placed directly in the peritoneal cavity. It consists of 2 17 m electric heating cables insulated with a silicon wrapping. Each cable is connected to a 24 V transformer and then to a 220 V electric outlet. One cable is distributed in the supramesocolic area and the other in the inframesocolic area and between the bowel loops. This device shows a favorable safety profile with no direct heat damage to the viscera, efficacy, and technical feasibility. It is now approved for use in people. The advantages of this technology in terms of cost, operating time, and simplicity are obvious.

SAFETY ISSUES

The introduction, handling, and management of chemotherapy in the operating room OR that come with HIPEC necessarily determine a change in surgical personnel habits and may bring a biased, unrealistic perception of added danger and risks. The staff involved in the procedure must be fully aware of the meaning of the potential risks and associated hazards to avoid unnecessary potential health problems or an irrational opposition to their participation in the program.

Education as a Safety Factor: Influence on Behavior

Ignorance may be the most dangerous health risk in the operating room. It is known from a behavioral standpoint (health belief model) that, even with the proper education, it is the individual who ultimately will or will not adhere to self-protective measures, influenced by his or her perception of susceptibility, severity, benefits, and efficacy of the barriers used.[21] Unrealistic optimism by which health care workers cannot believe they will become ill as a result of hazardous exposures should be avoided.

Appropriate education about cytoreductive surgery and HIPEC is a first, mandatory safety factor that must be observed by all personnel involved in the procedure.[22] The surgical oncologist leading the team should take responsibility to provide such education and training, as needed.

The educational program should cover the surgical technique, the intraperitoneal chemotherapy perfusion, the cytotoxic agents used, the effects of hyperthermia on these drugs and on the patient, and the indications, rationale, and results of the procedure. Then, they need to be educated on routes of exposure and risks of low-dose occupational exposure to cytotoxic agents. Additionally, they should be made aware of the potential risks associated with an increased amount of surgical smoke produced during cytoreductive surgery. Finally, we have to train the personnel on how to avoid these exposure hazards and how to perform a safe procedure.

Chemotherapy Exposure

During HIPEC, chemotherapy is always diluted, never pure, and absolute doses of drugs are in micrograms, so that it is not possible to have a major spill (defined as lesser than 5 g or 5 mL of undiluted cytotoxic agent by the US Occupational Safety Health Administration-OSHA). Although toxicity of these agents has been described for therapeutic dosages, long-term effects of prolonged, repeated occupational exposure to low doses remain unknown. For this reason, all precautions and guidelines for chemotherapy handling should be observed.[23]

The routes of exposure to chemotherapy during HIPEC are mainly direct skin contact and inhalation of aerosols or vapors, since accidental injection and ingestion are to be regarded anecdotal in this context. Direct contact of cytotoxic agents with skin or mucous membranes produces irritation or dermatitis. The use of the smoke evacuator under the plastic sheet during HIPEC administration using the coliseum technique, or the advent of the acrylic covers used in the semiopen methods, minimizes the exposure to potential aerosols.

Stuart and colleagues[24] were the first to evaluate the safety of operating room personnel during HIPEC. They administered mitomycin C using the coliseum technique. Urine from members of the operating team was assayed for chemotherapy levels. Air below and above the plastic sheet also was analyzed. Finally, sterile gloves commonly used in the operating room were examined for permeability to chemotherapy. All assessments of potential exposures were found to be negative, in compliance with established safety standards. Schmid and colleagues[25] arrived to the same conclusions regarding both mitomycin C detection levels and glove permeability assays. A Swedish study reported by Näslund Andréasson and colleagues[26] during HIPEC with oxaliplatin using the coliseum technique failed to detect any platinum in the urine or blood of the surgeon or the perfusionist involved in the procedure.

These studies confirm that, even in the method with a higher chance for surgical staff chemotherapy exposure, delivery of HIPEC is a safe procedure from the occupational risk standpoint provided adequate, standard protective measures are observed.

Surgical Smoke Exposure

Contrary to the exposure to chemotherapy, surgical staff tends to underappreciate the risks of electrosurgical smoke and the need to employ protective measures against it. Cytoreductive surgery uses high-voltage electrosurgery, both for visceral dissection and resection and for the electroevaporation of tumor nodules. The amount of smoke generated during this procedure exceeds that created during a regular surgical operation (eg, for colorectal cancer)[27] This fact added to the length of the operation (10–12 hours) may result in cumulative exposure.

Just by its physical effects, surgical smoke may produce headache, nausea, and eye and respiratory tract irritation to health care workers in the operating room. It also hampers the correct visualization of the surgical field. Surgical smoke contains ultrafine particles (UFPs), whose increase in the environment is related to lung dysfunction, cardiovascular changes, and mortality. Some dangerous substances have been identified in these UFPs like benzene, toluene, furfural, and polycyclic aromatic hydrocarbons (PAHs), some of which are carcinogenic or may cause ischemic heart disease. Additionally, smoke particles can bear viable microorganisms. In a Swedish study, the amount of UFPs detected during cytoreductive surgery was comparable to that in secondhand (sidestream) smoke of cigarettes. No single or cumulative values of PAHs in this context exceeded the occupational exposure limits.[27,28]

Investigations done by the Safety Work Agencies in Europe and the United States have shown that it is possible to control air contamination from electrosurgical smoke by keeping good ventilation of the operating room and by using a smoke evacuator at all times.[29,30]

Standard operating room ventilation procedures in effect for any type of major surgery are also valid and adequate in the operating room dedicated to HIPEC.[31]

A smoke evacuator should be ready for use from the beginning of the operation. This device must have a suction unit, an absorbent HEPA filter, and a disposable tube for smoke conduction with a rigid end.[30] Although several options are commercially available, this apparatus is unfortunately not among the regular equipment available in every operating room. Filters have a filling indicator; they should be changed frequently, and disposed of as biological hazardous material. The tip of the smoke evacuator tubing may be handled by the scrub nurse and kept about 5 cm from the origin of the smoke to catch every contaminating substance. Suction must work always while the smoke is being produced; synchronization of the smoke evacuator with the electrosurgical generator is of great help in this regard. Air suction with this device under the plastic sheet is also used as a protective measure during the administration of HIPEC by the coliseum technique.

Additionally, individual protective measures against surgical smoke may be used, including a high-power filtration mask and eye protection.

It should be noted that, although included in most safety guidelines, breathing through a high-power filtration mask (FFP-3) is neither comfortable nor easy, and some people just cannot stand them for prolonged periods of time. The consequences of not wearing them on the health of surgical workers if smoke evacuation and adequate ventilation are reinforced have not been assessed. Additionally, because no study to date has detected chemotherapy particles in the operating room air during the administration of open HIPEC,[23,30,31] the need to wear such a mask instead of a regular surgical mask is debatable.

Eye protection should be worn as a mechanical barrier not just for the smoke, but also for cytostatic agents and bodily fluid exposure, as part of a universal precaution protocol.

RECOMMENDED GUIDELINES FOR THE SAFE ADMINISTRATION OF HYPERTHERMIC INTRAPERITONEAL CHEMOTHERAPY
Recommended Individual Protective Measures and Environmental Measures

There are several recommended individual protective measures and environmental measures to minimize staff chemotherapy exposure during HIPEC[22]:

- Use of impervious, disposable surgical drapes; do not use textile cloth
- A correct laparotomy pad count should be obtained before initiation of HIPEC
- Operating room doors should be closed
- Signs should be placed outside the operating room advising that HIPEC is in progress
- Restriction of personnel circulation
- Placement of absorbent towels on the floor around surgical table for possible spills
- Use of disposable impervious gown (closed front, long sleeves, and closed cuffs)
- Use of disposable impervious shoe covers
- Use of double powderless latex gloving, outer 1 elbow length; change outer glove every 30 minutes
- Use eye protection (goggles)
- Use of FFP-3 is debatable
- Proper operating room ventilation and air conditioning
- Smoke evacuator is to be used continuously over surgical field (under plastic drape in coliseum technique)

- Leak-proof rigid containers labeled "cytotoxic agents" should be used for every material or bodily fluid to be discarded during or after HIPEC (and during the following 48 hours)

This is a list of generally recommended items but it is ultimately up to every institution and treatment program to define its own safety guidelines and reinforce them.

Further safety considerations that have to do with operating room staff selection and health checks, the management of chemotherapy spills, and the cleaning of the operating room after a HIPEC procedure.

Staff Selection and Health Checks

Any association between the participation in a HIPEC program and the chance of future newborn congenital defects, worsening of a blood dyscrasia, or even developing any health problem in the future should be avoided. Therefore, limitations for staff participation in the program must be established, among them: pregnant or nursing women, history of abortions or congenital malformation, individuals actively pursuing pregnancy (men or women), hematologic or teratogenic disease history, previous chemotherapy or radiotherapy treatments, usual work with radiographs or radiation therapy, active immunosuppressive treatment, allergy to cytotoxic drugs or latex, and severe dermatologic disease.

Regular health checks for health care workers involved in the delivery of HIPEC must be carried out. These should be done every 6 to 12 months, collecting information on the frequency of exposure to the procedure, any incident (eg, spillage or skin contact) during HIPEC, new symptoms (especially in skin, mucous membranes, or gastrointestinal tract, or hair loss). Blood work with at least a complete blood cell count and a biochemistry panel should be obtained. After learning all the pertinent data, an individualized assessment and follow-up instructions are to be provided.

Management of Direct Contact with Chemotherapy or Chemotherapy Spills

The US Occupational Safety and Health Administration (OSHA) categorizes chemotherapy spills as small or large using a threshold of 5 g or 5 mL of undiluted cytotoxic agent.[23]

If direct contact with cytotoxic agent occurs, contaminated clothing should be removed immediately and discarded in a hazardous waste container. Affected skin should be washed immediately with mild, additive-free soap without dyes or perfumes that may interact with the cytotoxic agent. If the affected area is the eye, it should be flooded immediately with water or isotonic saline for 5 minutes. The staff member should then report the incident to the occupational health office.

A small spill should be blotted dry using absorbent pads and wiped. The area should be washed 3 times with water and neutral soap. Then, the area can be cleaned in the routine manner. When clearing large spills, special care should be taken to avoid creating aerosols. To clean up any kind of spill, the personnel should wear the whole protective barrier garments already described, including a respirator mask for the large spills.

CLEANING UP THE OPERATING ROOM AFTER HYPERTHERMIC INTRAPERITONEAL CHEMOTHERAPY

Education about the meaning and risks of using chemotherapy in the operating room needs to extend to the cleaning personnel. Standard protective clothing described should be used. Special leak-proof bins should be used to discard all trash from the room. All bactericidal cleaning solutions should not be used to wash a contaminated area, because they may react with the cytotoxic agents and do not inactivate them. Water with neutral soap is adequate to clean up the operating room after HIPEC, 3 consecutive times; 70% isopropyl alcohol is also safe and effective.

Surgical instruments should be washed 3 times with water and pure soap before leaving the working area.

REFERENCES

1. Rajeev R, Turaga KK. Hyperthermic intraperitoneal chemotherapy and cytoreductive surgery in the management of peritoneal carcinomatosis. Cancer Control 2016;23:36–46.
2. Yan TD, Welch L, Black D, et al. A systematic review on the efficacy of cytoreductive surgery combined with perioperative intraperitoneal chemotherapy for diffuse malignancy peritoneal mesothelioma. Ann Oncol 2007;18:827–34.
3. Yan TD, Black D, Savady R, et al. A systematic review on the efficacy of cytoreductive surgery and perioperative intraperitoneal chemotherapy for pseudomyxoma peritonei. Ann Surg Oncol 2007;14:484–92.
4. Yan TD, Black D, Savady R, et al. Systematic review on the efficacy of cytoreductive surgery combined with perioperative intraperitoneal chemotherapy for peritoneal carcinomatosis from colorectal carcinoma. J Clin Oncol 2006;24:4011–9.
5. Glehen O, Gilly FN, Boutitie F, et al. Toward curative treatment of peritoneal carcinomatosis from nonovarian origin by cytoreductive surgery combined with perioperative intraperitoneal chemotherapy: a multi-institutional study of 1290 patients. Cancer 2010;116(24):5608–18.
6. Sticca RP, Dach BW. Rationale for hyperthermia with intraoperative intraperitoneal chemotherapy agents. Surg Oncol Clin N Am 2003;12:689–701.
7. Quenet F, Elias D (principal investigators): Protocole Prodige 7. ACCORD 15/0608. EudraCT N: 2006-006175-20. Essai de phase III évaluant la place de la chimiohyperthermie intrapéritonéale peropéraroire (CHIP) après résection maximale d'une carcinose péritonéale d'origine colorectale associée à une chimiothérapie sysstémique.
8. Elias D, Benizri E, Di Pietrantonio D, et al. Comparison of two kinds of intraperitoneal chemotherapy following complete cytoreductive surgery of colorectal peritoneal carcinomatosis. Ann Surg Oncol 2007;14:509–14.
9. Glehen O, Kwiatkowski F, Sugarbaker PH, et al. Cytoreductive surgery combined with perioperative intraperitoneal chemotherapy for the management of peritoneal carcinomatosis from colorectal cancer: a multi-institutional study. J Clin Oncol 2004;22:3284–92.
10. Sugarbaker PH. Technical handbook for the integration of cytoreductive surgery and perioperative intraperitoneal chemotherapy into the surgical management of gastrointestinal and gynecologic malignancy. 4th edition. Grand Rapids (MI): The Ludann Company; 2005. p. 52–6.
11. Fujimura T, Yonemura Y, Fujita H, et al. Chemo-hyperhtermic peritoneal perfusion for peritoneal dissemination in various intra-abdominal malignancies. Int Surg 1999;84:60–6.
12. Yonemura Y, Ninomiya I, Kaji M, et al. Prophylaxis with intraoperative chemohyperthermia against peritoneal recurrence of serosal invasion-positive gastric cancer. World J Surg 1995;19:450–5.
13. Rat P, Benoit L, Cheynel N, et al. Intraperitoneal chemohyperthermia with "overflow" open abdomen. Ann Chir 2001;126:669–71.

14. Sugarbaker PH. An instrument to provide containment of intraoperative intraperitoneal chemotherapy with optimized distribution. J Surg Oncol 2005;92:142–6.

15. Esquis P, Consolo D, Magnin G, et al. High intraabdominal pressure enhances the penetration and antitumor effect of intrapoeritoneal cisplatin on experimental peritoneal carcinomatosis. Ann Surg 2006;244:106–12.

16. Elias D, Antoun S, Goharin A, et al. Research on the best chemohyperthermia technique of treatment of peritoneal carcinomatosis after complete resection. Int J Surg Investig 2000;1:431–9.

17. Ortega-Deballon P, Facy O, Jambet S, et al. Which method to deliver hyperthermic intraperitoneal chemotherapy with oxaliplatin? An experimental comparison of open and closed techniques. Ann Surg Oncol 2010;17:1957–63.

18. Glehen O, Cotte E, Kusamura S, et al. Hyperthermic intraperitoneal chemotherapy: nomenclature and modalities of perfusion. J Surg Oncol 2008;98:242–6.

19. Sugarbaker PH, Clarke L. The approval process for hyperthermic intraoperative intraperitoneal chemotherapy. Eur J Surg Oncol 2006;32:637–43.

20. Ortega-Deballon P, Facy O, Magnin G, et al. Using a heating cable within the abdomen to make hyperthermic intraperitoneal chemotherapy easier: feasibility and safety study in a pig model. Eur J Surg Oncol 2010;36:324–8.

21. Näslund Andréasson S, editor. Work environment in the operating room during cytoreductive surgery and hyperthermic intraperitoneal chemotherapy: factors influencing the choice of protective equipment. Digital comprehensive summaries of Uppsala dissertations from the Faculty of Medicine 716. Uppsala (Sweden): Acta Universitatis Upsaliensis; 2011. p. 85.

22. González-Bayón L, González-Moreno S, Ortega-Pérez G. Safety considerations for operating room personnel during hyperthermic intraoperative intraperitoneal chemotherapy perfusion. Eur J Surg Oncol 2006;32:612–24.

23. Yodaiken RE, Bennett D. OSHA work practice guidelines for personnel dealing with cytotoxic (antineoplastic) drugs. Occupational Safety and Health Administration. Am J Hosp Pharm 1986;43:1193–204.

24. Stuart OA, Stephens AD, Welch L, et al. Safety monitoring of the coliseum technique for heated intraoperative intraperitoneal chemotherapy with mitomycin C. Ann Surg Oncol 2002;9:186–91.

25. Schmid K, Boettcher MI, Pelz JO, et al. Investigations on safety of hyperthermic intraoperative intraperitoneal chemotherapy (HIPEC) with mitomycin C. Eur J Surg Oncol 2006;32:1222–5.

26. Näslund Andréasson S, Anundi H, Thóren S-B, et al. Is platinum present in the blood and urine from treatment givers during hyperthermic intraperitoneal chemotherapy? J Oncol 2010;2010:649719.

27. Andréasson SN, Anundi H, Sahlberg B, et al. Peritonectomy with high voltage electrocautery generates higher levels of ultrafine smoke particles. Eur J Surg Oncol 2009;3:780–4.

28. Andréasson SN, Mahteme H, Sahlberg B, et al. Policyclic aromatic hydrocarbons in electrocautery smoke during peritonectomy procedures. In: Näslund Andréasson S, editor. Work environment in the operating room during cytoreductive surgery and hyperthermic intraperitoneal chemotherapy: factors influencing the choice of protective equipment. Digital comprehensive summaries of Uppsala dissertations from the Faculty of Medicine 716. Uppsala (Sweden): Acta Universitatis Upsaliensis; 2011. p. 35–8.

29. NIOSH Hazard Controls. Control of smoke from laser/electrical surgical procedures. Atlanta (GA): US Department of Health and Human Services. National Institute of Ocupational Safety and Health; 1996. Publication number 96-128.
30. Ross K. 3rd edition. Surgical smoke evacuators: a primer. Surgical services management, vol. 3. Denver (CO): AORN; 1997.
31. Ulmer BC. 3rd edition. Air quality in the operating room. Surgical services management, vol. 3. Denver (CO): AORN; 1997.

Learning Curve, Training Program, and Monitorization of Surgical Performance of Peritoneal Surface Malignancies Centers

Shigeki Kusamura, MD, PhD[a],
Santiago González-Moreno, MD, PhD[b], Eran Nizri, MD, PhD[c],
Dario Baratti, MD[a], Stefano Guadagni, MD[d],
Marcello Guaglio, MD[a], Luigi Battaglia, MD[e],
Marcello Deraco, MD[a],*

KEYWORDS

- Cytoreductive surgery • HIPEC • Learning curve • Surgical training
- Surgical performance

KEY POINTS

- Cytoreductive surgery (CRS) and hyperthermic intraperitoneal chemotherapy (HIPEC) is a complex procedure with a steep learning curve (LC).
- Using specific statistics with risk adjustment, it was observed that approximately 137 to 180 cases are necessary for the achievement of proficiency considering radicality and safety. Eighty-six to 100 cases were necessary to ensure short-term prognostic gains in rare peritoneal surface malignances (PSM).
- Centralization of PSM centers is advisable for rare diseases, such as pseudomyxoma peritonei (PMP) and peritoneal mesothelioma.
- Mentoring is a key factor to shorten the LC and ensure quality of the training in CRS and HIPEC.
- A well-structured training program was implemented in Europe to standardize the treatment, ease the setting up of new centers, and improve the quality of the services.

Disclosure Statement: The study represented in this article was partially supported by the Italian Association for Cancer Research. AIRC IG 2013 N.14445 and AIRC IG 2016 Id.19206

[a] Peritoneal Surface Malignancies unit, Fondazione IRCCS Istituto Nazionale dei Tumori di Milano, Via Venezian 1, Milano, Milan cap 20133, Italy; [b] Surgical Oncology, MD Anderson Cancer Center, Calle Arturo Soria, n°270, Madrid, Spain; [c] Department of General Surgery, Tel Aviv Sourasky Medical Center, Sackler Faculty of Medicine, Tel Aviv University, Weizmann Street 6, Tel Aviv, Israel; [d] Department of Biotechnological and Applied Clinical Sciences, Università degli Studi dell'Aquila, Via Giovanni di Vincenzo, 16/B, L'Aquila, Italy; [e] Colorectal Cancer unit, Fondazione IRCCS Istituto Nazionale dei Tumori di Milano, Via Venezian 1, Milano, MI, cap 20133, Italy
* Corresponding author.
E-mail address: marcello.deraco@istitutotumori.mi.it

INTRODUCTION

The advent of cytoreductive surgery (CRS) and hyperthermic intraperitoneal chemotherapy (HIPEC) changed dramatically the approach to peritoneal surface malignancies (PSM). The combined treatment allowed the achievement of durable oncologic results in clinical conditions that were formerly considered amenable only to palliative therapies. This combined treatment is currently accepted as the standard of care for pseudomyxoma peritonei (PMP) and peritoneal mesothelioma.[1–4] and is also applicable in selected cases of peritoneal metastasis (PM) from colorectal and advanced epithelial ovarian cancers.[5–8]

This new therapeutic modality has spread widely around the world and new PSM centers are continuously emerging. However, the annual overall (ie, from main etiologies) estimated incidence of PSM is about 709,941 cases.[9] The following clinical entities were considered in this evaluation: peritoneal mesothelioma, primary peritoneal carcinoma, desmoplastic small round cell tumor, PM from colorectal cancer, PM from gastric cancer, ovarian cancer, and pancreatic cancer. Considering the estimated number of main active PSM centers in the world of 150 (Santiago González-Moreno, personal communication, 2014) and even if liberally assuming a 10 times larger actual number of institutions, each center would need to treat more than 400 cases per year to provide an acceptable response to the global population demand. Therefore, more PSM units are required.

CRS and HIPEC is a resource consuming operation with an estimated cost of up to €39,000 per procedure.[10,11] Moreover, it is a high-risk intervention with perioperative morbidity and mortality rates of about 28.8% and 2.9%, respectively.[12] Consequently, the associated learning curve (LC) is intuitively expected to be steep. Furthermore, the availability of methods for quality control of established centers is of best interest of regional health care systems for the optimization of resources allocation. This article discusses (1) the available methods to monitor surgical performance in the learning and audit phase of a center development, (2) the factors associated with the surgical performance, (3) what type of training program to shorten the learning process of the surgeon, and (4) what aspects related to logistics and infrastructure of the center could be modulated to optimize the achievement of its proficiency.

THE LEARNING CURVE PROCESS

The process of setting up a new PSM is a complex issue whose main limiting factor is that of the LC. The LC could be conceived as the achievement of proficiency in the performance of surgical procedures. This encompasses not only the technical dexterity, but also the ability to select the right case for the surgery and the excellence in the management of the patient in the postoperative period in a multidisciplinary environment.[13] Several outcomes could be used for LC evaluation: completeness of cytoreduction rates, morbidity-mortality, prognosis, and quality of life. The LC could be applicable not only for individual surgeons but also for PSM institutions.

Different approaches have been used in the literature to assess LC and surveillance of surgical performance. The traditional method is represented by classic frequentist statistics without adjustments. The second approach is represented by statistical process control tests.

ASSESSMENT OF LEARNING CURVE USING TRADITIONAL FREQUENTIST STATISTICS

Traditional frequentist statistics assess the LC by arbitrarily splitting the cases into different groups. Mohamed and Moran and colleagues[14] reported single-surgeon LC in 100 consecutive cases of CRS and HIPEC for PSM dividing the series into three equal groups of consecutive cases and comparing outcomes across groups. They reported a drop in major morbidity and mortality rates from 27% to 0% and 18% to 3%, respectively, from the first to the last group of cases. Similarly, Smeenk and colleagues[15] reported on 323 procedures for PSMs at the Netherland Cancer Institute. The rate of complete cytoreductions increased from 35.6 to 65.1% ($P = .012$). The postoperative morbidity rate decreased from 71.2% to 34.1% ($P<.001$). The median duration of hospital stay decreased from 24 to 17 days. The mean simplified peritoneal cancer index (PCI) score decreased significantly over the study period ($P<.001$). Yan and colleagues[16] reported outcomes of one surgical team performing 140 cases of CRS/HIPEC, divided into two sequential time periods of 70 cases each. They demonstrated a reduction in severe morbidity (30%–10%), transfusion requirement, operative time, and ICU length of stay.

Overall, these studies suggest improved proficiency as case numbers increased; however, they failed to control for covariates known to affect surgical outcomes (confounders). Eventual improvement in surgical outcomes should not be attributed entirely to an actual improvement of the surgical proficiency because less complex cases could have been selected across the timeline of the center's experience. Thus, this arbitrarily splitting method, associated with classic frequentist statistics, is not appropriate in the assessment of surgical performance and LC of complex surgical procedures.

STATISTICAL PROCESS CONTROL TESTS

Although originally developed for quality control of military supplies during World War II, statistical process control tests have been largely used in medicine to monitor the safety of medical interventions, such as interventional cardiology, cardiac surgery, emergency medical services, and other procedures. Two tests are most frequently used: the cumulative sum and sequential probability ratio test (SPRT).[17–21]

The SPRT offers an advantage over other statistical process control methods by allowing formal hypothesis testing. This method incorporates selection of type I and II error rates and a threshold of an unacceptable odds ratio (OR) for an outcome. The SPRT is then able to determine whether the hypothesis has been accepted or rejected, or whether further information is required to determine the answer. The SPRT allows for adjustment of confounders by multivariate analysis. Moreover, by providing a graphic summary of changes in performance over time, SPRT can alert a surgeon to suboptimal performance. SPRT is also well suited to monitor surgical LCs.

The risk-adjusted SPRT (RA-SPRT) could be plotted to chart, across the case sequence, changes in the outcomes of interest. The latter should be variable of binary nature, such as rates of incomplete cytoreduction, rates of G3-5 morbidity, and short-term oncologic failure. To elaborate the SPRT, four parameters are defined: estimated probabilities of outcomes of interest for each case, a prespecified OR for the outcomes of interest, and type I and II error rates. Probability of type I and type II (a and b) error usually are set at 0.05. From these, two control limits (h0 and h1) and the cumulative sum of log-likelihood ratio with risk-adjustment are calculated according to equations outlined by Rogers and colleagues.[22] The estimated risk of an adverse outcome is expected to suffer a wide variation from case to case and does not depend exclusively on the expertise of the surgical team. Factors related to the characteristics of patients and tumors do exert an impact on the outcome of interest. Therefore, an adjustment for preoperative (baseline) risk is critical to ensure that unfavorable event rates that seem unusual are not erroneously attributed to insufficient proficiency. Accordingly, the probability of event is calculated using the logistic regression model, which is adjusted with independent risk factors of incomplete cytoreduction, G3-5 morbidity, or short-term oncologic. Then, the multivariate model's performance is evaluated by means of two parameters: discrimination and fitness. Discrimination is measured by the area under the receiver operating characteristic curve,[23] with values of 0.5 representing no discrimination and 1.0 representing perfect discrimination. Model fitness is assessed by the Hosmer-Lemeshow goodness-of-fit test,[24] with P values of greater than .05 indicating acceptable fit.

When creating the RA-SPRT curve, each case is plotted in sequence along the x-axis. When a success occurs a risk-adjusted log-likelihood ratio is subtracted from the cumulative score. When a failure occurs, the constant 1-s is added to the cumulative score. In practice there are four possible situations:

1. If a low-risk case happens to present an adverse outcome (G3-5 morbidity, incomplete cytoreduction, or early oncologic failure) the surgeon is penalized with a high positive score.
2. If a low-risk case presents a favorable outcome (uneventful postoperative period, complete cytoreduction, or absence of early oncologic failure) the surgeon is granted a low negative score.
3. If a high-risk case presents an adverse event the surgeon is penalized with a low positive score.
4. If a high-risk case presents a favorable outcome the surgeon is granted a high negative score.

The scores are plotted consecutively and cumulatively according to the case-sequence and this originates the RA-SPRT curve. An ascending slope in the RA-SPRT line indicates deterioration of performance, whereas a descending slope indicates improvement of performance. Unacceptable ORs for the outcomes of interest are set considering the highest and lowest rates of these outcomes available in the literature. The upper and lower control limits are respectively defined as h1 (reject line) and h0 (accept line). If the RA-SPRT curve crosses the upper decision limit (h1) from below, this means that the actual OR for outcome is equal to or higher than the prespecified OR with the probability of type I error of 0.05. If the line crosses the lower decision limit (h0 or accept line) from above, this indicates that the actual OR for the outcome being studied is less than the unacceptable OR with the probability of type II error of 0.05. When the line is between h0 and h1, no statistical inference could be made. Expertise is estimated to be achieved at point where the curve of RA-SPRT crosses the accept line (h0) for outcomes of interest. At the time of crossing to the lower boundary, the graph is reset to 0 to start the surveillance of surgical performance with audit intent.[20] Once the expertise is acquired, the surveillance continues to monitor any eventual deterioration of the performance. The RA-SPRT curve could assume a positive slope in the case of enrollment of new surgeons to the surgical team, introduction of new protocols, and the adoption of innovations or changes in surgical strategy based on new data obtained from other centers.

THE LEARNING CURVE OF CYTOREDUCTIVE SURGERY AND HYPERTHERMIC INTRAPERITONEAL CHEMOTHERAPY FOR PERITONEAL SURFACE MALIGNANCIES

Kusamura and colleagues[13] assessed the LC using RA-SPRT on 420 cases of PSM based on rates of incomplete cytoreduction and G3-5 morbidity (NCI-CTCAE.v3). They estimated the control limits setting the type I/II error rates at 0.05 and unacceptable ORs at 1.8 for incomplete cytoreduction and 1.4 for severe morbidity, based on the literature data. The RA-SPRT curve crossed the lower control limit at the 137th and 149th case, respectively, for incomplete cytoreduction and G3-5 morbidity. At those points, the actual ORs are lower than the prespecified ORs for outcomes being studied.

Subsequently Polanco and colleagues[25] reported similar results using the same methodology. The breaking point of the proficiency was located at the 180th case for severe morbidity.

HOW TO SHORTEN THE LEARNING CURVE: THE ROLE OF TUTOR

The results of Kusamura and colleagues[13] and Polanco and colleagues[25] confirm that a lengthy LC is required for the acquisition of proficiency in performing CRS and HIPEC. Considering the high morbidity rate and the high cost of the treatment (Santiago González-Moreno, personal communication, 2014), developing strategies to shorten the LC is critically important. Shortening the LC would imply a substantial reduction in the number of adverse events resulting from inexperience, and a reduction in costs associated with procedures performed by nonexperts.

The NCI of Milan, after having overcome its own LC, has provided technical and scientific assistance to a community-based hospital, located 250 km from Milan. The first step of the tutorial consisted of visits to the NCI of Milan by members of the emerging center. The second step was the development of study protocols, the definition of a multidisciplinary team, and logistic troubleshooting. The third step was the selection of initial cases and performance of CRS and HIPEC at the emerging center with the assistance of the tutor. The expert (D.M.) supervised Bentivoglio's operations participating in the surgeries during the first 2 years. The visits of the tutor to the Bentivoglio center were maintained on a regular basis every 2 months thereafter. The RA-SPRT curves were plotted for the two centers considering the following outcomes: incomplete cytoreduction rates, G3-5 morbidity, and procedure-related mortality (PRM).[26] The Bentivoglio center successfully managed to overcome the LC much earlier as compared with NCI of Milan regarding all three outcomes: 126 versus 141 for incomplete cytoreduction, 134 versus 158 for G3-5 morbidity, and 60 versus 144 for PRM. The authors concluded that surgical tutoring could substantially shorten the steep LC associated with CRS and HIPEC.

WHICH PARAMETER SHOULD BE USED TO EVALUATE LEARNING CURVE AND TO MONITOR SURGICAL PERFORMANCE?

Four outcomes have been used to evaluate LC and surgical performance: (1) incomplete cytoreduction rate, (2) severe morbidity, (3) PRM, and (4) early oncologic failure. Each has pros and cons.

Recently Voron and colleagues[27] evaluated the LC of a high-volume center in Paris. The analysis was conducted on a case mix of 290 PSM cases operated with CRS and HIPEC, prevalently composed by PM from colorectal cancer. The outcomes of interest were rates of incomplete cytoreduction and severe morbidity. The principal surgeon set up the PSM unit after having attended a long-lasting training program, with more than 200 procedures performed in another referral center. Therefore it was assumed that he was already proficient in performing the combined procedure in the beginning of the new center's activity. The RA-SPRT curves breach the lower boundary at 40th case to lower the risk of incomplete cytoreduction and 140 cases to lower the risk of severe morbidity. The authors highlighted the substantial difference in the number of cases that were necessary for the achievement of expertise between the two outcomes of interest. These results are in line with the concept that the ability to cytoreduce a PSM is more related to surgeons' technical dexterity, whereas severe morbidity is related to the expertise of the entire multidisciplinary team. Professionals from different disciplines, such as anesthesiologists, required their own time to acquire proficiency in managing the patient in the perioperative setting, and this learning process developed separately from the excellence of the principal surgeon. Thus, incomplete cytoreduction is a parameter to appraise the surgeons' LC, whereas severe morbidity is a parameter to appraise the institution's LC.

Another outcome for the evaluation of LC is the PRM. Li and colleagues[28] have recently discussed the interesting notion of failure to rescue (FTR) in patients suffering a complication following CRS and HIPEC. A total of 915 eligible CRS and HIPEC cases were identified from American College of Surgeons National Surgical Quality Improvement Program data set. FTR was defined as 30-day mortality in the setting of a complication. Overall, 382 patients (42%) developed more than one postoperative complication, and 88 patients (10%) suffered more than one major complication. The FTR rate was 4% and was independently associated with American Society of Anesthesiologists (ASA) class 4 (adjusted OR, 13.4; 95% confidence interval, 1.2–146.8) and major complications (adjusted OR, 66.0; 95% confidence interval, 8.4–516.6). This means that PRM is connected to the selection process performed in the preoperative period, or the ability of the surgeon to choose cases with a general clinical condition compatible with the extent of surgical trauma associated with this major operation.

Finally the prognostic outcome is the best parameter to evaluate LC and surgical performance. Survival has been deemed the ultimate testament to a learning process because it represents a single parameter that encompasses other aspects included in the concept of expertise, such as capacity to choose the right candidate for the combined treatment by means of a judicious preoperative evaluation, to cytoreduce PSM completely in a safe way, and to conduct postoperative care.[29] However SPRT requires the outcome of interest being binary so that a surrogate marker of prognosis with a yes/no format would be necessary. Such strategy has recently been used in a study that evaluated the quality of US transplant units.[30] More recently a multicentric study on LC of CRS and HIPEC was conducted in a cohort of PMP cases. The target outcome was early oncologic failure defined as progression of the disease or death within 2 years from the procedure.[28]

INSTITUTIONAL FACTORS AFFECTING LEARNING CURVE

In the previously mentioned multicentric study, 2451 cases of PMP treated by 47 surgeons in 33 PSM centers from around the world were considered for the LC analysis.[29] In the elaboration of multivariate model the authors included not only factors related to biology of the tumor, but also characteristics related to the surgeon's background and institutions' organization. The following factors were independent variables related to early oncologic failure: center volume, proportion of PMP, number of principal surgeons on the team, type of fellowship, previous systemic chemotherapy, histologic subtype, Peritoneal Cancer Index, completeness of cytoreduction, HIPEC, and early postoperative intraperitoneal chemotherapy.

The center volume was independently correlated with early oncologic failure in a nonlinear manner. Centers with annual caseload of more than 60 cases of PSM were associated with lower risk of early oncologic failure. Likewise, the higher the proportion of PMP in the center's experience in treating PSM the better was the outcome. Finally, the increased number of principal surgeons on the team was correlated with higher risk of early oncologic failure.

This study confirmed that the learning process and surgical performance are influenced by aspects related not only to the team's abilities and the complexity of the case, but also to characteristics of center organization. Only 8 of the 33 centers overcame the LC, and after a median of 100 (range, 78–284) procedures (**Fig. 1**).

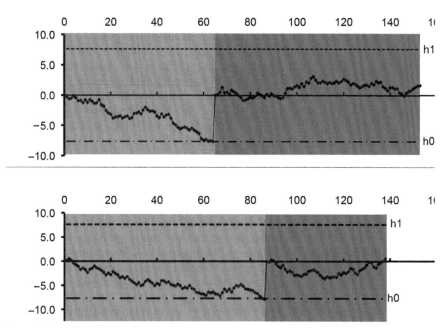

Fig. 1. The breaking point of the learning curve is the moment when the curve surpasses the lower boundary. Before this point is the learning phase (*red area*). After this point, the curve is reset to zero to start the audit phase (*blue area*).

CENTRALIZATION FOR RARE DISEASES

Kusamura and colleagues[31] have conducted the LC analysis on their center's experience with peritoneal mesothelioma. They adopted the early oncologic failure as target outcome and the breaking point of LC was 86 cases. Given the extremely low incidence of these conditions, it is virtually impossible for a center to gather experience on 100 cases of PMP or 86 of peritoneal mesothelioma, to be considered proficient in the treatment of such rare diseases, unless health care authorities set up mechanisms of regional centralization. Centralization could also be used for cost containment, because institutions that completed the LC are expected to be more economically efficient. Finally, centralization will ease regulation and quality control for the insurers. Considering that the approximate annual incidence of PMP is 1 to 2 million, it is estimated reasonably that 1 center for every 10 to 15 million inhabitants is ideal.

One could raise a criticism to this thesis arguing that cytoreduction and HIPEC could be applied uniformly to treat different diseases and that surgeons would not need specific training for rare diseases. This counterargument apparently makes sense but is unsustainable because of several weaknesses. Most PSM centers' experiences in the world are characterized by a predominance of peritoneal metastases from colorectal cancer, a clinical circumstance where the combined procedure is indicated in patients with less extensive and consequently less complex disease. PMP and peritoneal mesothelioma, in contrast to PM from colorectal cancer, are clinical circumstances where the extension of the disease is not a criterion to indicate CRS and HIPEC. A surgeon to become proficient in treating cases with PCI greater than 17[32] would need to gather experience in rare diseases. Moreover, the extension of the surgery should be modulated according not only to the PCI but also to the biologic characteristics of the disease. The surgeon should know how much to push the maximal surgical effort according to their knowledge regarding the biologic aggressiveness of the tumor. Furthermore, good prognostic outcome does not depend exclusively on excellent surgical performance but also on the work of the multidisciplinary team in the context of a multimodal treatment strategy where perioperative treatments could further improve survival results.[33] In summary, technical proficiency in CRS and HIPEC and acquaintance with the biology of the diseases are different qualities that are developed separately during the learning process in peritoneal surface oncology.

TRAINING PROGRAM

The ever-growing increase in the number of services offering the combined treatment has occurred in recent decades with neither a well-coded training program and nor regional government regulations. Therefore, it is likely that a significant number of recently emerged low-volume institutions claiming to have the knowhow to manage PSM might not be properly capacitated for this task, because their learning processes are still ongoing. Consequently, the current number of proficient centers in the world is unlikely able to response adequately to the demand of the population affected by PSM.

The European Society of Surgical Oncology in a joint venture initiative with Peritoneal Surface Oncology Group developed a well-structured training program in Peritoneal Surface Oncology in 2014.[34] The program is named European School of Peritoneal Surface Oncology and has the objective to offer a tutor-based fellowship to surgeons with strong interest in this field. During training the fellow should accomplish a series of theoretic and practical activities in a proficient center accredited by Peritoneal Surface Oncology International (PSOGI). With duration of 2 years, this nonprofit initiative has no pretension to follow the trainee along the entire duration of their LC. However, it intends to provide essentials that help the surgeon to set up a new center in their institution of origin and complete their training until the achievement of proficiency (**Fig. 2**).

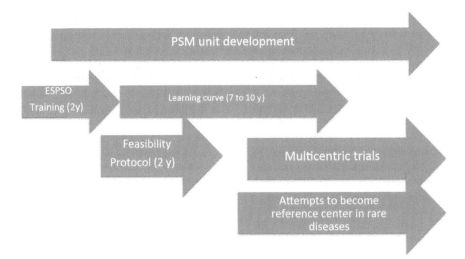

Fig. 2. Timeline of a center development. ESPSO, European School of Peritoneal Surface Oncology.

SUMMARY

The RA-SPRT is an effective and robust method to monitor surgical performance in the learning and audit phase of a center development. Several factors are associated with surgical performance and the most critical is mentoring of the trainee by an expert in CRS and HIPEC. Parameters related not only to patient and disease but also to logistics and infrastructure of the center could influence prognosis. The latter should be carefully adjusted to further optimize the achievement of center proficiency. Rare PSM, such as PMP and peritoneal mesothelioma, require further effort in the training process and their extremely low incidences make reasonable regional centralization. A well-structured tutor-based training program has been implemented in Europe. This initiative is expected to improve the standardization of the combined procedure and improve the quality of the services across the continent.

REFERENCES

1. Baratti D, Kusamura S, Nonaka D, et al. Pseudomyxoma peritonei: biological features are the dominant prognostic determinants after complete cytoreduction and hyperthermic intraperitoneal chemotherapy. Ann Surg 2009;249:243–9.
2. Yan TD, Deraco M, Baratti D, et al. Cytoreductive surgery and hyperthermic intraperitoneal chemotherapy for malignant peritoneal mesothelioma: multiinstitutional experience. J Clin Oncol 2009;27:6237–42.
3. Baratti D, Kusamura S, Deraco M. Diffuse malignant peritoneal mesothelioma: systematic review of clinical management and biological research. J Surg Oncol 2011;103:822–31. Review.
4. Chua TC, Moran BJ, Sugarbaker PH, et al. Early- and long-term outcome data of patients with pseudomyxoma peritonei from appendiceal origin treated by a strategy of cytoreductive surgery and hyperthermic intraperitoneal chemotherapy. J Clin Oncol 2012;30:2449–56.
5. Baratti D, Kusamura S, Pietrantonio F, et al. Progress in treatments for colorectal cancer peritoneal metastases during the years 2010-2015. A systematic review. Crit Rev Oncol Hematol 2016;100:209–22.
6. Esquivel J, Lowy AM, Markman M, et al. The American Society of Peritoneal Surface Malignancies (ASPSM) multiinstitution evaluation of the Peritoneal Surface Disease Severity Score (PSDSS) in 1,013 patients with colorectal cancer with peritoneal carcinomatosis. Ann Surg Oncol 2014;21:4195–201.
7. Van Driel WJ, Koole SN, Sikorska K, et al. A phase 3 trial of hyperthermic intraperitoneal chemotherapy (HIPEC) for ovarian cancer. N Engl J Med 2018;378(3):230–40. Available at: http://meetinglibrary.asco.org/record/152478/abstract.
8. Kusamura S, Sinukumar S, Baratti D, et al. Cytoreductive Surgery and HIPEC in the First-Line and Interval Time Points of Advanced Epithelial Ovarian Cancer. INDIAN JOURNAL OF GYNECOLOGIC ONCOLOGY 2017;15 supplement 1:11–20.
9. Nissan A, Stojadinovic A, Garofalo A, et al. Evidence-based medicine in the treatment of peritoneal carcinomatosis: past, present, and future. J Surg Oncol 2009;100:335–44.
10. Baratti D, Scivales A, Balestra MR, et al. Cost analysis of the combined procedure of cytoreductive surgery and hyperthermic intraperitoneal chemotherapy (HIPEC). Eur J Surg Oncol 2010;36:463–9.
11. Bonastre J, Jan P, de Pouvourville G, et al. Cost of an intraperitoneal chemohyperthermia (IPCH) related to cytoreductive surgery. Ann Chir 2005;130:553–61.

12. Chua TC, Yan TD, Saxena A, et al. Should the treatment of peritoneal carcinomatosis by cytoreductive surgery and hyperthermic intraperitoneal chemotherapy still be regarded as a highly morbid procedure?: a systematic review of morbidity and mortality. Ann Surg 2009;249:900–7.

13. Kusamura S, Baratti D, Deraco M. Multidimensional analysis of the learning curve for cytoreductive surgery and hyperthermic intraperitoneal chemotherapy in peritoneal surface malignancies. Ann Surg 2012;255:348–56.

14. Mohamed F, Moran BJ. Morbidity and mortality with cytoreductive surgery and intraperitoneal chemotherapy: the importance of a learning curve. Cancer J 2009;15:196–9.

15. Smeenk RM, Verwaal VJ, Zoetmulder FA. Learning curve of combined modality treatment in peritoneal surface disease. Br J Surg 2007;94:1408–14.

16. Yan TD, Links M, Fransi S, et al. Learning curve for cytoreductive surgery and perioperative intraperitoneal chemotherapy for peritoneal surface malignancy: a journey to becoming a nationally funded peritonectomy center. Ann Surg Oncol 2007;14:2270–80.

17. Andréasson H, Lorant T, Påhlman L, et al. Cytoreductive surgery plus perioperative intraperitoneal chemotherapy in pseudomyxoma peritonei: aspects of the learning curve. Eur J Surg Oncol 2014;40:930–6.

18. Matheny ME, Ohno-Machado L, Resnic FS. Risk-adjusted sequential probability ratio test control chart methods for monitoring operator and institutional mortality rates in interventional cardiology. Am Heart J 2008;155:114–20.

19. Chen TT, Chung KP, Hu FC, et al. The use of statistical process control (risk adjusted CUSUM, risk-adjusted RSPRT and CRAM with prediction limits) for monitoring the outcomes of out-of-hospital cardiac arrest patients rescued by the EMS system. J Eval Clin Pract 2011;17:71–7.

20. Grigg OA, Farewell VT, Spiegelhalter DJ. Use of risk-adjusted CUSUM and RSPRT charts for monitoring in medical contexts. Stat Methods Med Res 2003; 12:147–70.

21. Steiner SH, Cook RJ, Farewell VT. Risk-adjusted monitoring of binary surgical outcomes. Med Decis Making 2001;21:163–9.

22. Rogers CA, Reeves BC, Caputo M, et al. Control chart methods for monitoring cardiac surgical performance and their interpretation. J Thorac Cardiovasc Surg 2004;128:811–9.

23. Hanley JA, McNeil BJ. The meaning and use of the area under a receiver operating characteristic (ROC) curve. Radiology 1982;143:29–36.

24. Lemeshow S, Hosmer DW Jr. A review of goodness of fit statistics for use in the development of logistic regression models. Am J Epidemiol 1982;115:92–106.

25. Polanco PM, Ding Y, Knox JM, et al. Institutional learning curve of cytoreductive surgery and hyperthermic intraperitoneal chemoperfusion for peritoneal malignancies. Ann Surg Oncol 2015;22:1673–9.

26. Kusamura S, Baratti D, Virzì S, et al. Learning curve for cytoreductive surgery and hyperthermic intraperitoneal chemotherapy in peritoneal surface malignancies: analysis of two centres. J Surg Oncol 2013;107:312–9.

27. Voron T, Eveno C, Jouvin I, et al. Cytoreductive surgery with a hyperthermic intraperitoneal chemotherapy program: safe after 40 cases, but only controlled after 140 cases. Eur J Surg Oncol 2015;41:1671–7.

28. Li KY, Mokdad AA, Minter RM, et al. Failure to rescue following cytoreductive surgery and hyperthermic intraperitoneal chemotherapy. J Surg Res 2017;214: 209–15.

29. Kusamura S, Moran BJ, Sugarbaker PH, et al. Multicentre study of the learning curve and surgical performance of cytoreductive surgery with intraperitoneal chemotherapy for pseudomyxoma peritonei. Br J Surg 2014;101:1758–65.
30. Axelrod DA, Guidinger MK, Metzger RA, et al. Transplant quality assessment using a continuously updatable, risk-adjusted technique (CUSUM). Am J Transplant 2006;6:313–23.
31. Kusamura S, Baratti D, Hutanu I, et al. The importance of the learning curve and surveillance of surgical performance in peritoneal surface malignancy programs. Surg Oncol Clin N Am 2012;21:559–76.
32. Goéré D, Souadka A, Faron M, et al. Extent of colorectal peritoneal carcinomatosis: attempt to define a threshold above which HIPEC does not offer survival benefit: a comparative study. Ann Surg Oncol 2015;22:2958–64.
33. Asare EA, Compton CC, Hanna NN, et al. The impact of stage, grade, and mucinous histology on the efficacy of systemic chemotherapy in adenocarcinomas of the appendix: analysis of the National Cancer Data Base. Cancer 2016;122:213–21.
34. Available at: http://www.essoweb.org/school-of-peritoneal-surface-oncology-es/. Accessed March 21, 2018.

Evolving Treatment Strategies and Outcomes in Advanced Gastric Cancer with Peritoneal Metastasis

Fadi S. Dahdaleh, MD[a], Kiran K. Turaga, MD, MPH[b],*

KEYWORDS

- Advanced gastric cancer • Peritoneal metastasis • Chemotherapy
- Targeted therapy • Regional intraperitoneal chemotherapy • Cytoreductive surgery
- HIPEC

KEY POINTS

- Gastric cancer carries a high malignant potential compared with other epithelial malignancies and has a particular tendency to involve the peritoneum in its advanced stages.
- An important distinction must be made between macroscopic and microscopic peritoneal metastasis given the differences in treatment and prognosis.
- Effective systemic approaches for the treatment of advanced gastric cancer include cytotoxic chemotherapy and targeted therapies; however, their effect on peritoneal metastasis is not well-documented.
- The success of an approach that combines cytoreductive surgery with intraperitoneal chemotherapy in other epithelial malignancies has led investigators to explore this strategy in gastric cancer, with the ultimate goal of attaining long-term survival.
- The burden and extent of disease, as well as tumor biology, are important prognostic factors in determining candidates for peritoneal-directed therapies.

INTRODUCTION

Gastric cancer (GC) is the fourth most common malignancy and the second leading cause of cancer-related deaths worldwide, with only a quarter of patients surviving at 5 years.[1,2] Free tumor cells on cytologic-negative examination and macroscopic peritoneal metastasis (PM) are common manifestations of advanced GC because

Disclosure: The authors have nothing to disclose.
[a] Complex General Surgical Oncology, Section of General Surgery/Surgical Oncology, The University of Chicago Medicine, 5841 South Maryland Avenue, Room S214, MC 5094, Chicago, IL 60637, USA; [b] The University of Chicago Medicine, Section of General Surgery/Surgical Oncology, 5841 South Maryland Avenue, Room G207, MC 5094, Chicago, IL 60637, USA
* Corresponding author.
E-mail address: kturaga@surgery.bsd.uchicago.edu

Surg Oncol Clin N Am 27 (2018) 519–537
https://doi.org/10.1016/j.soc.2018.02.006
1055-3207/18/© 2018 Elsevier Inc. All rights reserved.

they are clinically evident in 11% of patients on initial presentation, are radiologically occult in 35% of cases intended for curative resection, and constitute recurrences in 30% of patients.[3-5] A distinction is made in the literature with regard to the treatment and prognosis of cytologic-negative disease and PM. When diagnosed, PM predicts a dismal prognosis, with median survival times of 3 to 4 months when left untreated and 10 months with conventional chemotherapy.[5-7] In contrast, cytologic-negative disease seems to respond to systemic therapy more readily with a reported median survival of up to 36 months in selected cases.[8-10] Importantly, long-term survival has rarely been reported in advanced GC with either cytologic-negative or PM when systemic approaches are used, which underscores the miniscule prospect for cure for those patients.[7,11,12] There have been major advances in the treatment of advanced GC with the introduction of novel cytotoxic chemotherapeutic regimens, molecular targeting agents, and immune checkpoint inhibitors.[13-15] In most published studies, however, peritoneal involvement is grouped with other forms of advanced GC, rendering the specific effect of these treatments on PM and cytologic-negative disease difficult to ascertain. The success of cytoreductive surgery (CRS) and hyperthermic intraperitoneal chemotherapy (HIPEC) in the treatment of PM in other epithelial malignancies has led investigators to explore this approach in GC and, perhaps encouragingly, survival beyond 5 years has been sporadically reported in highly selected patients.[16,17]

PATHOPHYSIOLOGY OF PERITONEAL INVOLVEMENT

It is commonly believed that PM occurs through the deposition of tumor cells either by the direct extension and subsequent cellular exfoliation, or through the traumatic dissemination of cancer cells during surgery.[18,19] Clinical validation of the concept of direct extension is perhaps provided by observing the higher rate of PM seen with increasing tumor stages (T-stages) and with the incidence of serosal invasion.[3] It is also hypothesized that during gastrectomy, cancer cells present within the lymphatic channels and blood vessels are shed, thereby contaminating the peritoneum.[20] In a study by Yu and colleagues,[21] cytologic-negative rates increased from 24% to 58% in lavage samples obtained at the beginning and end of gastrectomies. Free cancer cells then attach to the peritoneal surface; a process facilitated by the action of cytokines, which further aid in the deposition of fibrin layers, entrapping those cells. This new restrictive milieu is thought to hinder the penetrance of drugs delivered systemically and provides grounds for the early administration of intraperitoneal (IP) treatments.[22,23]

SYSTEMIC THERAPIES

The National Comprehensive Cancer Network recommends either systemic chemotherapy with fluoropyrimidine and platinum-based agents or best supportive care (BSC) for patients with metastatic GC, including PM and cytologic-negative disease.[24] Learning about specific practice patterns is challenging, however, given the sparsity of descriptive population studies. One study reported that 24% of patients with GC and PM underwent resection of their primary tumor, and only 23% of those received systemic chemotherapy.[5] Conversely, palliative chemotherapy was the treatment of choice in 65% of patients in another study, of which 80% had PM as their only documented site of metastasis.[25] Furthermore, the outcomes of patients with PM or cytologic-negative disease treated with systemic chemotherapy alone are difficult to determine because the literature typically groups patients with advanced GC in its different forms of metastasis into a single encompassing entity.[2,26,27] Finally, as the understanding of the biology and molecular profiling of GC advances, other treatments have emerged and, similarly, their efficacy in the treatment peritoneal disease has not been fully elucidated. This article reviews the systemically administered options.

TREATMENT OF CYTOLOGIC-POSITIVE DISEASE WITH SYSTEMIC CYTOTOXIC CHEMOTHERAPY

The prognostic and therapeutic significance of cytologic-negative disease in GC has been extensively studied and reviewed. Indeed, cytologic-negative status denotes worse outcomes than nonmetastatic disease and, currently, precludes consideration for curative resection.[10,24] Moreover, the relationship between gross PM and cytologic-negative disease has been established because evidence supports the notion that cytologic-negative disease is a likely precursor to PM. In 1 study, 81% of cytologic-negative subjects ultimately presented with PM following curative gastrectomy.[28] With that in mind, the efficacy of systemic therapy in cytologic-negative GC can be gauged by reviewing 2 key reports. First, in a study by Lorenzen and colleagues,[8] cytologic-negative subjects underwent combination therapy consisting of cisplatin, folinic acid, and fluorouracil (FU), followed by repeat laparoscopy. The investigators found that 7 out of 19 (37%) subjects converted to cytologic-negative status posttreatment. Interestingly, despite undergoing resection of their primary tumors following conversion, that group attained median survival times similar to those with stage IV disease treated with chemotherapy alone. Second, in a study by Mezhir and colleagues,[10] the outcomes of 93 cytologic-negative subjects were reviewed. In that cohort, 48 cytologic-negative subjects underwent repeat laparoscopies following systemic therapy and, compared with subjects with persistent cytologic-negative status, those who converted to cytologic-negative status (n = 27) had a significant improvement in disease-specific survival (2.5 years vs 1.4 years, P = .0003). The observed survival advantage in the latter study is likely due to by selection bias and it is difficult to reach a consensus based on these limited data.

TREATMENT OF PERITONEAL METASTASIS WITH SYSTEMIC CYTOTOXIC CHEMOTHERAPY

As previously noted, systemically administered cytotoxic chemotherapy regimens in advanced GC generally include fluoropyrimidines, anthracyclines, taxanes, and platinum. Indeed, several randomized trials have conclusively demonstrated a significant survival advantage afforded by chemotherapy when compared with BSC, with median survival times of 11 months as compared with 4.3 months with BSC.[27] Moreover, combination first-line regimens seem to offer a modest added improvement in survival when compared with single-agent therapy.[12,27,29] In a Cochrane review, trials comparing single-agent and combination chemotherapy in GC were identified, and the average median survival time of the combination group versus the single-agent group was 8.3 versus 6.7, respectively (hazard ratio 0.82; 95% CI 0.74–0.90).[27] Importantly, the investigators found that PM was among the factors predicting with a reduced probability of response to chemotherapy and concluded that equivalent benefit from chemotherapy is unlikely in all patients. Important randomized trials on first-line and second-line regimens are summarized in **Tables 1** and **2**, respectively. If one examines the available literature on the effect of systemic chemotherapy on advanced GC, it becomes evident that PM is rarely addressed separately. To the authors' knowledge, the only phase III trial that directly assessed the efficacy of systemic chemotherapy on PM came from Shirao and colleagues.[30] In this trial, 237 subjects with confirmed PM were randomized to receive FU or methotrexate plus FU. Therapy was discontinued at disease progression or unacceptable toxicities occurrences, and

Table 1
Randomized trials of first-line systemic chemotherapy in advanced and metastatic gastric cancer

Author, Year	Regimen	Number of Subjects	Median Survival (mo)	Proportion Surviving at >2 y	Effect on PM
Ohtsu et al,[69] 2003	FU vs CF vs UFTM	280	7.1 vs 7.3 vs 6.0	7% vs 7% vs 9% at 2 y	NR
Bouché et al,[70] 2004	LVFU vs LVFU + cisplatin vs LVFU + irinotecan	136	6.8 vs 9.5 vs 11.3	NR	NR
Van Cutsem et al,[71] 2006	DCF vs CF	445	9.2 vs 8.6 P = .02	18% vs 9% at 2 y	NR
Al-Batran et al,[72] 2007	FLO vs FLP	220	10.7 vs 8.8 (NS)	14% vs 16% at 2 y	NR
Cunningham et al,[15] 2008	ECF vs ECX vs EOF vs EOX	1002	9.9 vs 9.9 vs 9.3 vs 11.2	NR	NR
Dank et al,[73] 2008	IF vs CF	333	9.0 vs 8.7 (NS)	14% vs 10% at 2 y	NR
Koizumi et al,[74] 2008	CS vs S-1	298	13.0 vs 11.0	24% vs 15% at 2 y	S-1 had greater effect on OS in PM, degree NR
Kang et al,[75] 2009	XP vs FP	316	10.5 vs 9.3	NR	NR
Ajani et al,[76] 2010	CS vs CF	1053	8.6 vs 7.9 (NS)	4% vs 3% at 30 mo	NR
Guimbaud et al,[77] 2014	FOLFIRI vs ECX	416	9.5 vs 9.7 (NS)	11% vs 11% at 2 y	NR

Abbreviations: CF, cisplatin-fluorouracil; CS, cisplatin + S-1; DCF, docetaxel + cisplatin + fluorouracil; ECF, epirubicin + cisplatin + fluorouracil; ECX, epirubicin + cisplatin + capecitabine; EOF, epirubicin + oxaliplatin + fluorouracil; EOX, epirubicin + oxaliplatin + capecitabine; FLO, fluorouracil + leucovorin + oxaliplatin; FLP, fluorouracil + leucovorin + cisplatin; FOLFIRI, fluorouracil + leucovorin + irinotecan; FP, cisplatin + fluorouracil; FU, fluorouracil; IF, irinotecan + fluorouracil; LVFU, fluorouracil + leucovorin; NR, not reported; NS, not significant; SOX, S-1 + oxaliplatin; UFTM, uracil and tegafur + mitomycin; XP, cisplatin + capecitabine.

overall survival (OS) was not significantly different between the arms, with a median survival of 9.4 months in the FU arm and 10.6 months in the combination arm (P = .31). Interestingly, at 3 years, only 5 subjects were alive from the entire cohort.

TARGETED THERAPY IN ADVANCED GASTRIC CANCER

Advances in cancer molecular biology have led investigators to explore newer therapeutic targets with potentially more favorable side-effect profiles. Perhaps the most widely studied target in GC has been the human epidermal growth factor 2 (HER2). This receptor is overexpressed in approximately 20% of intestinal-type GC and has a wealth of evidence backing its role in tumorigenesis.[31–33] Indeed, the seminal Trastuzumab for Gastric Cancer (ToGA) trial demonstrated that the addition of trastuzumab to standard chemotherapy in tumors overexpressing HER2 led to a median OS time of 13.8 months.[34] Although peritoneal involvement was not specifically addressed in that trial, survival at 2 years was 21% and 0% at 3 years in the

Table 2
Randomized trials of second-line systemic chemotherapy in advanced and metastatic gastric cancer

Author, Year	Regimen	Number of Subjects	Median Survival (mo)	Proportion Surviving at >2 y	Effect on PM
Thuss-Patience et at,[78] 2011	Irinotecan vs BSC	40 randomized	4.0 vs 2.4 mo (closed early due to poor accrual)	0% vs 0% at 1 y	NR
Kang et at,[79] 2012	SLC vs BSC	202	5.3 vs 3.8	At 15 mo, 18% vs 5%	NR
Ford et at,[80] 2014	Docetaxel vs BSC	168	5.2 vs 3.6	4% vs 1% at 18 mo	NR
Nishina et at,[81] 2016	FU vs wPTX	100	7.7 vs 7.7 (NS)	1% vs 3% at 2 y	Study only included advanced GC with PM

Abbreviations: SLC, salvage chemotherapy (docetaxel or irinotecan); wPTX, weekly paclitaxel.

trastuzumab arm. Similar to cytotoxic therapy, most trials examining the effect of targeted therapy in this context do not focus on the response in PM or cytologic-negative disease (**Table 3**). Nevertheless, impressive results have been reported on the first-line and second-line fronts. Notably, in the RAINBOW trial, 45% of subjects in that cohort had documented PM and the addition of the vascular endothelial growth factor receptor 2 (VEGF-R2) inhibitor ramucirumab led to an OS of 35% at 16 months.[35] Other targets, such as the epidermal growth factor 1 and vascular endothelial growth factor, have similarly been investigated in clinical trials with variable results.[36–38]

IMMUNOTHERAPY IN ADVANCED GASTRIC CANCER

Fueled by transformative success in other solid malignancies, immunotherapy emerged as an attractive option for the treatment of advanced GC. Targeting the immune system in GC seemed particularly justifiable because pathologic chronic inflammation relates to more extensive genomic tumoral heterogeneity.[39–41] Indeed, Programmed death-ligand 1(PD-L1) expression has been found in approximately 40% of gastric and gastroesophageal junction cancers.[42] To date, formal results from randomized trials on the efficacy of immunotherapy in advanced GC have not yet been published; however, preliminary results boast response rates of 22% to 27% in subjects with PD-L1–positive (PD-L1+) tumors.[43] Notably, in KEYNOTE-12, Pembrolizumab for patients with PD-L1-positive advanced gastric cancer, and median OS was 11 months.[14] Similarly, nivolumab was investigated in the ONO-12 (ATTRACTION 2) phase III, randomized controlled trial, in which subjects with advanced GC refractory to 2 or more prior chemotherapy regimens were included.[44] Although the final results have not been reported, an encouraging improvement in OS (5.32 vs 4.14 months) was observed. As the trials continue to evolve, no data exist yet on the effect of immunotherapy on PM in advanced GC.

INTRAPERITONEAL-DIRECTED THERAPY

The treatment of peritoneal involvement has transformed over the past 2 decades, and surgical debulking in addition to IP therapy has drastically altered the natural history of

Table 3
Trials of first and second-line systemic targeted therapy in advanced and metastatic gastric cancer

Author, Year	Mode of Treatment	Type of Study	Number of Subjects	Intervention	Number of Subjects	Median Survival, mo	Proportion Surviving	Effect on PM
Bang et al,[34] 2010	First-line	RCT	594	Trastuzumab + (FU + cisplatin) or (capecitabine + cisplatin)	594	13.8 vs 11.1	21% and 14% at 2 y vs 0% and 0% at 3 y	Not discussed
Sun et al,[82] 2010	First-line	Phase II, single-arm	44	Sorafenib	44	13.6	NR	Not discussed
Bang et al,[83] 2011	Second-line	Phase II, single-arm	78	Sunitinib	78	6.8	24.2% at 1 y	NR
Ohtsu et al,[38] 2011	First-line	RCT	744	Bevacizumab + capecitabine + cisplatin vs capecitabine + cisplatin	744	12.1 vs 10.1 (NS)	0% vs 0% at 2 y	Not discussed
Martin-Richard et al,[84] 2013	Second-line	Phase II, single-arm	40	Sorafenib + oxaliplatin	40	6.5	18% at 20 mo	Rate of PM 15%, effect not discussed
Waddell et al,[85] 2013	First-line	RCT	533	EOC vs EOC + panitumumab	533	11.3 vs 8.8	3% vs 2% at 2 y	PM not discussed
Ohtsu et al,[86] 2013	Third-line	RCT	656	Everolimus vs placebo	656	5.4 vs 4.3	0% vs 0% at 2 y	Not discussed
Lordick et al,[36] 2013	First-line	RCT	904	Cetuximab + capecitabine + cisplatin vs capecitabine + cisplatin	904	9.4 vs 10.7 (NS)	5% vs 5% at 3 y	Rate of PM 25%, effect not discussed

Study	Line	Type	N	Regimen	N	OS (mo)	Survival	PM comment
Fuchs et al,[87] 2014	Second-line	RCT	355	Ramucirumab vs placebo	355	5.2 vs 3.8	7% vs 6% at 1 y, 0% vs 0% at 2 y	PM was found to be associated with reduced OS
Satoh et al,[88] 2014	Second-line	RCT	261	Lapatinib + paclitaxel vs paclitaxel alone	261	11.0 vs 8.9 (NS)	1% vs 2% at 35 mo	Not discussed
Wilke et al,[89] 2014	Second-line	RCT	655	Ramucirumab + paclitaxel vs placebo + paclitaxel	655	9.6 vs 7.4	35% vs 24% at 16 mo	Rate of PM 45%, effect not discussed
Chua et al,[90] 2015	First-line	Phase II, single-arm	30	Trastuzumab + cisplatin + S-1	30	14.6	NR	23.3% had PM, effect not discussed
Ryu et al,[91] 2015	First-line	Phase II, single-arm	55	Trastuzumab + XELOX	55	21	1 y 63%	27% had PM, effect not discussed
Li et al,[92] 2016	Third-line	RCT	267	Apatinib vs placebo	267	6.5 vs 4.7	1% vs 0% at 2 y	25% PM, effect not discussed

Abbreviations: EOC, epirubicin, oxaliplatin, capecitabine; RCT, randomized controlled trial; XELOX, capecitabine + oxaliplatin.

several malignancies.[45] This success has led investigators to apply the same therapeutic principles to GC, with the ultimate goal of achieving long-term survival. Over time, the aggressive biology of GC proved to be a nearly unsurmountable obstacle because early recurrences combined with significant operative morbidity dulled enthusiasm. Still, many investigators, Eastern Asian countries, persevered, gradually refining the process of patient selection and attaining better outcomes. Although those efforts are indeed remarkable, the evolution of IP-directed therapy has yielded an extremely heterogeneous body of literature. Specifically, studies vary with respect to enrollment criteria, agents used, timing, frequency and duration of therapy, extent of disease, and endpoints. Moreover, and perhaps most importantly, an answer to the fundamental question of whether IP-directed therapy provides a survival advantage over systemic therapy alone has not been adequately answered.

In an effort to organize the published literature, the authors elected to categorize studies according the timing of IP therapy administration; that is, preemptive and PM-directed.

PREEMPTIVE INTRAPERITONEAL THERAPY

Features of GC that render it high-risk for the development of PM have been identified and include advanced T-stage and node (N)-stages, young age, diffuse-mixed histology, and cytologic-negative disease.[3,28,46] This information, coupled with the dismal course of disease observed when PM occurs, has led investigators to devise strategies aimed at preventing PM from ensuing. Those reports can be traced back to the late 1980s when Koga and colleagues[47] examined the effect of using HIPEC with mitomycin C in subjects with advanced GC with serosal invasion undergoing gastrectomy. In that report, a historical and a prospective subset of subjects were found to have improved 3-year survival rates in the HIPEC-treated group (74% vs 53%, $P<.04$), although statistical significance was not reached when the prospectively treated group was analyzed independently.[48] Since that time, other investigators have attempted to improve on those results and the efficacy of adjuvant HIPEC in improving OS and reducing the rates of PM in high-risk subjects was confirmed (**Table 4**).

The largest trial to address the role of preemptive IP therapy in GC came from Kang and colleagues[49] in which subjects with serosal invasion identified at the time of primary resection were randomized to receive intravenous mitomycin C 3 to 6 weeks after surgery and oral doxifluridine after 4 weeks, continuing for 3 months, compared with intraoperative IP cisplatin, intravenous mitomycin C on postoperative day 1, followed by oral doxifluridine for 12 months, and 6 monthly intravenous cisplatin. In that study, the IP-treated group indeed had improved OS at 5 years (59% vs 50%); however, the investigators concluded it would be impossible to attribute those results to the IP portion alone, especially given the significant proportion of subjects who survived more than 5 years in the control arm. The notion of cytologic-negative disease behaving as a precursor to PM was tested in a provocative trial by Kuramoto and colleagues[50] in which 88 subjects with cytologic-negative disease were randomized to receive surgery alone, surgery plus IP chemotherapy, or surgery plus IP chemotherapy plus extensive peritoneal lavage (EPIL) with 10 L of normal saline. In that trial, all subjects received adjuvant systemic therapy. Interestingly, subjects in the EPIL group achieved an impressive median survival time of 35 months compared with 15 and 16 in the other groups; this, on subsequent analysis, was largely due to a decrease in peritoneal recurrences.

The only systematic review on this specific topic illustrates the diverse nature of the published literature, yet several points can be made.[51] First, most protocols deliver IP therapy intraoperatively. Second, cisplatin is the most common IP agent used in this

Table 4
Recent trials summarizing the use of preemptive intraperitoneal therapy in gastric cancer

Author, Year	Country	Inclusion Criteria	Agents Used	Number of Subjects	Median Survival (mo)	Proportion Surviving at >2 y
Kang et al,[49] 2014	Korea	Macroscopic serosal invasion	Mf vs iceMF	640	69.7 vs 54.3	9.3% vs 9.1% at 60 mo
Miyashiro et al,[93] 2011	Japan	Macroscopic serosal invasion, negative peritoneal lavage	IP cisplatin, IV cisplatin IV 5FU, oral FU (UFT)	135	NA	62.0% at 5 y
Topuz et al,[94] 2002	Turkey	Extend either up to the serosa or to adjacent organs	IP cisplatin 60 mg/m^2, mitoxantrone 12 mg/m^2, 5-FU 600 mg/m^2, and folinic acid 60 mg/m^2, instilled intraperitoneally	39	19 mo	30.7% at 5 y
Yonemura et al,[95] 2001	Japan	T2-4 lesions	MMC and cisplatin	48	NA	61% at 5 y
Kim and Bae,[96] 2001	Korea	Macroscopic serosal invasion	MMC	52	NA	32.7% at 5 y

Abbreviations: iceMFP, MF + cisplatin + IP cisplatin (unspecified) immediately postop; Mf, systemic mitomycin C and oral fluoropyrimidine; MMC, mitomycin.

setting, although mitomycin C does not seem to be inferior. Third, systemic therapy is frequently used in the adjuvant setting. Finally, a trend toward improved OS is observed in the IP-treated group. In that report, the investigators soundly conclude that a need to standardize the mode of therapy exists.

Currently, 3 phase-III randomized trials are studying the role of HIPEC in the treatment of advanced GC without PM. First, the French D2 Resection and HIPEC (Hyperthermic Intraperitoneal Chemoperfusion) in Locally Advanced Gastric Carcinoma (GASTRI-CHIP) study is designed to evaluate the effect of HIPEC with oxaliplatin on subjects with GC involving the serosa, lymph nodes, or with cytologic-negative status.[52] The protocol calls for treatment with neoadjuvant chemotherapy, followed by gastrectomy, before randomization to HIPEC versus observation. Second, in a multicenter open-label randomized phase III trial from Japan, subjects are planned to be randomized to receive standard IP lavage with 2 L normal saline versus extensive lavage with 10 L.[53] Finally, in a phase II trial by Badgwell and colleagues,[54,55] subjects with cytologic-negative or radiologically occult PM from GC were randomized to receive laparoscopic HIPEC with mitomycin C and cisplatin after completing systemic chemotherapy. Out of 19 subjects who met the selection criteria, complications were reported in 11% after 38 total procedures, and OS was 43.5% at 3 years with a median of 20.3 months.

INTRAPERITONEAL THERAPY FOR ESTABLISHED PERITONEAL METASTASIS

The surgical treatment of PM in GC was originally undertaken with the goal of palliating anticipated downstream complications such as bleeding, obstructions, and perforation.[56] Early encouraging results from such endeavors led investigators to progressively expand on the use of radical resections in the treatment of far-advanced GC.[57] Perhaps the first formal study on the role of CRS and HIPEC in subjects with GC came from Yonemura and colleagues[58] in 1996, in which 83 subjects with GC and PM underwent resections with the goal of clearing all macroscopic disease. In that report, an OS of 11% at 5 years was reported and, subsequently, similar efforts and outcomes were described.[59,60] Moreover, with the standardization of the technique of formal peritonectomy, complete cytoreduction became more common and improved oncologic outcomes were being reported.[22] Early on, almost all reports came from the East, calling into question the applicability of such an approach in Western centers. In 1 of the earlier reports from France and Belgium, the investigators reported their experience with 159 subjects with GC and PM.[61] Although the reported survival outcomes were encouraging (overall 1-year, 3-year, and 5-year survival were 43%, 18%, and 13%, respectively), the associated major morbidity and mortality rates were high at 27.8% and 6.5%. In fact, in their systematic review, Gill and colleagues[35] found that the overall 30-day mortality from CRS-HIPEC in GC was 5% and the rate of major complications was 21%, including a 5% to 33% reoperative rate.

The only phase III randomized trial assessing the impact of CRS-HIPEC on GC came from China, in which 68 subjects were randomized to either receive CRS with HIPEC versus CRS alone.[62] The 2 arms were matched with respect to median peritoneal carcinomatosis index scores (15) and CRS was attempted synchronously alongside resection of the primary tumor when possible. The 3-year survival in the CRS-HIPEC arm was 5.9% compared with 0% in the CRS-alone arm, and a similar trend was observed with regard to median survival (11 months vs 6.5 months, $P = .04$). Subgroup analysis revealed that the median OS was 12 months in the CC 0–1 subgroup (n = 20) and 8.2 months in CC, Completeness of Cytoreduction. 2 to 3 subgroup (n = 14). A summary of the relevant studies on the use of CRS-HIPEC in the treatment of established PM from GC is provided in **Table 5**.

Table 5
Studies on the outcomes of hyperthermic intraperitoneal chemotherapy or cytoreductive surgery in gastric cancer and peritoneal metastasis

Author, Year	Country	Number of Subjects	Type of IP Chemotherapy	Morbidity	Mortality	Survival
Fujimoto et al,[97] 1990	Japan	27	MMC	NA	NA	At 6 mo: 94% vs 57%
Yonemura et al,[98] 1991	Japan	41	MMC, cisplatin	12%	0%	At 3 y: 28.5%
Yonemura et al,[58] 1996	Japan	83	MMC, cisplatin, etoposide	—	—	At 5-y 11%, CCR0/1: 17%, CCR2: 2%
Fujimoto et al,[16] 1997	Japan	66	MMC	—	—	At 5 y: 42% vs 0%
Glehen et al,[60] 2004	France	49	MMC	27%	4%	At 5 y: 16%
Hall et al,[99] 2004	United States	74	MMC	35%	0%	At 2 y: 45%
Yonemura et al,[17] 2005	Japan	107	MMC, cisplatin, etoposide	21.5%	2.8%	At 5 y: 27%
Scaringi et al,[100] 2008	France	37	MMC, cisplatin	27%	3.8%	Median = 15 mo
Glehen et al,[61] 2010	France	159	MMC, oxaliplatin	27.8%	6.5%	At 5 y: 23%
Yang et al,[101] 2010	China	28	MMC	14.3%	0%	At 2 y: 43%
Yang et al,[62] 2011	China	68	MMC, cisplatin	14.7%	0%	At 3 y: 5.9%
Magge et al,[102] 2014	United States	23	MMC	52%	4.3%	At 3 y: 18%

It is noteworthy that in the ongoing Cytoreductive Surgery (CRS) With/Without HIPEC in Gastric Cancer With Peritoneal Carcinomatosis (GASTRIPEC) trial, subjects with advanced GC with synchronous PM are to receive perioperative chemotherapy (epirubicin, oxaliplatin, and capecitabine or cisplatin, or capecitabine and trastuzumab if HER-2 positive), followed by cytoreduction, and then will be randomized to receive HIPEC or no HIPEC.[63]

RECENT ADVANCES AND FUTURE DIRECTIONS

As experience with CRS-HIPEC in GC was gained, it became evident that enhanced patient selection is central to maximizing the derived survival benefit. In keeping with that principle, newer approaches using neoadjuvant systemic and IP chemotherapy were introduced, with the ultimate objective of minimizing tumor burden before attempting CRS.[64] In 1 popular technique, an IP port is used to deliver chemotherapy preoperatively alongside systemic agents.[65] When this was first evaluated clinically, the rate of cytologic-negative disease went from 82.2% pretreatment to 27.0% post-treatment and, impressively, a complete cytoreduction was possible in 70% of subjects. This translated to an OS of 40% at 2 years with a very low frequency of adverse events. An update from the same group demonstrated that, although neoadjuvant IP therapy was successful at converting the rate of cytologic-negative disease from 29% to 78%, the operative mortality rate was slightly higher than prior reports at 3.9%.[66] A recent report by Ishigami and colleagues[67] from Japan examined the utility of neoadjuvant IP and systemic chemotherapy in the treatment of cytologic-negative GC with or without PM. In that study, subjects were routed to receive IP paclitaxel plus S1 in addition to systemic paclitaxel. Curative gastrectomy was only undertaken after the resolution of PM and cytologic-negative status. Out of 100 subjects who met the selection criteria, gastrectomy was ultimately performed in 64 subjects and the median survival in that group was 30.5 months from the initiation of IP chemotherapy. Variations on the timing of neoadjuvant IP therapy, agents, and indications have been described since then, perhaps adding another layer of complexity to the applicability of the available data.[68]

SUMMARY

When peritoneal involvement is discovered in patients with GC, a comprehensive multidisciplinary evaluation is necessary given the variety of available options. Importantly, the distinction must be made between cytologic-negative disease and frank PM at the outset, given the disparate implications with respect to diagnosis, prognosis, and treatment. If metastasis is only in limited to cytologic-negative disease, available data would suggest that achieving cytologic-negative status could offer a small prospect for cure and curative resection is reasonable in selected cases. Conversely, to achieve favorable survival outcomes in patients with frank PM, interventions such as CRS-HIPEC must be carefully weighed in the treatment paradigm. The role of prophylactic IP therapy, neoadjuvant IP therapy, and second-look laparoscopy are rather interesting as results from ongoing trials are awaited.

REFERENCES

1. Jemal A, Bray F, Center MM, et al. Global cancer statistics. CA Cancer J Clin 2011;61(2):69–90.
2. Brenner H, Rothenbacher D, Arndt V. Epidemiology of stomach cancer. Methods Mol Biol 2009;472:467–77.
3. D'Angelica M, Gonen M, Brennan MF, et al. Patterns of initial recurrence in completely resected gastric adenocarcinoma. Ann Surg 2004;240(5): 808–16.
4. Ikoma N, Blum M, Chiang YJ, et al. Yield of staging laparoscopy and lavage cytology for radiologically occult peritoneal carcinomatosis of gastric cancer. Ann Surg Oncol 2016;23(13):4332–7.
5. Thomassen I, van Gestel YR, van Ramshorst B, et al. Peritoneal carcinomatosis of gastric origin: a population-based study on incidence, survival and risk factors. Int J Cancer 2014;134(3):622–8.
6. Sadeghi B, Arvieux C, Glehen O, et al. Peritoneal carcinomatosis from non-gynecologic malignancies: results of the EVOCAPE 1 multicentric prospective study. Cancer 2000;88(2):358–63.
7. Sarela AI, Miner TJ, Karpeh MS, et al. Clinical outcomes with laparoscopic stage M1, unresected gastric adenocarcinoma. Ann Surg 2006;243(2):189–95.
8. Lorenzen S, Panzram B, Rosenberg R, et al. Prognostic significance of free peritoneal tumor cells in the peritoneal cavity before and after neoadjuvant chemotherapy in patients with gastric carcinoma undergoing potentially curative resection. Ann Surg Oncol 2010;17(10):2733–9.

9. Badgwell B, Cormier JN, Krishnan S, et al. Does neoadjuvant treatment for gastric cancer patients with positive peritoneal cytology at staging laparoscopy improve survival? Ann Surg Oncol 2008;15(10):2684–91.

10. Mezhir JJ, Shah MA, Jacks LM, et al. Positive peritoneal cytology in patients with gastric cancer: natural history and outcome of 291 patients. Ann Surg Oncol 2010;17(12):3173–80.

11. Liu X, Cai H, Sheng W, et al. Long-term results and prognostic factors of gastric cancer patients with microscopic peritoneal carcinomatosis. PLoS One 2012; 7(5):e37284.

12. Shitara K, Ohtsu A. Advances in systemic therapy for metastatic or advanced gastric cancer. J Natl Compr Canc Netw 2016;14(10):1313–20.

13. Hecht JR, Bang YJ, Qin SK, et al. Lapatinib in combination with capecitabine plus oxaliplatin in human epidermal growth factor receptor 2-positive advanced or metastatic gastric, esophageal, or gastroesophageal adenocarcinoma: TRIO-013/LOGiC–a randomized phase III trial. J Clin Oncol 2016;34(5):443–51.

14. Muro K, Chung HC, Shankaran V, et al. Pembrolizumab for patients with PD-L1-positive advanced gastric cancer (KEYNOTE-012): a multicentre, open-label, phase 1b trial. Lancet Oncol 2016;17(6):717–26.

15. Cunningham D, Starling N, Rao S, et al. Capecitabine and oxaliplatin for advanced esophagogastric cancer. N Engl J Med 2008;358(1):36–46.

16. Fujimoto S, Takahashi M, Mutou T, et al. Improved mortality rate of gastric carcinoma patients with peritoneal carcinomatosis treated with intraperitoneal hyperthermic chemoperfusion combined with surgery. Cancer 1997;79(5):884–91.

17. Yonemura Y, Kawamura T, Bandou E, et al. Treatment of peritoneal dissemination from gastric cancer by peritonectomy and chemohyperthermic peritoneal perfusion. Br J Surg 2005;92(3):370–5.

18. Iitsuka Y, Kaneshima S, Tanida O, et al. Intraperitoneal free cancer cells and their viability in gastric cancer. Cancer 1979;44(4):1476–80.

19. Koga S, Kaibara N, Iitsuka Y, et al. Prognostic significance of intraperitoneal free cancer cells in gastric cancer patients. J Cancer Res Clin Oncol 1984;108(2):236–8.

20. Marutsuka T, Shimada S, Shiomori K, et al. Mechanisms of peritoneal metastasis after operation for non-serosa-invasive gastric carcinoma: an ultrarapid detection system for intraperitoneal free cancer cells and a prophylactic strategy for peritoneal metastasis. Clin Cancer Res 2003;9(2):678–85.

21. Yu XF, Ren ZG, Xue YW, et al. D2 lymphadenectomy can disseminate tumor cells into peritoneal cavity in patients with advanced gastric cancer. Neoplasma 2013;60(2):174–81.

22. Sugarbaker PH, Yu W, Yonemura Y. Gastrectomy, peritonectomy, and perioperative intraperitoneal chemotherapy: the evolution of treatment strategies for advanced gastric cancer. Semin Surg Oncol 2003;21(4):233–48.

23. Sugarbaker PH, Cunliffe WJ, Belliveau J, et al. Rationale for integrating early postoperative intraperitoneal chemotherapy into the surgical treatment of gastrointestinal cancer. Semin Oncol 1989;16(4 Suppl 6):83–97.

24. NCCN Clinical Practice Guidelines in Oncology. 2016. Available at: https://www.nccn.org/professionals/physician_gls/pdf/gastric_blocks.pdf. Accessed April 28, 2017.

25. Tan HL, Chia CS, Tan GH, et al. Gastric peritoneal carcinomatosis - a retrospective review. World J Gastrointest Oncol 2017;9(3):121–8.

26. Kamangar F, Dores GM, Anderson WF. Patterns of cancer incidence, mortality, and prevalence across five continents: defining priorities to reduce cancer

disparities in different geographic regions of the world. J Clin Oncol 2006; 24(14):2137–50.

27. Wagner AD, Unverzagt S, Grothe W, et al. Chemotherapy for advanced gastric cancer. Cochrane Database Syst Rev 2010;(3):CD004064.

28. Yonemura Y, Elnemr A, Endou Y, et al. Multidisciplinary therapy for treatment of patients with peritoneal carcinomatosis from gastric cancer. World J Gastrointest Oncol 2010;2(2):85–97.

29. Wagner AD, Grothe W, Haerting J, et al. Chemotherapy in advanced gastric cancer: a systematic review and meta-analysis based on aggregate data. J Clin Oncol 2006;24(18):2903–9.

30. Shirao K, Boku N, Yamada Y, et al. Randomized Phase III study of 5-fluorouracil continuous infusion vs. sequential methotrexate and 5-fluorouracil therapy in far advanced gastric cancer with peritoneal metastasis (JCOG0106). Jpn J Clin Oncol 2013;43(10):972–80.

31. Gravalos C, Jimeno A. HER2 in gastric cancer: a new prognostic factor and a novel therapeutic target. Ann Oncol 2008;19(9):1523–9.

32. Hofmann M, Stoss O, Shi D, et al. Assessment of a HER2 scoring system for gastric cancer: results from a validation study. Histopathology 2008;52(7): 797–805.

33. Tanner M, Hollmen M, Junttila TT, et al. Amplification of HER-2 in gastric carcinoma: association with Topoisomerase IIalpha gene amplification, intestinal type, poor prognosis and sensitivity to trastuzumab. Ann Oncol 2005;16(2):273–8.

34. Bang YJ, Van Cutsem E, Feyereislova A, et al. Trastuzumab in combination with chemotherapy versus chemotherapy alone for treatment of HER2-positive advanced gastric or gastro-oesophageal junction cancer (ToGA): a phase 3, open-label, randomised controlled trial. Lancet 2010;376(9742):687–97.

35. Gill RS, Al-Adra DP, Nagendran J, et al. Treatment of gastric cancer with peritoneal carcinomatosis by cytoreductive surgery and HIPEC: a systematic review of survival, mortality, and morbidity. J Surg Oncol 2011;104(6):692–8.

36. Lordick F, Kang YK, Chung HC, et al. Capecitabine and cisplatin with or without cetuximab for patients with previously untreated advanced gastric cancer (EXPAND): a randomised, open-label phase 3 trial. Lancet Oncol 2013;14(6): 490–9.

37. Song ZJ, Gong P, Wu YE. Relationship between the expression of iNOS,VEGF,-tumor angiogenesis and gastric cancer. World J Gastroenterol 2002;8(4):591–5.

38. Ohtsu A, Shah MA, Van Cutsem E, et al. Bevacizumab in combination with chemotherapy as first-line therapy in advanced gastric cancer: a randomized, double-blind, placebo-controlled phase III study. J Clin Oncol 2011;29(30): 3968–76.

39. Das S, Suarez G, Beswick EJ, et al. Expression of B7-H1 on gastric epithelial cells: its potential role in regulating T cells during Helicobacter pylori infection. J Immunol 2006;176(5):3000–9.

40. Fridman WH, Pages F, Sautes-Fridman C, et al. The immune contexture in human tumours: impact on clinical outcome. Nat Rev Cancer 2012;12(4):298–306.

41. Le DT, Durham JN, Smith KN, et al. Mismatch repair deficiency predicts response of solid tumors to PD-1 blockade. Science 2017;357(6349):409–13.

42. Geng Y, Wang H, Lu C, et al. Expression of costimulatory molecules B7-H1, B7-H4 and Foxp3+ Tregs in gastric cancer and its clinical significance. Int J Clin Oncol 2015;20(2):273–81.

43. Kelly RJ. Immunotherapy for esophageal and gastric cancer. Am Soc Clin Oncol Educ Book 2017;37:292–300.

44. Yoon-Koo Kang TS, Ryu MH, Chao Y, et al. Nivolumab (ONO-4538/BMS-936558) as salvage treatment after second or later-line chemotherapy for advanced gastric or gastro-esophageal junction cancer (AGC): a double-blinded, randomized, phase III trial. J Clin Oncol 2017;35(suppl 4S). abstract 2.

45. Dehal A, Smith JJ, Nash GM. Cytoreductive surgery and intraperitoneal chemotherapy: an evidence-based review-past, present and future. J Gastrointest Oncol 2016;7(1):143–57.

46. Aoyama T, Yoshikawa T, Hayashi T, et al. Risk factors for peritoneal recurrence in stage II/III gastric cancer patients who received S-1 adjuvant chemotherapy after D2 gastrectomy. Ann Surg Oncol 2012;19(5):1568–74.

47. Koga S, Hamazoe R, Maeta M, et al. Prophylactic therapy for peritoneal recurrence of gastric cancer by continuous hyperthermic peritoneal perfusion with mitomycin C. Cancer 1988;61(2):232–7.

48. Hamazoe R, Maeta M, Kaibara N. Intraperitoneal thermochemotherapy for prevention of peritoneal recurrence of gastric cancer. Final results of a randomized controlled study. Cancer 1994;73(8):2048–52.

49. Kang YK, Yook JH, Chang HM, et al. Enhanced efficacy of postoperative adjuvant chemotherapy in advanced gastric cancer: results from a phase 3 randomized trial (AMC0101). Cancer Chemother Pharmacol 2014;73(1):139–49.

50. Kuramoto M, Shimada S, Ikeshima S, et al. Extensive intraoperative peritoneal lavage as a standard prophylactic strategy for peritoneal recurrence in patients with gastric carcinoma. Ann Surg 2009;250(2):242–6.

51. Feingold PL, Kwong ML, Davis JL, et al. Adjuvant intraperitoneal chemotherapy for the treatment of gastric cancer at risk for peritoneal carcinomatosis: a systematic review. J Surg Oncol 2017;115(2):192–201.

52. Glehen O, Passot G, Villeneuve L, et al. GASTRICHIP: D2 resection and hyperthermic intraperitoneal chemotherapy in locally advanced gastric carcinoma: a randomized and multicenter phase III study. BMC Cancer 2014;14:183.

53. Kim G, Chen E, Tay AY, et al. Extensive peritoneal lavage after curative gastrectomy for gastric cancer (EXPEL): study protocol of an international multicentre randomised controlled trial. Jpn J Clin Oncol 2017;47(2):179–84.

54. Badgwell BD, Blum MA, Das P, et al. A phase II study of laparoscopic hyperthermic intraperitoneal chemoperfusion (HIPEC) for gastric carcinomatosis or positive cytology. American Society of Clinical Oncology 2016.

55. Badgwell B, Blum M, Das P, et al. Phase II trial of laparoscopic hyperthermic intraperitoneal chemoperfusion for peritoneal carcinomatosis or positive peritoneal cytology in patients with gastric adenocarcinoma. Ann Surg Oncol 2017; 24(11):3338–44.

56. Stern JL, Denman S, Elias EG, et al. Evaluation of palliative resection in advanced carcinoma of the stomach. Surgery 1975;77(2):291–8.

57. Fujimoto S, Shrestha RD, Kokubun M, et al. Intraperitoneal hyperthermic perfusion combined with surgery effective for gastric cancer patients with peritoneal seeding. Ann Surg 1988;208(1):36–41.

58. Yonemura Y, Fujimura T, Nishimura G, et al. Effects of intraoperative chemohyperthermia in patients with gastric cancer with peritoneal dissemination. Surgery 1996;119(4):437–44.

59. Sayag-Beaujard AC, Francois Y, Glehen O, et al. Intraperitoneal chemohyperthermia with mitomycin C for gastric cancer patients with peritoneal carcinomatosis. Anticancer Res 1999;19(2B):1375–82.

60. Glehen O, Schreiber V, Cotte E, et al. Cytoreductive surgery and intraperitoneal chemohyperthermia for peritoneal carcinomatosis arising from gastric cancer. Arch Surg 2004;139(1):20–6.
61. Glehen O, Gilly FN, Arvieux C, et al. Peritoneal carcinomatosis from gastric cancer: a multi-institutional study of 159 patients treated by cytoreductive surgery combined with perioperative intraperitoneal chemotherapy. Ann Surg Oncol 2010;17(9):2370–7.
62. Yang XJ, Huang CQ, Suo T, et al. Cytoreductive surgery and hyperthermic intraperitoneal chemotherapy improves survival of patients with peritoneal carcinomatosis from gastric cancer: final results of a phase III randomized clinical trial. Ann Surg Oncol 2011;18(6):1575–81.
63. Charite University B, Germany, Aid GC. Cytoreductive Surgery (CRS) with/without HIPEC in gastric cancer with peritoneal carcinomatosis. 2014. Available at: https://clinicaltrials.gov/show/NCT02158988. Accessed June 27, 2017.
64. Yonemura Y, Bandou E, Kinoshita K, et al. Effective therapy for peritoneal dissemination in gastric cancer. Surg Oncol Clin N Am 2003;12(3):635–48.
65. Yonemura Y, Endou Y, Shinbo M, et al. Safety and efficacy of bidirectional chemotherapy for treatment of patients with peritoneal dissemination from gastric cancer: selection for cytoreductive surgery. J Surg Oncol 2009;100(4): 311–6.
66. Canbay E, Mizumoto A, Ichinose M, et al. Outcome data of patients with peritoneal carcinomatosis from gastric origin treated by a strategy of bidirectional chemotherapy prior to cytoreductive surgery and hyperthermic intraperitoneal chemotherapy in a single specialized center in Japan. Ann Surg Oncol 2014; 21(4):1147–52.
67. Ishigami H, Yamaguchi H, Yamashita H, et al. Surgery after intraperitoneal and systemic chemotherapy for gastric cancer with peritoneal metastasis or positive peritoneal cytology findings. Gastric Cancer 2017;20(Suppl 1):128–34.
68. Yonemura Y, Ishibashi H, Hirano M, et al. Effects of neoadjuvant laparoscopic hyperthermic intraperitoneal chemotherapy and neoadjuvant intraperitoneal/systemic chemotherapy on peritoneal metastases from gastric cancer. Ann Surg Oncol 2017;24(2):478–85.
69. Ohtsu A, Shimada Y, Shirao K, et al. Randomized phase III trial of fluorouracil alone versus fluorouracil plus cisplatin versus uracil and tegafur plus mitomycin in patients with unresectable, advanced gastric cancer: the Japan Clinical Oncology Group Study (JCOG9205). J Clin Oncol 2003;21(1):54–9.
70. Bouché O, Raoul JL, Bonnetain F, et al. Randomized multicenter phase II trial of a biweekly regimen of fluorouracil and leucovorin (LV5FU2), LV5FU2 plus cisplatin, or LV5FU2 plus irinotecan in patients with previously untreated metastatic gastric cancer: a Federation Francophone de Cancerologie Digestive Group Study–FFCD 9803. J Clin Oncol 2004;22(21):4319–28.
71. Van Cutsem E, Moiseyenko VM, Tjulandin S, et al. Phase III study of docetaxel and cisplatin plus fluorouracil compared with cisplatin and fluorouracil as first-line therapy for advanced gastric cancer: a report of the V325 Study Group. J Clin Oncol 2006;24(31):4991–7.
72. Al-Batran SE, Hartmann JT, Probst S, et al. Phase III trial in metastatic gastroesophageal adenocarcinoma with fluorouracil, leucovorin plus either oxaliplatin or cisplatin: a study of the Arbeitsgemeinschaft Internistische Onkologie. J Clin Oncol 2008;26(9):1435–42.
73. Dank M, Zaluski J, Barone C, et al. Randomized phase III study comparing irinotecan combined with 5-fluorouracil and folinic acid to cisplatin combined with

5-fluorouracil in chemotherapy naive patients with advanced adenocarcinoma of the stomach or esophagogastric junction. Ann Oncol 2008;19(8):1450–7.

74. Koizumi W, Narahara H, Hara T, et al. S-1 plus cisplatin versus S-1 alone for first-line treatment of advanced gastric cancer (SPIRITS trial): a phase III trial. Lancet Oncol 2008;9(3):215–21.

75. Kang YK, Kang WK, Shin DB, et al. Capecitabine/cisplatin versus 5-fluorouracil/cisplatin as first-line therapy in patients with advanced gastric cancer: a randomised phase III noninferiority trial. Ann Oncol 2009;20(4):666–73.

76. Ajani JA, Rodriguez W, Bodoky G, et al. Multicenter phase III comparison of cisplatin/S-1 with cisplatin/infusional fluorouracil in advanced gastric or gastro-esophageal adenocarcinoma study: the FLAGS trial. J Clin Oncol 2010;28(9):1547–53.

77. Guimbaud R, Louvet C, Ries P, et al. Prospective, randomized, multicenter, phase III study of fluorouracil, leucovorin, and irinotecan versus epirubicin, cisplatin, and capecitabine in advanced gastric adenocarcinoma: a French intergroup (Federation Francophone de Cancerologie Digestive, Federation Nationale des Centres de Lutte Contre le Cancer, and Groupe Cooperateur Multidisciplinaire en Oncologie) study. J Clin Oncol 2014;32(31):3520–6.

78. Thuss-Patience PC, Kretzschmar A, Bichev D, et al. Survival advantage for irinotecan versus best supportive care as second-line chemotherapy in gastric cancer–a randomised phase III study of the Arbeitsgemeinschaft Internistische Onkologie (AIO). Eur J Cancer 2011;47(15):2306–14.

79. Kang JH, Lee SI, Lim DH, et al. Salvage chemotherapy for pretreated gastric cancer: a randomized phase III trial comparing chemotherapy plus best supportive care with best supportive care alone. J Clin Oncol 2012;30(13):1513–8.

80. Ford HE, Marshall A, Bridgewater JA, et al. Docetaxel versus active symptom control for refractory oesophagogastric adenocarcinoma (COUGAR-02): an open-label, phase 3 randomised controlled trial. Lancet Oncol 2014;15(1):78–86.

81. Nishina T, Boku N, Gotoh M, et al. Randomized phase II study of second-line chemotherapy with the best available 5-fluorouracil regimen versus weekly administration of paclitaxel in far advanced gastric cancer with severe peritoneal metastases refractory to 5-fluorouracil-containing regimens (JCOG0407). Gastric Cancer 2016;19(3):902–10.

82. Sun W, Powell M, O'Dwyer PJ, et al. Phase II study of sorafenib in combination with docetaxel and cisplatin in the treatment of metastatic or advanced gastric and gastroesophageal junction adenocarcinoma: ECOG 5203. J Clin Oncol 2010;28(18):2947–51.

83. Bang YJ, Kang YK, Kang WK, et al. Phase II study of sunitinib as second-line treatment for advanced gastric cancer. Invest New Drugs 2011;29(6):1449–58.

84. Martin-Richard M, Gallego R, Pericay C, et al. Multicenter phase II study of ox-aliplatin and sorafenib in advanced gastric adenocarcinoma after failure of cisplatin and fluoropyrimidine treatment. A GEMCAD study. Invest New Drugs 2013;31(6):1573–9.

85. Waddell T, Chau I, Cunningham D, et al. Epirubicin, oxaliplatin, and capecitabine with or without panitumumab for patients with previously untreated advanced oesophagogastric cancer (REAL3): a randomised, open-label phase 3 trial. Lancet Oncol 2013;14(6):481–9.

86. Ohtsu A, Ajani JA, Bai YX, et al. Everolimus for previously treated advanced gastric cancer: results of the randomized, double-blind, phase III GRANITE-1 study. J Clin Oncol 2013;31(31):3935–43.

87. Fuchs CS, Tomasek J, Yong CJ, et al. Ramucirumab monotherapy for previously treated advanced gastric or gastro-oesophageal junction adenocarcinoma (REGARD): an international, randomised, multicentre, placebo-controlled, phase 3 trial. Lancet 2014;383(9911):31–9.

88. Satoh T, Xu RH, Chung HC, et al. Lapatinib plus paclitaxel versus paclitaxel alone in the second-line treatment of HER2-amplified advanced gastric cancer in Asian populations: TyTAN–a randomized, phase III study. J Clin Oncol 2014; 32(19):2039–49.

89. Wilke H, Muro K, Van Cutsem E, et al. Ramucirumab plus paclitaxel versus placebo plus paclitaxel in patients with previously treated advanced gastric or gastro-oesophageal junction adenocarcinoma (RAINBOW): a double-blind, randomised phase 3 trial. Lancet Oncol 2014;15(11):1224–35.

90. Chua C, Tan IB, Yamada Y, et al. Phase II study of trastuzumab in combination with S-1 and cisplatin in the first-line treatment of human epidermal growth factor receptor HER2-positive advanced gastric cancer. Cancer Chemother Pharmacol 2015;76(2):397–408.

91. Ryu MH, Yoo C, Kim JG, et al. Multicenter phase II study of trastuzumab in combination with capecitabine and oxaliplatin for advanced gastric cancer. Eur J Cancer 2015;51(4):482–8.

92. Li J, Qin S, Xu J, et al. Randomized, double-blind, placebo-controlled phase III trial of apatinib in patients with chemotherapy-refractory advanced or metastatic adenocarcinoma of the stomach or gastroesophageal junction. J Clin Oncol 2016;34(13):1448–54.

93. Miyashiro I, Furukawa H, Sasako M, et al. Randomized clinical trial of adjuvant chemotherapy with intraperitoneal and intravenous cisplatin followed by oral fluorouracil (UFT) in serosa-positive gastric cancer versus curative resection alone: final results of the Japan Clinical Oncology Group trial JCOG9206-2. Gastric Cancer 2011;14(3):212–8.

94. Topuz E, Basaran M, Saip P, et al. Adjuvant intraperitoneal chemotherapy with cisplatinum, mitoxantrone, 5-fluorouracil, and calcium folinate in patients with gastric cancer: a phase II study. Am J Clin Oncol 2002;25(6):619–24.

95. Yonemura Y, de Aretxabala X, Fujimura T, et al. Intraoperative chemohyperthermic peritoneal perfusion as an adjuvant to gastric cancer: final results of a randomized controlled study. Hepatogastroenterology 2001;48(42):1776–82.

96. Kim JY, Bae HS. A controlled clinical study of serosa-invasive gastric carcinoma patients who underwent surgery plus intraperitoneal hyperthermo-chemoperfusion (IHCP). Gastric Cancer 2001;4(1):27–33.

97. Fujimoto S, Shrestha RD, Kokubun M, et al. Positive results of combined therapy of surgery and intraperitoneal hyperthermic perfusion for far-advanced gastric cancer. Ann Surg 1990;212(5):592–6.

98. Yonemura Y, Fujimura T, Fushida S, et al. Hyperthermo-chemotherapy combined with cytoreductive surgery for the treatment of gastric cancer with peritoneal dissemination. World J Surg 1991;15(4):530–5 [discussion: 535–6].

99. Hall JJ, Loggie BW, Shen P, et al. Cytoreductive surgery with intraperitoneal hyperthermic chemotherapy for advanced gastric cancer. J Gastrointest Surg 2004;8(4):454–63.

100. Scaringi S, Kianmanesh R, Sabate JM, et al. Advanced gastric cancer with or without peritoneal carcinomatosis treated with hyperthermic intraperitoneal chemotherapy: a single western center experience. Eur J Surg Oncol 2008; 34(11):1246–52.

101. Yang XJ, Li Y, Yonemura Y. Cytoreductive surgery plus hyperthermic intraperitoneal chemotherapy to treat gastric cancer with ascites and/or peritoneal carcinomatosis: results from a Chinese center. J Surg Oncol 2010;101(6): 457–64.
102. Magge D, Zenati M, Mavanur A, et al. Aggressive locoregional surgical therapy for gastric peritoneal carcinomatosis. Ann Surg Oncol 2014;21(5): 1448–55.

Peritoneal Metastases from Malignant Mesothelioma

Claire Yue Li, MD[a], H. Richard Alexander Jr, MD[b],*

KEYWORDS

- Diffuse malignant peritoneal mesothelioma • Peritoneal metastases
- Operative cytoreduction • Hyperthermic intraoperative peritoneal chemotherapy
- Early postoperative intraperitoneal chemotherapy

KEY POINTS

- Diffuse malignant peritoneal mesothelioma (MPM) is a rare cancer that is ultimately fatal in almost all afflicted individuals.
- Morbidity and mortality from MPM is due to its propensity to progress locoregionally within the abdominal cavity.
- The Widely accepted first time treatment in properly selected patients is Operative cytoreduction and regional Chemotherapy.
- MPM is considered a chemotherapy-resistant malignancy.

INTRODUCTION

Diffuse malignant peritoneal mesothelioma or MPM is a rare cancer that is ultimately fatal in almost all afflicted individuals. MPM represents approximately 15% to 20% of all mesothelioma diagnoses, with most being the pleural variant; there are approximately 500 to 700 new cases of MPM diagnosed annually in the United States. Male and female individuals have an equal incidence of the disease.[1,2] It is a diffuse malignancy arising from the mesothelial lining of the peritoneum; morbidity and mortality from MPM is due to its propensity to progress locoregionally within the abdominal cavity. Patients with MPM most commonly present with nonspecific abdominal symptoms that usually lead to diagnosis when the condition is relatively advanced. Historically, median overall survival for patients with MPM without treatment is approximately less than 1 year.[3] MPM is considered a chemotherapy-resistant malignancy; the couplet of systemic pemetrexed and cisplatin has an overall response rate of approximately 25% and a median overall survival of approximately 1 year.[4,5] The

Disclosure: The authors have nothing to disclose.
[a] Department of Surgery, New York Presbyterian Hospital, 170 William Street, New York, NY 10038, USA; [b] Rutgers Cancer Institute of New Jersey, Department of Surgery, Rutgers Robert Wood Johnson Medical School, New Brunswick, NJ, USA
* Correspondence author.
E-mail address: richard.alexander@rutgers.edu

Surg Oncol Clin N Am 27 (2018) 539–549
https://doi.org/10.1016/j.soc.2018.02.010
1055-3207/18/© 2018 Elsevier Inc. All rights reserved.
surgonc.theclinics.com

available data, almost all retrospective in nature, have shown that in selected patients, operative cytoreduction (CRS) and regional chemotherapy administered as hyperthermic intraoperative peritoneal chemotherapy (HIPEC) or early postoperative intraperitoneal chemotherapy (EPIC) is associated with long-term survival.[6–8]

The first reported case of MPM was more than 100 years ago.[9] In 1908, 2 pathologists working in Birmingham, England, Drs James Miller and William Wynn, published a case report of a 32-year-old male miller who presented with weight loss and ascites. Over the course of 7 months, he underwent repeated paracenteses to drain large amounts of viscous ascites. He was eventually explored and in addition to copious ascites, the visualized peritoneum was noted to be studded with innumerable soft, friable tissue nodules that varied in size. Sometime later, an autopsy confirmed the diffuse nature of the process as neoplastic tissue was noted diffusely covering the liver, spleen, and viscera; however, on microscopic analysis, the tumor cells appeared to infiltrate these organs rather than arise from them. Of particular interest was the absence of tumor cells in the lymphatics or any hematogenous metastases indicating this process, even at an advanced stage, remained localized to the abdominal cavity. Fifty years later, a review of the literature identified only 13 pathologically confirmed cases of MPM.[10] However, after that publication's description of the tumor's pathologic features, there was a marked increase in the number of documented cases in the medical literature accompanied by an initial understanding of the risk factors and clinical features of the condition. At the time of Moertel's[11] review of the subject in 1972, there were at least 169 cases documented in the literature. Despite the initial description of MPM in the early twentieth century, it was not until the end of the last century that results of clinical trials and treatment strategies specifically for patients with MPM were reported.[12,13]

There are several risk factors that have been implicated in the development of MPM; data indicating a strong association between asbestos exposure and the development of disease have been known for many years.[14,15] Radiation also has been implicated as a factor associated with increased risk of developing peritoneal mesothelioma.[16] The lifetime risk of developing mesothelioma among asbestos workers has been shown to be as high as 10% and the latency period can be as long as 30 years.[17,18]

Recently a mutation in the BRCA Associated Protein-1 (BAP-1) has been shown to be present in high frequency in patients with MPM; in BAP-1 mutant mice there is an increased susceptibility to the development of MPM after low-dose asbestos exposure, suggesting that individuals with germline BAP-1mutations may be at increased risk of developing MPM.[19,20] Although loss of BAP-1 protein expression has been shown in almost 80% of MPM tissues in one study, the clinical utility of BAP-1 mutation analysis in patients or assessment of protein expression in tumors has not yet been defined.[21]

CLINICAL PRESENTATION, DIAGNOSIS, AND STAGING

MPM has a heterogeneous tumor biology; some patients live for many years even with evidence of disease, whereas others suffer rapid tumor progression and succumb quickly even after an apparent successful initial therapeutic intervention. The most common presenting symptoms are vague abdominal pain and increasing abdominal girth secondary to ascites (**Fig. 1**).[22] Other reported signs and symptoms are weight loss, dyspnea, chest pain, and palpable abdominal mass on physical examination (**Fig. 2**).[3,23] The age at initial presentation ranges widely from 40 to 65 years, and due to the vague and slowly progressive nature of symptoms, the average time to diagnosis is approximately 5 months.[3,6,24] More than half of patients diagnosed with MPM are women.[8]

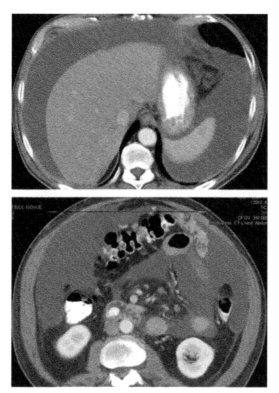

Fig. 1. Computed tomography scan of a patient with MPM showing typical findings of diffuse ascites and a subtle omental mass. Note the lack of nodularity along the peritoneal surfaces.

Most cases of MPM present with diffuse peritoneal involvement and clinical manifestations that are related to ascites or tumor progression within the abdominal cavity. Very rarely, patients with MPM present with localized disease, such as a circumscribed mass that may invade locally and extend into adjacent organs. Patients

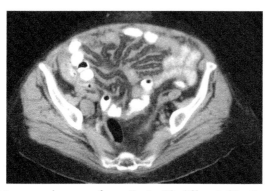

Fig. 2. Computed tomography scan of a patient with diffuse infiltrative MPM distributed extensively along the small bowel mesentery. This type of radiographic picture usually indicates that cytoreduction will not be successful.

may complain of localized abdominal pain or a palpable abdominal or pelvic mass. In a recently reported series of 35 patients with MPM in Turkey, the median age was 59 years.[3] Patients received either palliative systemic chemotherapy or supportive care and the overall survival was 16 months. On multivariate analysis, patients who were older than 60 years, individuals exposed to asbestos for more than 20 years, and those who had a poor performance status at diagnosis were more likely to have shortened survival.

A diagnosis of MPM should be considered in any individual with evidence of a diffuse malignant process in the abdominal cavity on clinical and radiographic evaluation and can be confirmed pathologically with tissue biopsy or, less commonly, on cytologic analysis. Either computed tomography–guided core needle biopsy or laparoscopic biopsy should provide sufficient tissue for diagnosis. Although a diagnosis of MPM can be made on cytologic evaluation, fluid cytology is often inconclusive and has a low yield.[25] Additionally, cytology does not allow for assessment of true tissue invasion through the peritoneum into underlying stroma or fat,[26] both of which are histologic features associated with aggressive tumor biology and shortened survival.[27,28]

Accurate tumor immunohistochemistry is critical for the definitive diagnosis of MPM; however, no single marker is specific for mesothelioma. Instead, a panel of markers is generally used to differentiate MPM from more common tumors, such as adenocarcinoma or peritoneal serous carcinoma. Positive antibody staining for at least 2 markers including cytokeratin 5/6, calretinin, and WT-1 and negative staining for cancinoembryonic antigen, Ber-Ep4, LeuM1, and Bg8 are recommended to establish a diagnosis of MPM.[26,29]

Because of the propensity of the disease to be confined to the peritoneum, extensive staging evaluation for distant metastases has low utility. The extent of tumor in the abdomen is codified using the peritoneal cancer index (PCI); a score of 0 (no gross disease) to 3 (extensive disease) is assigned to 9 quadrants of the abdominal cavity and 4 segments of small bowel and mesentery.[30] The total PCI score therefore ranges from 0 to 39 with a higher score reflecting a more advanced tumor burden. A tumor-node-metastasis (TNM) staging system for MPM has been proposed but is not widely used in patients with MPM.[31] The staging system stratifies PCI into quartiles (1–10, 11–20, 21–30, >30) as a surrogate for T-stages 1 to 4; N codifies the absence or presence of intra-abdominal lymph node metastases, and M describes the absence or presence of extra-abdominal disease. Based on this system, stages were enumerated based on survival. Those with T1 N0 M0 disease demonstrated a 5-year survival of 87% and grouped as stage I. Patients with T2 N0 M0 or T3 N0 M0 demonstrated similar 5-year survival of 53% and are designated as stage II. Five-year survival for patients with T4, N1, and/or M1 disease are similarly poor at 29% and are categorized as stage III.

The measurement of serum levels of cancer antigen 125 has been shown to be prognostic in one study,[32] but not routinely used in patient selection for operation. Its best use is as a component of surveillance for recurrence after treatment.

SYSTEMIC CHEMOTHERAPY

MPM is generally considered to be a chemotherapy-resistant cancer with reported response rates of approximately 25% and overall survival of approximately 1 year. One of the earliest studies evaluating systemic chemotherapy specifically for patients with MPM was published by Antman and colleagues[13] in 1983. In this study, 18 patients with MPM were treated with a doxorubicin-containing regimen. There was evidence of a response in 6 (43%) of 14 patients who had measurable disease. The median survival in the 6 responding patients was 22 months, whereas survival for the remaining 8 patients was 5 months. Unfortunately, despite its modest clinical benefit, these doxorubicin-containing regimens were associated with significant toxicity.

Two phase II studies evaluating the efficacy of pemetrexed-based chemotherapeutic regimens in patients with MPM have been conducted. In 2005, Jänne and colleagues[4] reported the results of an expanded access program that evaluated pemetrexed alone or in combination with cisplatin for 98 patients with MPM who were deemed surgically unresectable. The response rates for chemotherapy-naïve patients versus those who had previously received chemotherapy were similar (25.0% and 23.3%, respectively). The median survival was 13 months for patients who received the combination regimen and the disease control rate (CR + PR + SD) was 71%. Pemetrexed and cisplatin was also shown to have a favorable safety profile, and this regimen has been widely adopted as the preferred initial chemotherapeutic regimen for patients with MPM with surgically unresectable disease.[33]

The results of a second phase II trial evaluated the efficacy of pemetrexed and gemcitabine in surgically unresectable and chemotherapy-naïve patients with MPM.[5] The median overall survival was 26.8 months with an estimated 1-year survival rate of 67.5%. The median time to disease progression was 10.4 months, and the rate of disease control was 67%. Unfortunately, the toxicity associated with this regimen was significant; 25% of patients did not finish the planned course of therapy and there was 1 treatment-related death. Despite the similar disease control rates and the longer median overall survival for patients in this study compared with those who received the pemetrexed and cisplatin combination in the previous study, the severe toxicity associated with this regimen limits its clinical utility for patients with MPM.

A recent prospective random assignment trial in patients with pleural mesothelioma demonstrated a statistically significant but 2.5-month clinically marginal improvement in overall survival when bevacizumab was combined with pemetrexed and cisplatin compared with the chemotherapy couplet alone.[34] The role of this biologic agent in patients with peritoneal mesothelioma is not known, and its use may complicate any planned operative intervention around treatment.

The benefit of systemic chemotherapy in the neoadjuvant or adjuvant setting around CRS and HIPEC has not been established. Two large retrospective and, therefore, uncontrolled studies did not show any benefit to the use of systemic chemotherapy before or after CRS and HIPEC.[35,36] In general, the use of chemotherapy before or after a planned CRS and HIPEC procedure should be individualized and reserved for those who may not be medically optimized for immediate operative intervention or whose histopathology indicates a very high risk for early recurrence and progression.

OPERATIVE CYTOREDUCTION AND REGIONAL CHEMOTHERAPY

CRS with some type of regional perioperative chemotherapy has become the preferred first-line treatment for appropriately selected patients with MPM. Perioperative regional chemotherapy that has been delivered as either HIPEC or EPIC are the most commonly used surgical treatments in select patients with MPM, extending overall survival from a median of 6 months in treatment-naïve patients to 34 to 92 months for those undergoing operation.[6,37–39] In a meta-analysis of 20 publications with data on outcomes of 1047 patients with MPM treated with operative CRS reported a 5-year actuarial overall survival of 42%.[8] The percentage of patients who successfully had a complete or near-complete cytoreduction ranged from 46% to 93% with a median of 67%. In this analysis, the use of EPIC and the use of cisplatin were associated with prolonged survival.

The available primary data reporting outcomes of patients treated with CRS and HIPEC are derived from retrospective single-center institutional reviews, 2 large multicenter reviews, and a Surveillance, Epidemiology, End Results (SEER) database analysis (**Table 1**). Several factors that have been consistently shown to be important in patent selection and outcome are a good patient performance status, a disease burden and tumor distribution that is favorable for a complete or near-complete cytoreduction, young age, female gender, epithelioid histology, and absence of preoperative thrombocytosis.[6,38,40,41] Numerous studies have shown that age older than 60 years, male gender, biphasic or sarcomatoid histology, deep tissue invasion, solid tumor masses present on small bowel or its mesentery on preoperative cross-sectional imaging, and pretreatment thrombocytosis are all associated with decreased likelihood of a complete cytoreduction, early recurrence and progression after operation, and shortened survival.[24,28,37,42] In an institutional analysis of 100 patients with MPM who underwent CRS and HIPEC, patients with preoperative thrombocytosis had a median survival of 13 months versus 58 months for those with normal platelet counts (**Fig. 3**).[41]

In a recent analysis of 1591 patients with MPM patients identified in the SEER database, several important findings were reported.[24] Factors associated with shortened survival included male gender, advanced age, high-grade (biphasic) histology, large burden of disease at presentation, and the lack of use of surgical resection. Notably, the study included patients with MPM diagnosed between 1973 and 2006, and in patients undergoing surgical resection, there was a significant improvement in overall survival over time; most likely, this was a consequence of improved patient selection.

Table 1				
Results of selected series of cytoreduction and HIPEC for patients with MPM				
Study	**n**	**Median OS, mo**	**5-y OS**	**Favorable Prognostic Factors**
Yan et al,[40] 2009 Multicenter international	405	53	47%	Epithelioid histology Negative LNs Optimal CCR Use of HIPEC
Baratti et al,[38] 2013 Single institution	108	63	N/A	Low mitotic count (Ki-67) Epithelioid histology Optimal CCR
Alexander et al,[6] 2013 Multicenter US	211	38	41%	Histologic grade Optimal CCR Age <60 y Use of cisplatin
Magge et al,[37] 2014 Single institution	65	46	39%	Young age Female gender Optimal CCR Absence of operative complications
Li et al,[41] 2017 Single institution	100	33	36%	Lack of thrombocytosis Optimal CCR
Schaub et al,[32] 2012 Single institution	104	N/A	46%	Low PCI Histologic grade Low preoperative CA-125
Helm et al,[8] 2015 SEER database	1047	N/A	42%	Use of cisplatin Use of EPIC

Abbreviations: CA, cancer antigen; CCR, completeness of cytoreduction; EPIC, early postoperative intraperitoneal chemotherapy; HIPEC, hyperthermic intraoperative peritoneal chemotherapy; LN, lymph nodes; N/A, not available; OS, overall survival; PCI, peritoneal cancer index; SEER, Surveillance, Epidemiology, End Results.

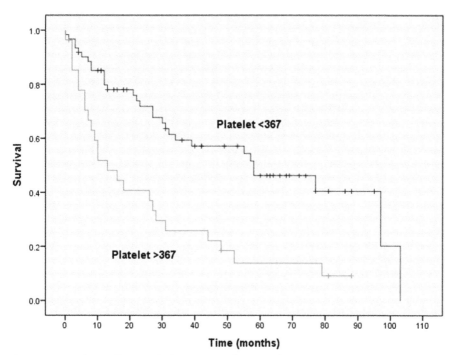

Fig. 3. Actuarial overall survival of patients with MPM after cytoreduction comparing those with baseline thrombocytosis versus normal platelet counts. Thrombocytosis is a surrogate for aggressive tumor biology; even after a complete or near-complete cytoreduction, survival is significantly shorter in patients with baseline thrombocytosis. (*From* Li YC, Khashab T, Terhune J, et al. Preoperative thrombocytosis predicts shortened survival in patients with malignant peritoneal mesothelioma undergoing operative cytoreduction and hyperthermic intraperitoneal chemotherapy. Ann Surg Oncol 2017;24(8):2263; with permission.)

The largest multicenter retrospective study included results from 29 centers for 405 patients treated in both the United States and Europe.[40] The perioperative treatments administered were not controlled and varied considerably with respect to type of chemotherapeutic agent, duration of treatment, and magnitude of hyperthermia (see **Table 1**). The actuarial median and 5-year overall survivals were 53 months and 47%, respectively. Factors that were independently associated with improved outcome included favorable histologic subtype (epithelioid), absence of lymph node metastases, completeness of cytoreduction, and the administration of HIPEC.

A more recent second retrospective review of outcomes of 211 patients with MPM treated at 3 centers in the United States revealed outcomes consistent with the other multicenter study.[6] The actuarial median and 5-year overall survival were 38 months and 41%, respectively (**Fig. 4**). Factors that were independently associated with improved outcome were age younger than 60, completeness of cytoreduction, favorable tumor histology, and the use of cisplatin versus mitomycin c administered via HIPEC. It was also noted that in patients who had a suboptimal cytoreduction (ie, completeness of cytoreduction [CCR] >1), that HIPEC with any agent conferred no apparent clinical benefit.

Treatment morbidity from CRS and HIPEC can be considerable, and should be considered in any patient for whom CRS and HIPEC are contemplated. Outcomes with a focus on morbidity in 65 patients with MPM who underwent CRS and HIPEC

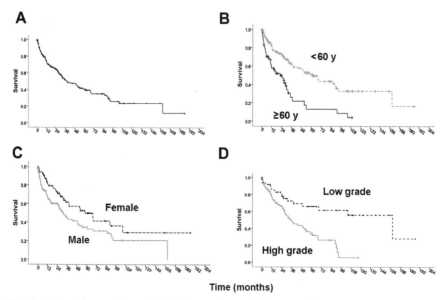

Fig. 4. Actuarial overall survival in 211 patients with MPM after CRS and HIPEC (*A*) and based on age (*B*), gender (*C*), and histologic grade (*D*). (*From* Alexander HR Jr, Bartlett DL, Pingpank JF, et al. Treatment factors associated with long-term survival after cytoreductive surgery and regional chemotherapy for patients with malignant peritoneal mesothelioma. Surgery 2013;153(6);783; with permission.)

at a high-volume treatment center has been reported.[37] In this cohort, the mean age was 54 years, median PCI was 12, optimal cytoreduction was achieved in 56 patients (86%), and the median overall survival was 46 months, all suggesting that this was a representative experience. The mean operating time was approximately 440 minutes; the estimated blood loss was 600 mL, and the median length of hospital stay was 12 days. Major postoperative morbidity (grade III/IV) occurred in 23 patients (35%), and the 60-day mortality rate was 6%. On multivariate analysis, postoperative sepsis was a significant factor associated with shortened survival. Importantly, other studies have reported operative mortality rates of less than 2%.[6,38] Together these data suggest that careful patient selection and expertise in patient management are essential to optimize outcomes in patients with MPM undergoing CRS and HIPEC.

SUMMARY AND FUTURE ADVANCES

Operative cytoreduction with regional intraperitoneal chemotherapy has become accepted as the preferred first-line treatment in selected patients with MPM. Factors important in patient selection include performance status, high likelihood of achieving a complete or near-complete cytoreduction, favorable tumor histology, favorable tumor distribution in the abdomen, and lack of baseline thrombocytosis. Operative morbidity is largely comparable to other routinely performed oncologic abdominal procedures. The use of chemotherapy perioperatively has not been shown to be beneficial in uncontrolled retrospective analyses and it is therefore used very selectively in patients not suited for immediate operation or who are at very high risk of early recurrence.

Current research evaluating novel targets such as mammalian target of rapamycin or the phosphoinsitide-3-kinase pathways or the use of immune checkpoint inhibitors are under active clinical testing.[43,44]

REFERENCES

1. Price B, Ware A. Time trend of mesothelioma incidence in the United States and projection of future cases: an update based on SEER data for 1973 through 2005. Crit Rev Toxicol 2009;39(7):576–88.
2. Moolgavkar SH, Meza R, Turim J. Pleural and peritoneal mesotheliomas in SEER: age effects and temporal trends, 1973-2005. Cancer Causes Control 2009;20(6): 935–44.
3. Kaya H, Sezgi C, Tanrikulu AC, et al. Prognostic factors influencing survival in 35 patients with malignant peritoneal mesothelioma. Neoplasma 2014;61(4):433–8.
4. Jänne PA, Wozniak AJ, Belani CP, et al. Open-label study of pemetrexed alone or in combination with cisplatin for the treatment of patients with peritoneal mesothelioma: outcomes of an expanded access program. Clin Lung Cancer 2005;7(1):40–6.
5. Simon GR, Verschraegen CF, Janne PA, et al. Pemetrexed plus gemcitabine as first-line chemotherapy for patients with peritoneal mesothelioma: final report of a phase II trial. J Clin Oncol 2008;26(21):3567–72.
6. Alexander HR Jr, Bartlett DL, Pingpank JF, et al. Treatment factors associated with long-term survival after cytoreductive surgery and regional chemotherapy for patients with malignant peritoneal mesothelioma. Surgery 2013;153(6):779–86.
7. Yan TD, Edwards G, Alderman R, et al. Morbidity and mortality assessment of cytoreductive surgery and perioperative intraperitoneal chemotherapy for diffuse malignant peritoneal mesothelioma–a prospective study of 70 consecutive cases. Ann Surg Oncol 2007;14(2):515–25.
8. Helm JH, Miura JT, Glenn JA, et al. Cytoreductive surgery and hyperthermic intraperitoneal chemotherapy for malignant peritoneal mesothelioma: a systematic review and meta-analysis. Ann Surg Oncol 2015;22(5):1686–93.
9. Miller J, Wynn WH. Malignant tumor arising from endothelium of peritoneum, and producing mucoid ascitic fluid. J.Path.& Bact 1908;12:267–78.
10. Winslow DJ, Taylor HB. Malignant peritoneal mesotheliomas: a clinicopathological analysis of 12 fatal cases. Cancer 1960;13:127–36.
11. Moertel CG. Peritoneal mesothelioma. Gastroenterology 1972;63(2):346–50.
12. Antman KH, Blum RH, Greenberger JS, et al. Multimodality therapy for malignant mesothelioma based on a study of natural history. Am J Med 1980;68:356–62.
13. Antman K, Pomfret F, Aisner J, et al. Peritoneal mesothelioma: natural history and response to chemotherapy. J Clin Oncol 1983;1:386–91.
14. Selikoff IJ, Churg J, Hammond EC. Relation between exposure to asbestos and mesothelioma. N Engl J Med 1965;272:560–5.
15. Selikoff IJ, Hammond EC, Seidman H. Latency of asbestos disease among insulation workers in the United States and Canada. Cancer 1980;46:2736–40.
16. Antman KH, Corson JM, Li FP, et al. Malignant mesothelioma following radiation exposure. J Clin Oncol 1983;1:695–700.
17. Boffetta P. Epidemiology of peritoneal mesothelioma: a review. Ann Oncol 2007; 18(6):985–90.
18. Spirtas R, Heineman EF, Bernstein L, et al. Malignant mesothelioma: attributable risk of asbestos exposure. Occup Environ Med 1994;51(12):804–11.
19. Alakus H, Yost SE, Woo B, et al. BAP1 mutation is a frequent somatic event in peritoneal malignant mesothelioma. J Transl Med 2015;13:122.
20. Napolitano A, Pellegrini L, Dey A, et al. Minimal asbestos exposure in germline BAP1 heterozygous mice is associated with deregulated inflammatory response and increased risk of mesothelioma. Oncogene 2016;35(15):1996–2002.

21. Singhi AD, Krasinskas AM, Choudry HA, et al. The prognostic significance of BAP1, NF2, and CDKN2A in malignant peritoneal mesothelioma. Mod Pathol 2016;29(1):14–24.
22. Sugarbaker PH, Acherman YI, Gonzalez-Moreno S, et al. Diagnosis and treatment of peritoneal mesothelioma: the Washington Cancer Institute experience. Semin Oncol 2002;29(1):51–61.
23. Antman K, Shemin R, Ryan L, et al. Malignant mesothelioma: prognostic variables in a registry of 180 patients, the Dana Farber Cancer Institute and Brigham and Women's Hospital experience over two decades, 1965-1985. J Clin Oncol 1988; 6:147–53.
24. Miura JT, Johnston FM, Gamblin TC, et al. Current trends in the management of malignant peritoneal mesothelioma. Ann Surg Oncol 2014;21(12):3947–53.
25. Manzini Vde P, Recchia L, Cafferata M, et al. Malignant peritoneal mesothelioma: a multicenter study on 81 cases. Ann Oncol 2010;21(2):348–53.
26. Husain AN, Colby TV, Ordonez NG, et al. Guidelines for pathologic diagnosis of malignant mesothelioma: 2017 update of the consensus statement from the international mesothelioma interest group. Arch Pathol Lab Med 2018;142(1):89–108.
27. Lee M, Alexander HR, Burke A. Diffuse mesothelioma of the peritoneum: a pathological study of 64 tumours treated with cytoreductive therapy. Pathology 2013; 45(5):464–73.
28. Liu S, Staats P, Lee M, et al. Diffuse mesothelioma of the peritoneum: correlation between histological and clinical parameters and survival in 73 patients. Pathology 2014;46(7):604–9.
29. Comin CE, Saieva C, Messerini L. h-caldesmon, calretinin, estrogen receptor, and Ber-EP4: a useful combination of immunohistochemical markers for differentiating epithelioid peritoneal mesothelioma from serous papillary carcinoma of the ovary. Am J Surg Pathol 2007;31(8):1139–48.
30. Jacquet P, Sugarbaker PH. Clinical research methodologies in diagnosis and staging of patients with peritoneal carcinomatosis. Cancer Treat Res 1996;82: 359–74.
31. Yan TD, Deraco M, Elias D, et al. A novel tumor-node-metastasis (TNM) staging system of diffuse malignant peritoneal mesothelioma using outcome analysis of a multi-institutional database*. Cancer 2011;117(9):1855–63.
32. Schaub NP, Alimchandani M, Quezado M, et al. A novel nomogram for peritoneal mesothelioma predicts survival. Ann Surg Oncol 2013;20(2):555–61.
33. Obasaju CK, Ye Z, Wozniak AJ, et al. Single-arm, open label study of pemetrexed plus cisplatin in chemotherapy naive patients with malignant pleural mesothelioma: outcomes of an expanded access program. Lung Cancer 2007;55(2): 187–94.
34. Zalcman G, Mazieres J, Margery J, et al. Bevacizumab for newly diagnosed pleural mesothelioma in the Mesothelioma Avastin Cisplatin Pemetrexed Study (MAPS): a randomised, controlled, open-label, phase 3 trial. Lancet 2016; 387(10026):1405–14.
35. Deraco M, Baratti D, Hutanu I, et al. The role of perioperative systemic chemotherapy in diffuse malignant peritoneal mesothelioma patients treated with cytoreductive surgery and hyperthermic intraperitoneal chemotherapy. Ann Surg Oncol 2013;20(4):1093–100.
36. Kepenekian V, Elias D, Passot G, et al. Diffuse malignant peritoneal mesothelioma: evaluation of systemic chemotherapy with comprehensive treatment through the RENAPE Database: multi-institutional retrospective study. Eur J Cancer 2016;65:69–79.

37. Magge D, Zenati MS, Austin F, et al. Malignant peritoneal mesothelioma: prognostic factors and oncologic outcome analysis. Ann Surg Oncol 2014;21(4): 1159–65.
38. Baratti D, Kusamura S, Cabras AD, et al. Diffuse malignant peritoneal mesothelioma: long-term survival with complete cytoreductive surgery followed by hyperthermic intraperitoneal chemotherapy (HIPEC). Eur J Cancer 2013;49(15): 3140–8.
39. Sugarbaker PH, Chang D. Long-term regional chemotherapy for patients with epithelial malignant peritoneal mesothelioma results in improved survival. Eur J Surg Oncol 2017;43(7):1228–35.
40. Yan TD, Deraco M, Baratti D, et al. Cytoreductive surgery and hyperthermic intraperitoneal chemotherapy for malignant peritoneal mesothelioma: multiinstitutional experience. J Clin Oncol 2009;27(36):6237–42.
41. Li YC, Khashab T, Terhune J, et al. Preoperative thrombocytosis predicts shortened survival in patients with malignant peritoneal mesothelioma undergoing operative cytoreduction and hyperthermic intraperitoneal chemotherapy. Ann Surg Oncol 2017;24(8):2259–65.
42. Low RN, Barone RM. Combined diffusion-weighted and gadolinium-enhanced MRI can accurately predict the peritoneal cancer index preoperatively in patients being considered for cytoreductive surgical procedures. Ann Surg Oncol 2012; 19(5):1394–401.
43. Kanteti R, Dhanasingh I, Kawada I, et al. MET and PI3K/mTOR as a potential combinatorial therapeutic target in malignant pleural mesothelioma. PLoS One 2014;9(9):e105919.
44. Maio M, Scherpereel A, Calabro L, et al. Tremelimumab as second-line or third-line treatment in relapsed malignant mesothelioma (DETERMINE): a multicentre, international, randomised, double-blind, placebo-controlled phase 2b trial. Lancet Oncol 2017;18(9):1261–73.

Peritoneal Metastases from Appendiceal Cancer

Konstantinos I. Votanopoulos, MD, PhD[a],*, Perry Shen, MD[a],
Aleksander Skardal, PhD[b], Edward A. Levine, MD[a]

KEYWORDS

- Appendiceal cancer • Pseudomyxoma peritonei • Low-grade mucinous tumors
- Low-grade lesions

KEY POINTS

- The early symptoms of appendiceal cancer may mimic the clinical picture of appendicitis.
- Most patients are diagnosed incidentally during surgical exploration or late when peritoneal or systemic dissemination has already occurred, as colonoscopy rarely will diagnose an appendiceal cancer.
- Systemic/extraperitoneal metastases are distinctly unusual for appendiceal mucinous lesions.

INTRODUCTION

Appendiceal neoplasms are diagnosed in approximately 1% of all appendectomy specimens.[1] The early symptoms of appendiceal cancer may be nonspecific, or they may mimic the clinical picture of appendicitis. Not surprisingly, most patients are diagnosed incidentally during surgical exploration or late when peritoneal or systemic dissemination has already occurred, as colonoscopy rarely will diagnose an appendiceal cancer.

The common pathway of all appendiceal tumors regardless of grade and cell of origin involves invasion of the appendiceal wall, luminal obstruction, and perforation with subsequent dissemination of malignant epithelial cells throughout the peritoneal cavity (**Figs. 1** and **2**). Systemic/extraperitoneal metastases are distinctly unusual for appendiceal mucinous lesions. The subsequent course of disease for a mucinous lesion depends on the grade of appendiceal primary as defined by Bradley and colleagues.[2]

Disclosure: K.I. Votanopoulos, P. Shen, and E.A. Levine have nothing to disclose.
[a] Surgical Oncology Service, Department of General Surgery, Wake Forest University School of Medicine, Winston-Salem, NC 27157, USA; [b] Wake Forest Institute for Regenerative Medicine, Wake Forest School of Medicine, Medical Center Boulevard, Winston-Salem, NC 27157, USA
* Corresponding author. Department of General Surgery, Surgical Oncology Service, Wake Forest University School of Medicine, Medical Center Boulevard, Winston-Salem, NC 27157.
E-mail address: kvotanop@wakehealth.edu

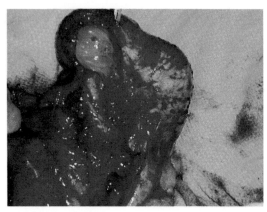

Fig. 1. Ruptured appendiceal mucocele.

Patients with low-grade mucinous tumors (LGA) will typically progress slowly over years and can possibly develop pseudomyxoma peritonei, which describes accumulation of mucinous ascites within the peritoneal cavity. Approximately 7% of the low-grade lesions have lymph node involvement, and up to 16% will dedifferentiate into higher-grade lesions during the course of the disease.[3–5]

High-grade lesions (HGA) are more likely to metastasize systemically, resulting in a poorer prognosis. The variability of HGA clinical presentation stems from the variability in biologic behavior and grade of the primary lesions: moderately differentiated, poorly differentiated, as well as signet ring cell histologies that are all included in the HGA group.[2]

Pseudomyxoma peritonei (PMP) is a descriptive term, referring to the presence of muscinous ascites. Mucinous ascites is by for most commonly associated with mucinous appendiceal neoplasms. However, pseudomyxoma can be produced by several primary tumor types, including appendiceal, colon, ovarian, mucinous pancreatic, and low-grade urachal primaries among others. The prognosis of patients with PMP of nonappendiceal origin depends on the primary tumor type, while the surgical selection for cytoreductive surgery (CRS)/hyperthermic intraperitoneal chemotherapy (HIPEC) for non-LGA PMP patients follows different selection criteria.

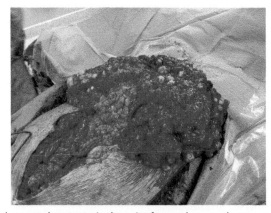

Fig. 2. Eviscerated omental metastatic deposits form a low-grade appendiceal primary.

Not every appendiceal primary is associated with mucin production or ascites. Patients often present with solid peritoneal disease that has no phenotypic difference from any other gastrointestinal malignancy with peritoneal dissemination. In addition, not every PMP or appendiceal cancer is associated with long-term survival. Such factors as histologic grade, tumor biology of the primary lesion, age, functional status, and extent of disease at the time of diagnosis determine the disease-free survival and overall survival of these patients.

The authors' group's approach to peritoneal dissemination from appendiceal tumors has been optimal CRS with the goal of removal of all gross disease if feasible. This typically entails selective peritonectomy and multivisceral resection followed by HIPEC. LGA primaries will be treated with CRS/HIPEC without systemic chemotherapy, while HGA primaries usually are treated with upfront systemic chemotherapy prior to CRS/HIPEC. Selected patients (approximately 10%) who recur may again be candidates to undergo repeat CRS with HIPEC as dictated by their performance status, clinical staging, and symptoms.[6]

Preoperative Patient Evaluation

Selection criteria

Appropriate patient selection is of paramount importance in the management of patients with PSD. All patients presenting to the authors' multidisciplinary clinic have a complete history and physical examination followed by imaging with either MRI of the abdomen and pelvis or computed tomography (CT) of the chest, abdomen, and pelvis (with oral and intravenous contrast). The authors also will obtain baseline blood counts renal and hepatic functions as well as tumor markers including CEA, CA19–9, and CA125. All patients undergo pathologic review of previous biopsy or resected tissue.

In general, the authors use the following eligibility criteria for any patient presenting with documented peritoneal surface malignancy:

1. Patients should be medically with electrocorticography (ECOG) performance status of no more than 2
2. Absence of metastatic disease outside the abdomen
3. The primary lesion is resectable (or has been previously resected)
4. The peritoneal disease is resectable
5. Parenchymal hepatic metastases if present are easily resectable
6. There is no bulky retroperitoneal disease

In cases of appendiceal cancer specifically, the authors' selection criteria are modified based on the grade of the appendiceal primary.

For low-grade appendiceal cancer a cytoreduction is attempted regardless of the volume of disease. LGA primaries progress as sclerotic metastases and as space-occupying lesions within the peritoneal cavity, which are uniformly fatal if left untreated, typically resulting in death from bowel obstruction. LGA tumor biology is typically indolent, and even in cases of incomplete cytoreduction patients receive the benefit of symptomatic control and improved overall survival that can often be measured in years.[7] In addition a multi-institutional retrospective review of 2298 patients with LGA with peritoneal carcinomatosis index (PCI) from 31 to 39 had a 10-year survival of 68% when a complete cytoreduction was achieved.[8] However, even if not completely debulkable, there is frequently benefit to cytoreduction of low-grade lesions. The decision to proceed with heated intraperitoneal chemotherapy after incomplete cytoreduction depends on the volume of residual disease and the amount of ascites. In general, patients with voluminous ascites are perfused, because

HIPEC with CRS will control the production of ascites in approximately 90% of the patients.[9] In patients without symptomatic ascites, but with excessive post-CRS residual disease, the perfusion is aborted.

In high-grade appendiceal primaries, the PCI along with the specific distribution of the peritoneal disease is taken into consideration before proceeding with cytoreduction. Patients with imaging showing disease not amenable to complete cytoreduction are not taken into the operating room for CRS. These patients are treated with systemic chemotherapy followed by restaging imaging, potentially supplemented with a laparoscopic exploration, to evaluate resectability. Generally, HGA patients are preferably treated with upfront chemotherapy with the possible exception of the patient who presents with limited metastatic disease (PCI <10) that is amenable to nonmorbid resection. In case of postchemotherapy presence of ascites, these patients will be evaluated with diagnostic laparoscopy to determine resectability. Ascites, hydronephrosis, and bowel obstruction are regarded as signs of inability to achieve complete CRS due to volume and distribution of disease.[5,9,10] Such patients may be candidates for palliative procedures (such as stoma and/or gastrostomy tube placement), followed by second-line systemic therapy.

Preoperative imaging

All patients have a thin-cut contrast-enhanced CT of the thorax, abdomen, and pelvis or MRI, ideally within 30 days of the scheduled operation.

CT is the authors' modality of choice for low-grade appendiceal malignancies to obtain a rough estimate of the distribution of disease and avoid surprises of possible extra-abdominal involvement. Even though MRI with gadolinium has increased sensitivity in identifying smaller peritoneal implants, the authors believe that this additional information has no impact on the clinical decision-making algorithm for low-grade appendiceal patients. In addition, it increases the cost of the preoperative evaluation and patient discomfort. The authors use MRI more frequently for the long term follow-up of CT-negative patients who have elected not to proceed with CRS/HIPEC or surveillance of completely cytoreduced patients. MRI with dilute oral barium and delayed enhanced intravenous gadolinium for mucinous appendiceal lesions when compared with intraoperative findings has been shown to be superior to CT scan in detecting peritoneal metastasis, with a sensitivity of 82% to 89%.[11]

The strength of the CT is its fundamental ability to detect anatomic details and differences in tissue density. Unfortunately, in peritoneal carcinomatosis, one often encounters subcentimeter lesions spread in a carpet- or plaque-like fashion. Comparison of intraoperative findings with CT findings showed a CT scan sensitivity between 25% and 37%, with a negative predictive value that ranged between 47% and 51%, while the CT sensitivity for lesions less than 1 cm was between 9% and 24%.[12] In a similar study, the false-negative rate for the CT to detect small bowel lesions was 60%.[13] Therefore, the authors explain to their patients that what is seen in the preoperative imaging is rarely what one gets in the operating room. There is also significant variability among radiologists in the interpretation of the extent of peritoneal carcinomatosis, making it advantageous for the surgeon who treats PSD to develop expertise in the interpretation of abdominal imaging.[8] Despite thorough preoperative imaging, approximately 5% to 10% of patients are deemed not to be operative candidates on exploration.

Positron emission tomography (PET) has approximately 10% sensitivity in low-volume peritoneal carcinomatosis.[14]

For LGA primaries specifically, PET offers no additional information given the low proliferation index of these lesions and the almost universally false-negative or indeterminate reading of the final examination. For HGA primaries, PET has a place in cases of debatable disease outside the peritoneal cavity or in evaluating specific peritoneal lesions for local recurrence. PET with or without CT has serious limitations in predicting the extent of carcinomatosis, and is rarely if ever obtained in the authors' institution.[15]

Colonoscopy for Appendiceal Tumors

Colonoscopy itself for identification of appendiceal cancer is diagnostic less than 5% of the time, with most endoscopists describing a smooth, submucosal cecal mass at the appendiceal orifice with or without free-flowing intraluminal mucin. The authors do offer colonoscopy in patients with low-grade appendiceal primaries who have not had one in the previous 5 years, because close to 44% of patients with appendiceal primaries have synchronous colonic polyps. Given the potential of these patients for long survival, the authors prefer to address a colonic resection at the time of CRS-HIPEC. For high-grade nonmucinous appendiceal tumors, a colonoscopic examination does not commonly alter the course of the disease and is requested in selected patients based on age and volume of disease.[16]

Tumor Markers

All patients have preoperatively drawn CEA, CA125, and CA19-9. The likelihood of having increased tumor markers has been observed to be equivalent in low- and high-grade lesions. It has been shown that normal preoperative levels of all three are associated with increased likelihood to obtain a complete cytoreduction, probably functioning as a marker of low-volume disease. In addition, normal preoperative CA125 (in male and female patients) has been shown to be associated with prolonged overall survival. Postoperatively, tumor markers are obtained in 3- to 6-month intervals. Levels are taken into consideration along with diagnostic imaging findings and the presence or not of symptoms in evaluating patients for possible recurrence. Patients with voluminous disease and normal preoperative levels rarely benefit from further testing for those markers after HIPEC. A decision to offer a repeat cytoreduction is never based exclusively on the laboratory tumor marker values.[17]

Clinical Outcomes

Clinical outcomes of appendiceal peritoneal surface malignancies after optimal cytoreduction depend primarily on histology, the extent of peritoneal disease at the time of diagnosis, the completeness of resection, and functional status of the patient.[18–20] Appendiceal primaries can be grouped based on their ability to produce mucin. In general, mucin-producing primaries have a better biologic behavior than their nonmucin-producing counterparts.

Ronnett and Sugarbaker had classified pseudomyxoma patients in 3 groups in terms of survival: (1) disseminated peritoneal adenomucinosis (DPAM) with 5- and 10-year survival of 75% and 68%; (2) mucinous carcinomatosis with intermediate or discordant features (peritoneal mucinous carcinomatosis [PMCA] I/D) with 5- and 10-year survival of 50% and 21%; and (3) PMCA with 5- and 10-year survival of 14% and 3%, respectively.[21] In the authors' clinical experience, DPAM was prognostically indistinguishable from what Ronnett had defined as PMCA I/D. Therefore, the authors concluded that categorizing mucinous appendiceal primaries into low- and high-grade lesions is more predictive of overall survival and response to CRS-HIPEC, with 5-year survival for the low- and high-grade mucinous cohorts of 62.5% and 37.7%, respectively.[2] DPAM and intermediated primaries also had similar outcomes in a review of 2298 patients with PMP ($P<.001$).[8] In the Wake Forest classification, low-grade mucinous carcinoma peritonei includes all cases formerly classified as DPAM, well-differentiated mucinous carcinomatosis, PMCA I/D, and well-differentiated variants of mucinous adenocarcinoma or low-grade appendiceal mucinous neoplasms. High-grade mucinous carcinoma peritonei applies to cases histologically recognized as either moderately or poorly differentiated adenocarcinoma, PMCA, and cases with signet-ring cell component.[2] Within the HGA cases and the cohort with signet features, invasion of signet cell into tissue is associated with worse survival than floating signet cells in mucin, with median survival of 0.5 years versus 2.4 years ($P = .03$), respectively.[22]

Patients who develop PMP from appendiceal primaries have been considered the best candidates for CRS-HIPEC, with 5-year survival ranging between 60% and 97% and 15-year overall survival up to 59%.[19,20,23–25] Similarly, 5-year survival of 45% for the high-grade group has been reported for patients with PCI greater than 20 who had a complete cytoreduction. High-grade mucinous patients with PCI less than 20 who had a complete cytoreduction achieved a 5-year survival of 66%.[26] However, high-grade nonmucinous appendiceal primaries that include appendiceal adenocarcinoma, goblet cell, and carcinoid tumors derive significantly less benefit from a CRS-HIPEC procedure, with a 3-year survival of approximately 15%. In the authors' experience, goblet cell patients with low-volume disease (PCI <11) and without nodal involvement experience a median survival of 29 months after complete CRS/HIPEC.[27]

The completion of CRS is probably the most dominant driver of survival outcomes.[18] What is defined as complete CRS is different for LGA and HGA primaries. CCO and CC1 (or R1 and R2a) resection have similar but not identical outcomes for LGA primaries, while CC1 resection in HGA lesions have similar survival with CC2 resections. In the authors' series of 481 CRS/HIPEC cases for LGA and HGA appendiceal primaries, a complete CRS had superior outcomes compared with those who underwent incomplete CRS (respective medians of 175, 73, 29, and 17 months for R0/R1, R2a, R2b, and R2c resections $P<.001$).[5] This finding confirms data from the authors' institution and others that demonstrate a significant survival advantage for patients undergoing R0/R1 resection compared with those with R2 resections.[19,20] The extent of disease, as described by the PCI at the time of CRS/HIPEC, seems to be a significant factor in overall survival even in cases where a complete cytoreduction was achieved. Elias and colleagues[19] reported that in 206 patients with pseudomyxoma treated with complete cytoreduction, the 5-year survival was 57% for patients with a PCI greater than 19% and 83% for patients with PCI less than 19 ($P 5 .004$). These data underline the importance of earlier diagnosis and treatment. At the same time, increased PCI by itself should not function as an exclusion criterion for operative treatment, given that increased PCI is not incompatible with prolonged survival, especially in low-grade lesions.[8]

For HGA lesions, PCI is predictive in a linear fashion of the ability to achieve complete macrosocopic CRS. Unlike colon cancer, where a complete CRS for PCI greater than 17 is not associated with a survival benefit, it is unknown if a similar PCI threshold exists for HGA primaries.[28] Colon cancer and HGAs, however, are distinct entities with different sequencing profiles.[29] Currently, the authors will proceed with a CRS/HIPEC, regardless of the recorded PCI at exploration, as long a complete CRS is feasible and safe. On the other hand, an incomplete CRS for HGA should not be attempted, as it offers no survival benefit, while it is associated with operative morbidity and delays or inability to receive systemic chemotherapy.[5,9]

Low-grade mucinous lesions, without excluding DPAM, may also present with positive lymph nodes in less than 10% of cases.[5] The authors do not perform a right hemicolectomy routinely in LGA patients unless the right colon cannot be stripped from peritoneal disease. Lymph node involvement, besides being a predictor of surgical morbidity, is also a negative prognostic feature for both LGA and HGA primaries. Thus nodal metastases in this setting seem to function as a surrogate of aggressive tumor biology. In the authors' hands, node-positive patients with a complete cytoreduction exhibit median survival that is less than the median survival of their node-negative counterparts for both LGA (85 months vs not reached [82% alive at 90 months]) and HGA primaries (30 vs 153 months) ($P<.001$). In addition, in the authors' experience, node positivity was a more important than grade predictor of survival, as the node-positive LGA patients had worse long-term survival than the node-negative HGA subjects, even after an R0/R1 complete cytoreduction.[5]

Systemic chemotherapy for PSD of low-grade appendiceal neoplasms is considered largely ineffective. This has been related to the inability of systemically delivered drugs to reach effective intraperitoneal concentrations and the slow growth kinetics of the low-grade malignant cells. A phase 2 study in advanced unresectable low-grade appendiceal primaries with concurrent mitomycin C and capecitabine showed a response in 38% of the patients in the form of either stabilization or radiologic reduction in the volume of disease.[30] Lack of progression of disease of LGA primaries while on chemotherapy should be interpreted cautiously, and is likely a solid treatment goal, because lack of progression is common for these lesions regardless of chemotherapy treatment. Further, in determining chemotherapy responses, it should be kept in mind that the mucin does not respond to chemotherapy, only the cells producing it. In the authors' experience, administration of postoperative chemotherapy had no effect on OS for LGA primary lesions.

For high-grade lesions, it seems that systemic chemotherapy might improve progression-free survival, with the overall survival benefit being derived from the ability to achieve a complete cytoreduction.[31] Chemotherapy with folinic acid, fluorouracil and oxaliplatin (FOLFOX) in the neoadjuvant setting for high-grade appendiceal mucinous lesions was related to progression of disease in 50% of patients who had surgical exploration. Tumor response was observed in 29% of the examined specimens.[32] More recently, the authors have also utilized FOLFOXIRI based on the superior response rates seen in treating marginally resectable hepatic lesions in colorectal cancer.

Preoperative ECOG performance status is a significant prognosticator of survival. In the authors' experience in patients with 1000 HIPEC procedures from a variety of primaries, ECOG was predictive of survival in univariate and multivariate analysis ($P<.0001$ hazard ratio [HR] 2.8 for ECOG 2 – HR 4.3 for ECOG 3 or 4).[18] This is also true for appendiceal primaries, specifically where for each stepwise increase in ECOG score, the risk of death is increased 8.8-fold.[10] The authors use the performance status routinely as a selection criterion for CRS/HIPEC.

Age itself has not been found to be significant in predicting survival.[19,20] The authors do not use age as an exclusion criterion for CRS-HIPEC, but rather as another factor to be considered before the procedure. In the authors' series with patients older than 70, complete CRS was associated with a median survival of 33 months for appendiceal primaries. It is important to mention that in elderly population, the completeness of cytoreduction was significant predictor of survival ($P = .007$) only when surgical complications were not included as a covariate. With complications included in modeling only, the institutional experience ($P = .001$) and the absence of complication itself

(P = .001) were predictive of survival, suggesting challenges in rescuing a surgical complication in elderly patients, possibly as a result of comorbidities and diminished physiologic reserves.[33]

For all appendiceal patients who had a CRS-HIPEC for PSD, approximately 10% ultimately have a repeat cytoreduction to treat recurrent disease. Patients selected in the authors' institution for repeat HIPEC are those who have maintained an ECOG 0 to 1 functional status, have adequate nutritional reserves, and have had an interval between the 2 procedures lasting a least a year. The survival of these patients depends predominantly on the completion status of the second CRS and the interval between the 2 operations.[6] In the authors' experience, each additional month between cytoreductions was related to a reduction of the risk of cancer-related death by 2.6%, while the median survival was 1.3 years for less than a 1-year interval, 3.7 years for a 1- to 2-year interval, and 7 years for an interval greater than 2 years interval, P < .001. Incomplete (R2a,b) first cytoreduction is not an absolute contraindication to an attempted second cytoreduction for low-grade appendiceal primaries, because 20% of these patients achieve a complete R0/R1 repeat cytoreduction. Successful complete repeat CRS/HIPEC for recurrent carcinomatosis from HGA is a rare event with a handful of cases recorded in the authors' database over the last 26 years.[34]

Despite similar morbidity and mortality between repeat CRS/HIPEC procedures, it is the authors' experience that each surgical exploration alters the mechanical properties of the LGA peritoneal disease, with much more sclerotic features and plane obliteration upon subsequent surgeries.

FUTURE DIRECTIONS

The variability of outcomes of appendiceal primaries cannot be predicted by the current classification systems that in a nutshell are based on the presence or not of mucin and grade. By using hierarchical clustering analysis of tumor expression profiles, the authors had previously identified a 139-gene cassette that distinguished 2 LGA molecular subtypes (based on low vs high expression of the gene cassette) that correlated with survival. In multivariate analysis inclusive of molecular subtype, grade, R status of resection, ECOG, and age, only the molecular subtype (P = .0007), grade (P<.001), and ECOG (P = .007) remained significant, while R status of resection was not.[35] This raises the question of which patient will not benefit from a CRS, because of either indolent disease or too aggressive disease.

The authors are working with their biomedical engineering department and reconstructing individual patients' own appendiceal tumors in the form of 3-dimensional organoids that are inclusive of stroma and tumor cells. They replicate the tumor microenvironment by microengineering 3-dimensional tumor organoids directly from fresh appendiceal tumors with biofabrication time of less than 1 week and a take rate of approximately 90%. These organoids are housed in microfluidic devices – resulting in tumor-on-a-chip system – enabling parallel real-time screening of multiple chemotherapy drugs while linking multiple patient-derived tissues and tumor together in a systems approach[36,37] (**Fig. 3**).

These systems are currently lacking clinical correlation data. Upon establishment of clinical correlation, they can potentially match patients, based on in vitro efficacy, with the best available drug or combination of drugs, in the neoadjuvant, adjuvant, or intraperitoneal setting. Another possibility is identifying patients who will not benefit from surgery or chemotherapy, therefore sparing them from unnecessary morbidity while reducing health care cost at the single patient level.

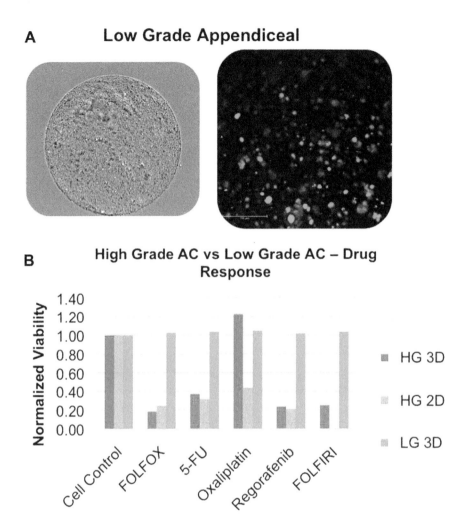

Fig. 3. (A) LGA organoids from patient derived tumor specimen. (left) 2-dimensional image of an LGA organoid. (Right) 3 dimensional (B) Subsequent LGA and HGA organoid chemosensitivity results.

REFERENCES

1. Collins DC. 71,000 human appendix specimens. A final report, summarizing forty years' study. Am J Proctol 1963;14:265–81.

2. Bradley RF, Stewart JH 4th, Russell GB, et al. Pseudomyxoma peritonei of appendiceal origin: a clinicopathologic analysis of 101 patients uniformly treated at a single institution, with literature review. Am J Surg Pathol 2006;30:551–9.

3. Chua TC, Al-Zahrani A, Saxena A, et al. Secondary cytoreduction and perioperative intraperitoneal chemotherapy after initial debulking of pseudomyxoma peritonei: a study of timing and the impact of malignant dedifferentiation. J Am Coll Surg 2010;211:526–35.

4. Foster JM, Gupta PK, Carreau JH, et al. Right hemicolectomy is not routinely indicated in pseudomyxoma peritonei. Am Surg 2012;78:171–7.

5. Votanopoulos KI, Russell G, Randle RW, et al. Peritoneal surface disease (PSD) from appendiceal cancer treated with cytoreductive surgery (CRS) and hyperthermic intraperitoneal chemotherapy (HIPEC): overview of 481 cases. Ann Surg Oncol 2015;22:1274–9.

6. Votanopoulos KI, Ihemelandu C, Shen P, et al. Outcomes of repeat cytoreductive surgery with hyperthermic intraperitoneal chemotherapy for the treatment of peritoneal surface malignancy. J Am Coll Surg 2012;215:412–7.

7. Miner TJ, Shia J, Jaques DP, et al. Long-term survival following treatment of pseudomyxoma peritonei: an analysis of surgical therapy. Ann Surg 2005;241:300–8.

8. Chua TC, Moran BJ, Sugarbaker PH, et al. Early- and long-term outcome data of patients with pseudomyxoma peritonei from appendiceal origin treated by a strategy of cytoreductive surgery and hyperthermic intraperitoneal chemotherapy. J Clin Oncol 2012;30:2449–56.

9. Randle RW, Swett KR, Swords DS, et al. Efficacy of cytoreductive surgery with hyperthermic intraperitoneal chemotherapy in the management of malignant ascites. Ann Surg Oncol 2014;21(5):1474–9.

10. Stewart JH 4th, Shen P, Russell GB, et al. Appendiceal neoplasms with peritoneal dissemination: outcomes after cytoreductive surgery and intraperitoneal hyperthermic chemotherapy. Ann Surg Oncol 2006;13:624–34.

11. Low RN, Barone RM, Gurney JM, et al. Mucinous appendiceal neoplasms: preoperative MR staging and classification compared with surgical and histopathologic findings. AJR Am J Roentgenol 2008;190:656–65.

12. de Bree E, Koops W, Kroger R, et al. Peritoneal carcinomatosis from colorectal or appendiceal origin: correlation of preoperative CT with intraoperative findings and evaluation of interobserver agreement. J Surg Oncol 2004;86:64–73.

13. Dromain C, Leboulleux S, Auperin A, et al. Staging of peritoneal carcinomatosis: enhanced CT vs. PET/CT. Abdom Imaging 2008;33:87–93.

14. Sobhani I, Tiret E, Lebtahi R, et al. Early detection of recurrence by 18FDG-PET in the follow-up of patients with colorectal cancer. Br J Cancer 2008;98:875–80.

15. Rohani P, Scotti SD, Shen P, et al. Use of FDG-PET imaging for patients with disseminated cancer of the appendix. Am Surg 2010;76:1338–44.

16. Trivedi AN, Levine EA, Mishra G. Adenocarcinoma of the appendix is rarely detected by colonoscopy. J Gastrointest Surg 2009;13:668–75.

17. Ross A, Sardi A, Nieroda C, et al. Clinical utility of elevated tumor markers in patients with disseminated appendiceal malignancies treated by cytoreductive surgery and HIPEC. Eur J Surg Oncol 2010;36:772–6.

18. Levine EA, Stewart JH 4th, Shen P, et al. Intraperitoneal chemotherapy for peritoneal surface malignancy: experience with 1,000 patients. J Am Coll Surg 2014; 218:573–85.

19. Elias D, Gilly F, Quenet F, et al. Pseudomyxoma peritonei: a French multicentric study of 301 patients treated with cytoreductive surgery and intraperitoneal chemotherapy. Eur J Surg Oncol 2010;36:456–62.

20. Smeenk RM, Verwaal VJ, Antonini N, et al. Survival analysis of pseudomyxoma peritonei patients treated by cytoreductive surgery and hyperthermic intraperitoneal chemotherapy. Ann Surg 2007;245:104–9.

21. Ronnett BM, Zahn CM, Kurman RJ, et al. Disseminated peritoneal adenomucinosis and peritoneal mucinous carcinomatosis. A clinicopathologic analysis of 109 cases with emphasis on distinguishing pathologic features, site of origin, prognosis, and relationship to "pseudomyxoma peritonei". Am J Surg Pathol 1995; 19:1390–408.

22. Sirintrapun SJ, Blackham AU, Russell G, et al. Significance of signet ring cells in high-grade mucinous adenocarcinoma of the peritoneum from appendiceal origin. Hum Pathol 2014;45:1597–604.

23. Sugarbaker PH, Chang D. Results of treatment of 385 patients with peritoneal surface spread of appendiceal malignancy. Ann Surg Oncol 1999;6:727–31.

24. Yan TD, Links M, Xu ZY, et al. Cytoreductive surgery and perioperative intraperitoneal chemotherapy for pseudomyxoma peritonei from appendiceal mucinous neoplasms. Br J Surg 2006;93:1270–6.

25. Chua TC, Yan TD, Smigielski ME, et al. Long-term survival in patients with pseudomyxoma peritonei treated with cytoreductive surgery and perioperative intraperitoneal chemotherapy: 10 years of experience from a single institution. Ann Surg Oncol 2009;16:1903–11.

26. El Halabi H, Gushchin V, Francis J, et al. The role of cytoreductive surgery and heated intraperitoneal chemotherapy (CRS/HIPEC) in patients with high-grade appendiceal carcinoma and extensive peritoneal carcinomatosis. Ann Surg Oncol 2012;19:110–4.

27. Randle RW, Griffith KF, Fino NF, et al. Appendiceal goblet cell carcinomatosis treated with cytoreductive surgery and hyperthermic intraperitoneal chemotherapy. J Surg Res 2015;196:229–34.

28. Faron M, Macovei R, Goere D, et al. Linear relationship of peritoneal cancer index and survival in patients with peritoneal metastases from colorectal cancer. Ann Surg Oncol 2016;23:114–9.

29. Levine EA, Blazer DG 3rd, Kim MK, et al. Gene expression profiling of peritoneal metastases from appendiceal and colon cancer demonstrates unique biologic signatures and predicts patient outcomes. J Am Coll Surg 2012;214:599–606 [discussion: 606–7].

30. Farquharson AL, Pranesh N, Witham G, et al. A phase II study evaluating the use of concurrent mitomycin C and capecitabine in patients with advanced unresectable pseudomyxoma peritonei. Br J Cancer 2008;99:591–6.

31. Lieu CH, Lambert LA, Wolff RA, et al. Systemic chemotherapy and surgical cytoreduction for poorly differentiated and signet ring cell adenocarcinomas of the appendix. Ann Oncol 2012;23:652–8.

32. Sugarbaker PH, Bijelic L, Chang D, et al. Neoadjuvant FOLFOX chemotherapy in 34 consecutive patients with mucinous peritoneal carcinomatosis of appendiceal origin. J Surg Oncol 2010;102:576–81.

33. Votanopoulos KI, Newman NA, Russell G, et al. Outcomes of Cytoreductive Surgery (CRS) with hyperthermic intraperitoneal chemotherapy (HIPEC) in patients older than 70 years; survival benefit at considerable morbidity and mortality. Ann Surg Oncol 2013;20:3497–503.

34. Konstantinidis IT, Levine EA, Chouliaras K, et al. Interval between cytoreductions as a marker of tumor biology in selecting patients for repeat cytoreductive surgery with hyperthermic intraperitoneal chemotherapy. J Surg Oncol 2017;116(6):741–5.

35. Levine EA, Votanopoulos KI, Qasem SA, et al. Prognostic molecular subtypes of low-grade cancer of the appendix. J Am Coll Surg 2016;222:493–503.

36. Skardal A, Devarasetty M, Forsythe S, et al. A reductionist metastasis-on-a-chip platform for in vitro tumor progression modeling and drug screening. Biotechnol Bioeng 2016;113:2020–32.

37. Skardal A, Devarasetty M, Soker S, et al. In situ patterned micro 3D liver constructs for parallel toxicology testing in a fluidic device. Biofabrication 2015;7:031001.

Peritoneal Metastases from Colorectal Cancer
Treatment Principles and Perspectives

Diane Goéré, MD, PhD*, Isabelle Sourrouille, MD,
Maximiliano Gelli, MD, Léonor Benhaim, MD, PhD,
Matthieu Faron, MD, Charles Honoré, MD, PhD

KEYWORDS

- Peritoneal metastases • Carcinomatosis • Colorectal cancer • HIPEC

KEY POINTS

- Peritoneal metastases are a common site of recurrence of colorectal cancer.
- Diagnosis is difficult and often made at an advanced stage.
- A better understanding of the prognostic factors and of the risk factors made new therapeutic approaches possible.

INTRODUCTION

Colorectal cancer (CRC) is the third most common cancer worldwide,[1] and up to 20% of the patients have synchronous distant dissemination at diagnosis,[2] among whom 4% exhibit isolated peritoneal spread.[3] In the modern era, about three-quarters of the patients presenting with CRC are treated with a curative intent, and 5-year survival rates range from 71.2% to 90.1%.[2] Unfortunately, despite a curative colorectal resection, many patients with initial stage II or III disease will develop local or distant recurrence.[4–7] The peritoneum is the third most common site of recurrence after the liver and lung,[4] with peritoneal metastasis (CRPM) occurring in about 8% to 20% of cases.[6] CRPM is most of the time diagnosed at a very advanced stage because no symptoms are fully specific, and is associated with a poor survival. However, the prognosis of patients with CRPM has been widely improved with the development of a new therapeutic approach consisting of a complete cytoreductive surgery (CRS) of the peritoneal disease followed with hyperthermic intraperitoneal chemotherapy (HIPEC).

Disclosure: The authors have nothing to disclose.
Department of Visceral and Oncological Surgery, Gustave Roussy, Cancer Campus, Villejuif Cedex 94805, France
* Corresponding author.
E-mail address: diane.goere@gustaveroussy.fr

COLORECTAL PERITONEAL METASTASES: INCIDENCE, DIAGNOSIS, PROGNOSIS
Incidence

Besides the hematogenous and lymphatic dissemination, colorectal tumor cells can spread directly into the peritoneum via the transcoelomic route and cause CRPM. Occurring either synchronously or metachronously to the primary tumor, CRPM is diagnosed in 8% to 20% of the patients with CRC.[8] In a recent Swedish registry, which analyzed 11,124 patients with CRC treated between 1995 and 2007, CRPM was diagnosed in 8.3%.[3] In another recent analysis of 5671 patients operated on for CRC,[6] and followed up at least 5 years, 1042 (18%) developed metastases, which were located in the peritoneum in 197 patients (19%), presenting as the unique metastatic site in up to 40% of those cases. This point is important to be underlined because, in these patients, a potential curative treatment must be discussed.

Diagnosis

Clinical presentation

Given that no symptoms are fully specific of CRPM, serious symptoms progressively arise leading to diagnosis at a very advanced stage.[9] Two main events can lead to suspicion of CPRM: the presence of an ascites occurring in 28% to 30% of patients with synchronous CRPM and/or a small bowel obstruction, which concerns 8% to 20% of the patients at the time of diagnosis.[8]

Imaging

The accuracy of imaging is quite disappointing in the diagnosis of CRPM.

Computed tomography The sensitivity of computed tomography (CT) scan of the abdomen and pelvis for the diagnosis of CRPM is 90% for peritoneal implants larger than 5 cm but drops to less than 25% for lesions smaller than 5 mm[10] **(Fig. 1)**. Many factors other than size influence the sensitivity of CT in CRPM diagnosis: the aspect of the peritoneal lesions (nodular or beach), their location (on the outskirts of solid organ or in the center of bowel loops), and the experience of the radiologist.[11] However, it has been recently reported (in 48 patients operated on CRPM from different origins) that preoperative evaluation of the small bowel could be done with high sensitivity (92%) and specificity (96%) using CT-enteroclysis.[12]

PET PET scan with ¹⁸Fluorodeoxyglucose (¹⁸FDG) is equally sensitive for the positive diagnosis of peritoneal metastasis (PM) ranging from 57% to 86.4%[13] and seems quite superior for the detection of PM located in the mesentery and the small bowel

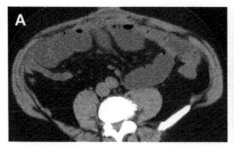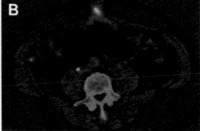

Fig. 1. (*A*) CT scan showing small bowel obstruction due to CRPM, (*B*) PET scan showing multiple peritoneal localizations.

surface.[14] The resolution is improved when the imaging is coupled to a CT scan (FDG-PET/CT).

MRI The CRPM detection with MRI is still being evaluated but is promising, especially with the use of diffusion-weighted sequences. Diffusion suppresses fluid hypersignal and consecutively allows a better detectability of tumoral implants. Standard T2-weighted sequence also easily depicts mucinous deposits.[15] However, a strict protocol and an experienced radiologist are required.

With the globally low sensitivity of actual imaging, the diagnosis is usually made at an advanced stage. However, some preoperative radiological aspects can arouse suspicion of a CRPM: ascitis, ovarian metastases, a tumor invading neighboring organs, a parietal peritoneal thickening, a peritoneal enhancement either smooth or nodular, a small bowel involvement with wall thickening and bowel distortion, an omental involvement such as soft tissue permeation of fat, enhancing nodules, or omental cake.[16] All of these imaging modalities strongly underestimate the real extent of the peritoneal disease. Because radiologic tests lack sensitivity for PM when peritoneal extension is discovered during surgery, it is mandatory to precisely describe location, number, and size of the peritoneal implants.

CPRM is thus very difficult to diagnose, whether in a clinical or a radiological way, mostly if the practitioner does not think about it. That is why knowing risk factors of developing CPRM is essential to help to diagnose it earlier on imaging examinations, or to propose new therapeutics in these patients.

Patients at Risk

Numerous studies have retrospectively reported on factors linked to the primary CRC that exert an influence on the onset of recurrences in general, but only very few have focused on peritoneal recurrences[17,18] (**Box 1**). Notwithstanding, multiple factors have been identified that give rise to a high risk of developing CRPM. A predictive score of metachronous CRPM has been established, after

---

Box 1
Patients with primary colorectal cancer identified to be at high risk for locoregional recurrence and/or peritoneal metastases

1. Visible evidence of peritoneal metastates

2. Ovarian cysts showing adenocarcinoma suggested to be of gastrointestinal origin

3. Perforated cancer

4. Positive cytology either before or after cancer resection

5. Positive lateral margins of excision

6. Adjacent organ involvement or cancer-induced fistula

7. T3 mucinous cancer

8. T4 cancer or positive "imprint cytology" of the primary cancer

9. Cancer mass ruptured with the excision

10. Obstructed cancer

From Sugarbaker PH, Sammartino P, Tentes A. Proactive management of peritoneal metastases from colorectal cancer: the next logical step toward optimal locoregional control. Colorectal Cancer 2012;1(2):115–23; with permission.

follow-up of 8044 patients, with a maximal incidence of 60.7% when all the risks factors are present.[19] In a recent review of the literature published between 1940 and 2011, Honoré and colleagues[20] selected 16 clinical studies, 3 prospective and 13 retrospective, that analyzed the risk of CRPM after resection of CRC. The low quality of the methodology of these studies has to be underlined. Some risk factors of developing CRPM were synchronous CRPM resected with the primary tumor, history of ovarian metastases, perforated tumor, serosal and/or adjacent organ invasion, histologic mucinous subtype, and positive peritoneal cytology, with a reported incidence of peritoneal relapse ranging from 8% to 75%.

Prognosis

For the last 2 decades, prognosis of CRPM has nevertheless been widely improved, and modern systemic chemotherapies actually enable a median survival of 12.7 to 24 months.[21] However, patients with CRPM have reduced overall survival (OS) compared with patients with metastatic CRC without peritoneal involvement, and CRPM are still often considered a terminal disease without any cure possible.[21]

Recently, Franko and colleagues[22] reported the outcome of patients with CRPM from a pooled analysis of 14 prospective randomized trials from the Analysis and Research in Cancers of the Digestive System database that included 10,553 patients treated with systemic chemotherapy. Among them, 9178 (87%) patients had nonperitoneal metastatic CRC (4385 with one site of metastasis, 4793 with 2 or more sites of metastasis), 194 (2%) patients had isolated CRPM, and 1181 (11%) had CRPM and other organ involvement. These groups were similar in age, ethnic origin, and use of targeted treatment. Patients with non-PM in one disease site had better survival than those with peritoneal-only involvement (liver-only metastases-adjusted hazard ratio [HR] 0.79, 95% confidence interval [CI] 0.65–0.95; $P = .012$; lung-only metastases 0.61, 0.49–0.76; $P<.0001$; lymph node as the only disease site 0.73, 0.58–0.92; $P = .008$). The median survival of patients with isolated CRPM reached 16.3 (CI 95% 1.5–18.8) months compared with 24.6 (CI 95% 22.7–26.4) months for patients with isolated lung metastases and 19.1 (CI 95% 18.3–19.8) months for patients with isolated liver metastases (**Fig. 2**). Thus, peritoneal involvement confers a worsened prognosis that could be due to biological (greater proportion of BRAF-mutated tumors) and histologic particularities (greater proportion of the signet-ring cell histologic subtype) but also to lower chemosensitivity compared with other metastatic sites.

Similar results were reported by the Dutch Colorectal Cancer Group.[23] In the CAIRO study, median OS was 10.4 months for patients with CRPM compared with 17.3 months for patients with no CRPM ($P<.001$), and in CAIRO2, median OSs were 15.2 months and 20.7 months, respectively ($P<.001$). The investigators concluded that standard chemotherapy with or without biologic agents is less effective in patients with CRPM and that the poor outcome of patients with CRPM could not be explained by under treatment or increased susceptibility to toxicity, but rather by a relative resistance to treatment secondary to a different biologic behavior of tumors that spread to the peritoneal cavity. In another report, Chua and colleagues[24] reviewed the therapeutic options of 2492 patients with metastatic colon cancer from 19 studies between 1995 and 2009. They reported a survival of only 12.5 months (5–24) for patients having undergone palliative surgery and/or systemic chemotherapy versus a survival of 33 months (20–63) for patients who underwent a more comprehensive treatment strategy with CRS/HIPEC.

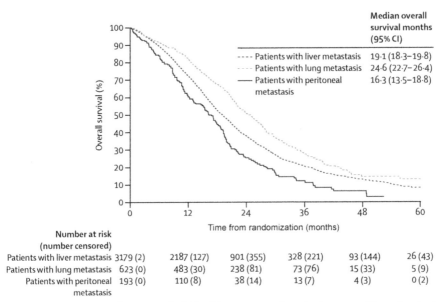

Fig. 2. OS in patients with metastatic CRC with metastases in a single organ. (*From* Franko J, Shi Q, Meyers JP, et al. Prognosis of patients with peritoneal metastatic colorectal cancer given systemic therapy: an analysis of individual patient data from prospective randomised trials from the Analysis and Research in Cancers of the Digestive System (ARCAD) database. Lancet Oncol 2016;17(12):1709–19; with permission.)

Thus, besides these drugs' improvements, the development of a new therapeutic concept that combines a CRS of the visible peritoneal tumorous deposits combined with HIPEC was able to improve the median survival up to 63 months (**Fig. 3**).[21] Therefore, the National Comprehensive Cancer Network has included this

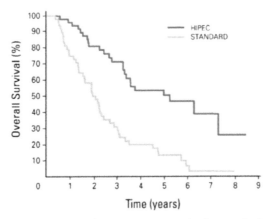

Fig. 3. OS cytoreductive surgery and HIPEC versus standard systemic chemotherapy in patients with colorectal PM. (*From* Elias D, Lefevre JH, Chevalier J, et al. Complete cytoreductive surgery plus intraperitoneal chemohyperthermia with oxaliplatin for peritoneal carcinomatosis of colorectal origin. J Clin Oncol 2009;27(5):681–5; with permission.)

therapeutic option in the last version[25] and stated that "complete cytoreductive surgery and/or intraperitoneal chemotherapy can be considered in experienced centers for selected patients with limited peritoneal metastases for whom R0 resection can be achieved."

COMPLETE CYTOREDUCTIVE SURGERY PLUS HYPERTHERMIC INTRAPERITONEAL CHEMOTHERAPY: OBJECTIVES AND RESULTS

Principles and Objectives

The combination of maximal cytoreductive surgery with HIPEC to treat peritoneal pseudomyxoma was first described by Spratt in 1980,[26] but the main initiator of this combined treatment of peritoneal disease was P.H. Sugarbaker.[27] The purpose of surgery is to treat all the macroscopic (ie, visible) disease, and the purpose of HIPEC is to treat immediately after resection the remaining microscopic (ie, nonvisible) residual disease. It is essential that surgery resect all the tumor implants exceeding 1 mm, because the drug's penetration in the tissue and in the tumoral deposits is small, less than 1 to 2 mm.

Schematically, there are 2 main trends worldwide for HIPEC: one uses mitomycin C over 60 to 90 minutes at 41°C with a closed-abdomen technique, and the other uses oxaliplatin (460 mg/m^2 of oxaliplatin in 2 L/m^2 of iso-osmotic 5% dextrose) over 30 minutes (strictly 30 minutes as soon as the minimal temperature of 42°C had been reached throughout the abdominal cavity, plus 5–8 minutes before to heat the infusate from 38°C to 42°C), at a homogeneous temperature of 43°C (range: 42°C–44°C) with an open-abdomen technique. A bidirectional (intraperitoneal plus systemic) intraoperative chemotherapy, which combines intraperitoneal oxaliplatin preceded by an intravenous infusion of 5-fluorouracil (5-FU; 400 mg/m^2) with leucovorin (20 mg/m^2), is now mostly used for CRPM[28]; current evidence does not show that one is superior to the other.[29]

Regarding the potential beneficial effect on survival of HIPEC, until now, only one randomized study has been conducted, a multicentric French trial,[30] which compared CRS plus HIPEC to CRS without HIPEC. This trial is closed for inclusion, and final results on OS should be available in 2018.

Short-Term Results

Morbidity and mortality

CRS plus HIPEC is considered to be a procedure leading to a high morbidity and mortality. However, over the years, an improvement in the patient selection, surgical techniques, and perioperative management has led to a reduction in the morbidity and especially in the mortality. Mortality has greatly decreased and is currently less than 5%, similar to that observed after major surgery (hepatobiliary, esogastric, pancreatic). Various studies report morbidity rates of 23% to 45%.[31] Morbidity can be divided into surgery-related complications, such as anastomotic leakage, bleeding, and wound infection, and chemotherapy-related complications, such as neutropenia, cardiac arrhythmia, or renal insufficiency.

Predictive factors for postoperative complications

Many predictors of postoperative complications have been described, based on the patient status and the extent of the disease.

Regarding the patient status, more than the age,[32] frailty appears to be a strong predictor of severe morbidity (grade 4 in the Dindo-Clavien classification)[33] and mortality after CRS and HIPEC. In a recent study, frailty was assessed using the Modified Frailty Index among 1171 patients who underwent CRS and HIPEC.[34] For nonfrail, mildly frail, and severely frail patients, worsening frailty correlated with an increase in grade 4 morbidity (6.7% vs. 10.9% vs. 33.3%; P = .004) and mortality (1.3% vs. 3.3% vs. 33.3%; P<.001), respectively. Interestingly, it has been demonstrated that sarcopenia was significantly correlated with the occurrence of intraperitoneal chemotherapy-related major morbidity, but not to surgery-related complications.[35]

Regarding the disease, the most widely known factor is the extent of the peritoneal disease measured with the peritoneal cancer index (PCI), with an increased risk of grade 4 morbidity when the PCI is greater than 12.[36] In the study reported by Saxena and colleagues,[37] an extensive disease involvement in the left hemidiaphragm was the only significant predictor of severe morbidity on multivariate analysis, probably because this procedure results in respiratory complications, and in a higher risk of pancreatic leak, bleeding, intra-abdominal abscess, due to the dissection of the hilum of the spleen. Two recent studies have pointed out that performing a distal pancreatectomy during HIPEC procedure was associated with a high rate of pancreatic leaks (21%–75%) and a higher risk of complications.[38] However, the need for a distal pancreatectomy should not be considered a contraindication for CRS/HIPEC procedures, but has to be considered and balanced with other predictors for complications. It has also been reported that splenectomy increases the risk of major postoperative complications (59 vs. 35.9%, P = .041) and that efforts should be done to preserve the spleen.[39] On the other hand, genitourinary reconstruction can be done safely at the time of CRS and HIPEC and does not adversely influence surgical morbidity.[40]

In conclusion, morbidity rate remains high after CRS/HIPEC, but morbidity and mortality is similar to that observed after major surgery for cancer (major hepatectomy, esophagectomy, duodenopancreatectomy).

Prevention of complications is mainly based on a careful selection of the patients and of the adequacy between the extent of the surgery and the general condition of the patient. Moreover, reduction of the postoperative mortality requires early diagnosis and active management of complications, which means that complications must always be looked into, and an abdominal complication must be considered in the first place when the postoperative evolution is not usual.

Long-Term Results

The benefit of the CRS/HIPEC above systemic chemotherapy (5-FU leucovorin) has been confirmed in a phase 3 randomized study.[41] One hundred 5 patients of CRPM were randomized to CRS/HIPEC with mitomycin C followed by systemic chemotherapy with 5-FU and leucovorin or to systemic chemotherapy alone with the same agents. Palliative surgery for prophylaxis or therapy for tumor-related complications was allowed in the control group. The median OS was significantly improved from 12.6 to 22.2 months (P = .028). Moreover, these results were obtained despite that one-half of the patients in the experimental arm were ultimately not good candidates for HIPEC because their CRPM could not be completely surgically resected. These results were confirmed after longer follow-up, at 8 years.[42] In the subgroup of patients with complete macroscopic cytoreduction (CCR-0/1), the median survival increased up to 48 months, confirming that the CRS plays a pivotal role regarding the efficacy of the combined treatment. The 5-year survival rate of these patients was 45%. However, the main criticism of this trial has been that modern chemotherapeutic agents have not been used and that it fails to clarify whether the survival benefit that is gained is from CRS and HIPEC both or CRS alone.

The benefit of CRS and HIPEC over modern systemic chemotherapy has also been demonstrated in the study of Elias and colleagues.[21] In this study, 48 patients with isolated CRPM received palliative systemic oxaliplatin- or irinotecan-based chemotherapy and were compared with 48 patients who underwent additional CRS and HIPEC with oxaliplatin. There was no difference in systemic chemotherapy, with a mean of 2.3 lines per patient. Median follow-up was 95.7 months in the standard group versus 63 months in the HIPEC group. Two-year and 5-year OS rates were 81% and 51% for the HIPEC group, respectively, and 65% and 13% for the standard group, respectively. Median survival was 23.9 months in the standard group versus 62.7 months in the HIPEC group ($P<.05$). They concluded that although patients with isolated, resectable CRPM achieve a median survival of 24 months with modern chemotherapies, and only surgical cytoreduction plus HIPEC is able to prolong median survival to roughly 63 months, with a 5-year survival rate of 51%.

Therefore, long-term survival and even cure can be obtained after CRS/HIPEC for CRPM. In the study reported by Goéré and colleagues,[43] a cure rate of 16% was obtained after CRS/HIPEC. This rate of cure was comparable to that reported after resection of colorectal liver metastases,[44] suggesting that prognosis of selected patients who underwent CCRS plus HIPEC could benefit from this aggressive treatment as well as patients operating on liver metastases. This point was confirmed in a recent study, with a 5-year OS rate not statistically different between patients operated on liver metastases from CRC and those who had CCRS plus HIPEC (38.5% and 36.5%, respectively).[45]

Prognostic Factors

Elias and colleagues[46] reported the results of a study of that included 523 patients from 23 centers in 4 French-speaking countries that underwent CRS and HIPEC between 1990 and 2007. Independent prognostic variables on multivariate analysis were completeness of CRS, extent of CRPM evaluated by the PCI, lymph node positivity, and the use of adjuvant chemotherapy. The investigators concluded that the combined modality of treatment has a low postoperative morbidity and mortality and provides a good long-term survival in patients with PCI scores lower than 20.

Recently, a meta-analysis of 25 cohort studies was reported, with the aim of identifying factors to select patients for CRS and HIPEC.[47] Among 10 preoperatively assessable clinicopathologic parameters, the investigators demonstrated that concurrent liver metastasis (HR 1.30, CI 95% 1.13–2.83), lymph node metastases (HR 1.88, CI 95% 1.48–2.39), Eastern Cooperative Oncology Group (ECOG) score (HR 1.51, CI 95% 1.13–1.49), tumor differentiation (HR 1.78, CI 95% 1.26–2.53), and signet-ring cell histology (HR 2.01, CI 95% 1.27–3.17) were all negative prognostic variables on OS after CRS and HIPEC. On the other hand, any definitive conclusion about neoadjuvant chemotherapy, onset of CRPM, and mucinous histology could be drawn.

Completeness of cytoreductive surgery

The impact of the completeness of cytoreductive surgery is very high in this combined treatment. This point is clearly apparent in all of the studies reported by experienced as well as inexperienced centers. In the French study,[46] at a median follow-up of 45 months, the median OS was 30.1 months. The 5-year OS was 27% and the 5-year disease-free survival was 10%. The 5-year survival was 29% in patients with no residual disease, and 14% in patients with residual disease less than 2.5 mm, and the group of patients with residual disease greater than 2.5 mm had no 5-year survivors.

Extent of the disease

The extent of the disease evaluated with the PCI is the other main prognostic factor. In the study from Elias and colleagues,[46] patients with a PCI less than 20 had a better long-term survival with CRS and HIPEC. In another retrospective study of 180 patients published by Goéré and colleagues,[48] the investigators showed that when the PCI was greater than 17, the combined modality treatment offered no significant survival benefit compared with palliative systemic chemotherapy alone (**Fig. 4**). Recently, the same team has demonstrated that there was a perfect correlation between the PCI and OS.[49] Better survival was obtained after CRS and HIPEC in patients with a PCI lower than 12, and worsened prognosis in patients with a PCI higher than 17; the investigators concluded that a PCI greater than 17 should be a contraindication to CRS and HIPEC. Between 12 and 17, other parameters have to be taken into account, such as the presence of extra-PM, general performance status, and chemosensitivity.

Association to extraperitoneal metastases

Several studies have focused on comparing patients with and without concurrent liver metastases; all these studies confirmed that the synchronous presence of liver metastases has a negative impact on survival.[50] However, it has also been demonstrated that long-term survival could be obtained in such patients, when the both metastatic diseases (peritoneal and hepatic) were limited. In the series of Chua and colleagues,[51] 3-year OS reached 55% after resection of liver metastases and CRPM in patients with a very limited disease (mean PCI = 8 and mean number of liver metastases = 2). In the matched-control study reported by Maggiori and colleagues,[52] complete resection of both types of disease results in interesting prolonged survival up to 40 months, when the extent of peritoneal disease was limited (PCI <12) and when the number of liver metastases was not greater than 3 (**Fig. 5**).

Thus, CRS/HIPEC associated with synchronous complete resection (and/or thermoablation) of liver metastases is a feasible therapeutic option and should be proposed in selected patients with a limited disease.

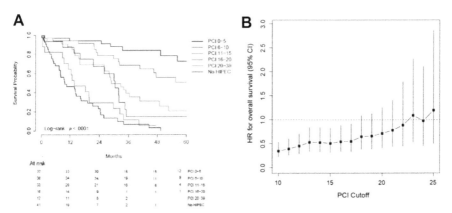

Fig. 4. (*A*) OS curves of patients undergoing HIPEC according to PCI, compared with palliative treatment, (*B*) evolution of the HR for OS between the patients in the curative group and those in the palliative group according to each value of peritoneal carcinomatosis (PCI: 10–25). (*From* Goere D, Souadka A, Faron M, et al. Extent of colorectal peritoneal carcinomatosis: attempt to define a threshold above which HIPEC does not offer survival benefit: a comparative study. Ann Surg Oncol 2015;22(9):2958–64; with permission.)

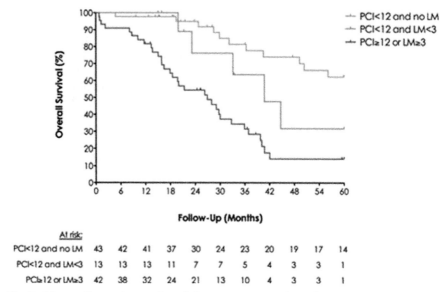

Fig. 5. OS according to the number of Liver Metastases and PCI after curatively intended surgery. (*From* Maggiori L, Goere D, Viana B, et al. Should patients with peritoneal carcinomatosis of colorectal origin with synchronous liver metastases be treated with a curative intent? A case-control study. Ann Surg 2013;258(1):116–21; with permission.)

Occurrence of major postoperative complications

After abdominal surgical procedures, it has been demonstrated that occurrence of postoperative complications worsens the prognosis.[53] As well, Simkens and colleagues[54] pointed out the fact that severe postoperative complications (grade ≥3) after CRS and HIPEC were strong independent factors correlated with impaired survival (22.1 months for patients with severe complications compared with 31.0 months in patients without; $P = .02$). Occurrence of a severe complication was also significantly associated with a higher risk of early recurrence (odds ratio 2.3; $P = .046$). The same conclusions have been reported in a previous study of 101 patients who underwent CRS and HIPEC for CRPM.[55] Five-year disease-specific survival was 14.3% for patients who experienced major complications and 52.3% for those who did not ($P = .001$). Five-year OS was 11.7% for patients who experienced major complications, and 58.8% for those who did not ($P = .003$). At multivariate analysis, major morbidity was correlated to both worse overall and disease-specific survival.

It is therefore essential to ensure that the rate of complications remain low; for this, better selection of the patients on their general condition, their ability to support this type of treatment, and the extent of resection procedures is crucial.

Signet-ring cell histology

Adenocarcinoma is the most frequently diagnosed type of CRC, followed by mucinous adenocarcinoma (10%–15%) and signet-ring cell carcinoma (1%). However, because of their peritoneal metastatic tendency, mucinous and signet-ring cell carcinomas are more frequently observed in CRPM. This point was confirmed in a recent study of 5516 patients with synchronous CRPM diagnosed between 2005 and 2014.[56] The most prevalent histologic subtype was adenocarcinoma (71.8%); mucinous was observed in 21.2%, and signet-ring cell was observed in 7.0%. In total, 445 patients (8.1%)

were treated with CRS and HIPEC, including 6.2% of the patients with an adenocarcinoma subtype, 13.3% with mucinous, and 11.2% with signet-ring cell histology ($P<.001$). Median OS in patients treated with CRS plus HIPEC was 32.8 months (95% CI 27.8–37.8), compared with 12.7 months (95% CI 12.1–13.2) in the systemic therapy group and 3.0 months (95% CI 2.7–3.2) in the supportive care–only group. All 3 histologic subgroups benefited equally from CRS and HIPEC in terms of relative survival gain. However, the absolute survival gain in signet-ring cell patients was 18 months, considerably lower than in adenocarcinoma (gain 30.0 months) and mucinous (gain 35.4 months) patients. This may be explained by the more aggressiveness of the signet-ring cell histology subgroup, with a rapid spread and more advanced primary tumor stage. The negative impact on survival of signet-ring cell histology has also been demonstrated in the study from Winer and colleagues[57] with a median OS of 12 months after CRS/HIPEC. Interestingly, the prognosis was worse in patients with signet-ring cell CRPM compared with patients with signet-ring cell appendiceal PM.

However, actually, signet-ring cell histology type is not considered to be exclusion criteria for performing CRS/HIPEC; its negative impact on prognosis has to be considered in the final decision and balanced with the other prognostic factors.

SELECTING PATIENTS FOR CYTOREDUCTIVE SURGERY/HYPERTHERMIC INTRAPERITONEAL CHEMOTHERAPY

Patient selection is an extremely crucial aspect of planning for treatment of patients with CRPM. A consensus statement from representatives from the major peritoneal surface malignancy centers from around the world listed 8 clinical and radiographic variables associated with increased chances of achieving a complete cytoreduction[58]:

- ECOG performance status 2 or less
- No evidence of extra-abdominal disease, or
- Up to 3 small, resectable parenchymal hepatic metastases
- No evidence of biliary obstruction
- No evidence of ureteral obstruction
- No evidence of intestinal obstruction at more than one site
- Limited small bowel involvement: no evidence of gross disease in the mesentery with several segmental sites of partial obstruction
- Small-volume disease in the gastro-hepatic ligament.

Recently, a new prognostic score named COMPASS (colorectal peritoneal metastases prognostic surgical score) has just been developed by Simkens and colleagues.[59] The 4 following clinically relevant factors on OS were identified:

- High PCI score, which had the strongest association with OS (HR 1.11 per additional PCI point, $P<.001$);
- Signet-ring cell histology versus other histology (13.0 [95% CI 11.2–17.8] versus 35.8 [95% CI 27.6–44.1] months, $P<.001$);
- N2 versus N0/N1 regional lymph node metastases (26.3 [95% CI 18.8–33.7] versus 42.2 [95% CI 33.9–50.4] months, $P<.001$)
- Higher age (HR 1.24 per additional 10 years, $P=.142$).

After an internally validated model, a nomogram was constructed (**Fig. 6**) to predict adequately the OS with CRPM before performing CRS and HIPEC. This nomogram could be a useful tool to assist in the decision of CRS and HIPEC.

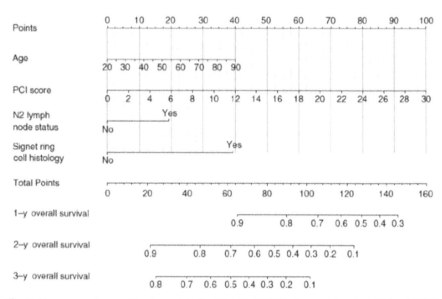

Fig. 6. Nomogram to predict adequately the OS with CRPM before performing CRS and HIPEC. (*From* Simkens GA, van Oudheusden TR, Nieboer D, et al. Development of a prognostic nomogram for patients with peritoneally metastasized colorectal cancer treated with cytoreductive surgery and HIPEC. Ann Surg Oncol 2016;23(13):4214–21; with permission.)

Concerning age, a negative impact on morbidity and mortality has been demonstrated.[32] However, age is not more considered a clear contraindication for CRS/HIPEC; the most important contraindication is that age and general status have to be balanced with the extent of the disease and of the surgery, and the expected survival according to the other clinical factors. Usually, patients older than 70 years are not considered for CRS/HIPEC, except in the case of a very good health status, a limited peritoneal disease, or accessibility to R0 resection without major surgical procedures.

Thus, indications for CRS/HIPEC are based on absolute and relative contraindications.

Absolute contraindications for CRS/HIPEC are as follows:

- Poor general status
- Presence of extra-PM (except 3 liver metastases easily resectable)
- PCI greater than 17 to 20.

Relative contraindications for CRS/HIPEC are as follows:

- Subocclusive syndrome due to more than one digestive stenosis
- Peritoneal disease progressing under systemic chemotherapy
- Presence of more than 3 resectable liver metastases.

THE ROLE OF PREOPERATIVE AND POSTOPERATIVE SYSTEMIC CHEMOTHERAPY

Preoperative chemotherapy has an uncertain place in the treatment of CRPM. Pathologic response to preoperative chemotherapy has been reported, leading to an improved survival.[60] On the other hand, Passot and colleagues[61] did not observed any significant difference in terms of OS between patient responders or stable and progressive (P = .452) and concluded that in patients with CRPM without extra-CRPM, failure of neoadjuvant systemic chemotherapy should not constitute an absolute contraindication to a curative procedure combining CRS and HIPEC.

The potential benefit of early postoperative systemic chemotherapy was evaluated in a recent retrospective study of 221 patients (chemotherapy group, n = 151; surveillance group, n = 70). The median OS after surgery was 43.3 months with no difference between postoperative chemotherapy and surveillance groups. In multivariate analysis, a low PCI (P<.0001) and a long delay between diagnosis of CRPM and HIPEC (P = .001) were associated with increased OS. The investigators concluded that early postoperative systemic chemotherapy does not improve OS after CRS and HIPEC for CRPM and may be a subgroup of patients that may benefit more from CT, but it remains to be defined.[62]

Finally, the time of systemic chemotherapy may not be crucial as suggested in the study from Kuijpers and colleagues.[63] Among 73 patients who underwent CRS and HIPEC for PM from lymph node–positive CRC, 14 patients received pre–CRS-HIPEC chemotherapy only, 32 patients underwent post-CRS-HIPEC chemotherapy only, 9 patients received chemotherapy both pre-CRS/HIPEC and post-CRS/HIPEC, and 16 patients did not receive any systemic chemotherapy according to the time of administration of systemic chemotherapy. Progression-free survival (PFS) and OS were significantly higher in patients who received systemic chemotherapy (PFS: median 15 vs. 4 months, P = .024; OS: median 30 vs. 14 months, P = .015). Some different chemotherapy timings did not differ significantly in either survival or recurrence patterns.

Nowadays, any data from the literature with a high level of evidence can help to decide to perform or not perform preoperative or postoperative chemotherapy. Some evidence should be provided by the CAIRO6 trial currently enrolling patients, and which evaluates the potential benefit in term of OS of perioperative systemic chemotherapy before CRS/HIPEC (ClinicalTrials.gov identifier: NCT02758951).

STRATEGIES TO PREVENT PERITONEAL METASTASES

Different proactive approaches have recently been proposed to anticipate the diagnosis of PM at an earlier stage and even more so to deliver prophylactic HIPEC to patients at high risk of developing PM based on the principle of treating occult microscopic peritoneal disease.[64]

The following 2 main attitudes can be distinguished:

1. Treat patients at high risk of developing PM before the macroscopic appearance of PM, meaning performing adjuvant intraperitoneal chemotherapy during the resection of the primary tumor;
2. Treat patients at high risk of developing PM after a delay after resection of the primary during a systematic second-look surgery.

In that way, the potential benefit of early administration of intraperitoneal chemotherapy has been studied. These studies were based on the fact that intraperitoneal chemotherapy could be considered nothing more than an alternative route of administration of a well-known and efficient treatment to maximize local drug delivery and reduce the risk of peritoneal recurrence. The first studies reported before the 2000s that compared systemic adjuvant chemotherapy-based on 5-FU to intraperitoneal administration of 5-FU either intraoperatively or immediately in the postoperative period failed to demonstrate a survival benefit and showed a potential but inconstant reduction of peritoneal recurrences.[65] Tentes and colleagues[66] investigated the role of different administration methods comparing HIPEC (oxaliplatin or mitomycin C) to normothermic postoperative intraperitoneal chemotherapy with 5-FU over 5 days in 107 patients with locally advanced T3 or T4 stage CRC. Three-year OS was similar between the 2 groups (100 vs. 72%), but the incidence of overall recurrences was lower in the HIPEC group (2.5 vs. 28%, $P = .009$) with a decreased rate of peritoneal recurrence ($P = .001$), which led the investigators to conclude that HIPEC can control viable cells during primary surgery. Adjuvant intraperitoneal chemotherapy immediately after the resection of the primary tumor has also been evaluated in patients at higher risk of developing CRPM. Noura and colleagues[67] evaluated adjuvant intraperitoneal mitomycin C in patients with stage II and III CRC with positive peritoneal lavage cytology. The rate of peritoneal recurrence was significantly lower in patients receiving adjuvant intraperitoneal chemotherapy (1/24 vs. 6/12, $P = .036$). The fact that approximately one-third of patients presented with stage IV CRC at the time of the diagnosis limits the interpretation of the long-term results of this study.

The potential benefit of adjuvant HIPEC has been evaluated in a nonrandomized study that compared 25 patients who received adjuvant HIPEC after resection of T3/4 mucinous or signet-ring cell histology CRC to a control group of 50 patients.[68] Before HIPEC, patients underwent omentectomy with resection of the liver round ligament and appendectomy associated with bilateral oophorectomy in postmenopausal patients. Again, the peritoneal relapse rate was significantly lower in the group of patients who had received adjuvant HIPEC (54% vs. 22%, $P<.03$) as well as the disease-free survival (37 months vs. 22 months, $P<.01$). These data emphasized that a standard surgical approach, associated with prophylactic HIPEC, could achieve better locoregional control, thus reducing peritoneal recurrences and significantly improving outcomes, without increasing morbidity. Consequently, the investigators started a pilot study[69] of adjuvant HIPEC in high-risk patients with CRC invading the visceral serosa (T4a) or directly invading adjacent organs (T4b), or positive peritoneal washing cytology, or resected ovarian metastases or minimal CRPM. As well, Dutch Colorectal Cancer Group started the COLOPEC trial in 2015,[70,71] which is now closed for inclusion. The aim of this study was to evaluate the efficacy of early adjuvant HIPEC using oxaliplatin, delivered either during colon resection (the same procedure or with an interval of <10 days after it) or after 5 to 8 weeks in patients operated on for a T4 (T4N0–2M0) or a perforated colon cancer. The main end point was the peritoneal recurrence-free survival at 18 months determined by CT or laparoscopy. Similarly, at Zhejiang University, a randomized control study[72] is comparing adjuvant HIPEC and surveillance alone in patients at high risk of peritoneal recurrence. Inclusion criteria are a history of resected minimal PM, ovarian metastases, a T4 identified by intraoperative pathologic diagnosis, or intra-abdominal tumor rupture, and the primary end point is 3-year disease-free survival. Interestingly, among the secondary end points, the investigators analyze the quality of life in the experimental arm, a crucial aspect when surgery is compared with noninterventional procedures.

Because of the poor performance of imaging to diagnose CRPM at an early stage, Elias and colleagues[73] reproposed in 2008 the concept of "systematic second-look surgery and HIPEC" in the absence of any sign of recurrent disease after completion of adjuvant chemotherapy in high-risk patients. Criteria for a high risk of developing CRPM were defined as follows: complete resection of limited synchronous CRPM, synchronous ovarian metastases, and a perforated primary tumor. This strategy attempted to identify PM undetected at preoperative workup in more than 50% of the patients. Curative treatment consisting of CRS followed by HIPEC was performed in patients with CRPM detected during this second-look surgery and systematically in patients with a history of CRPM. This strategy resulted in 5-year OS and disease-free survival rates of 90% and 44%, respectively.[73] As expected, morbidity and mortality were low in these patients with limited peritoneal disease, 9.7% and 2.4% respectively. Interestingly, the role of prophylactic HIPEC in the patients without any PM was highlighted by the lower rate of peritoneal recurrence in patients who were systematically treated with HIPEC, compared with that of patients who were not (0 vs 43%).[73] Delhorme and colleagues[74] recently confirmed the role of systematic second-look surgery after resection of a colorectal carcinoma, in high-risk patients according to Elias' criteria. After 12 cycles of adjuvant chemotherapy, PM was detected intraoperatively in 71% of patients with a median PCI of 10. Based on these encouraging results, a French collaborative group performed a multicentric prospective randomized phase 3 trial comparing mandatory second-look surgery with HIPEC to standard follow-up[75] after 6 months of systemic chemotherapy in patients at high risk of developing CRPM. Inclusion criteria for defining patients at "high risk" for CRPM were synchronous and limited CRPM completely resected during primary surgery, synchronous ovarian metastases, and perforated primary tumor. The main objective of this study was to evaluate disease-free survival at 3 years. Other end points were peritoneal recurrence and 3-year and 5-year OS. This study is closed to accrual (the target accrual, 150 patients, has been reached), and preliminary data will be available in 2018.

Both strategies have their advantages and disadvantages. An argument in favor of prophylactic HIPEC during resection of the primary is that only a one-stage procedure is planned with consequently fewer peritoneal and/or visceral resections, because so far, the patient does not exhibit any visible CRPM. However, 2 major problems have to be taken into consideration. First, the preoperative identification of high-risk CRC is not always feasible. Currently, these patients correspond to those with pT4 CRC, a mucinous lesion or a perforated tumor, or with positive peritoneal washing cytology. Except for the perforated tumor, it is quite difficult to appraise the other risk factors preoperatively. Then, if the risk of PM is identified intraoperatively, it is complicated to perform HIPEC in the absence of a specific informed consent for ethical reasons. Second, CRC surgery is, at present, in jeopardy in peripheral, referral, and academic hospitals, and in most cases, access to the HIPEC technique is not immediately available. That explains why patients are referred to centers that perform HIPEC after resection of the primary tumor. However, in patients at high risk of synchronous CRPM, synchronous resection of the primary and of the peritoneal disease followed by HIPEC should be proposed as a first-line treatment for patients, at the time of diagnosis of CRPM. In order to be able to refer these patients under the best possible conditions, it might be proposed to systematically perform a staging laparoscopy to patients at high risk of having synchronous CRPM, because it is carried to patients at risk of synchronous CRPM of gastric carcinoma.

The second-look surgery with HIPEC seems to be more appropriate in standard clinical practice. Another important issue remains the optimal timing of this second-look strategy. In the French PROPHYLOCHIP trial, the patients were operated on (second-look procedure) after completion of adjuvant systemic chemotherapy, which is 6 to 12 months after resection of the primary tumor. This topic is directly questioned in the COLOPEC trial, which compared 2 different delays for systematic HIPEC (immediately after resection of the primary tumor or after an interval of 5–8 weeks).

Finally, the authors consider that both approaches might be incorporated in a unique strategy in order to increase the chances of cure of patients presenting with limited occult peritoneal disease (second look with HIPEC) and whenever possible to prevent metachronous PM in high-risk patients (prophylactic HIPEC) with a limited impact on quality of life.

SUMMARY

The prognosis of patients with CRPM has changed dramatically since the introduction of CRS/HIPEC, with a clear increase in survival. A better understanding of the prognostic factors and of the risk factors for developing CRPM made it possible to refine the criteria for selecting patients for this combined treatment and to define new therapeutic approaches based on proactive attitudes. However, most studies and analyzes are from retrospective series; thus, the results of randomized prospective studies available soon will further improve the management of these patients.

REFERENCES

1. Parkin DM, Bray F, Ferlay J, et al. Global cancer statistics, 2002. CA Cancer J Clin 2005;55(2):74–108.
2. Howlader N, Noone A, Krapcho M, et al. SEER cancer statistics review, 1975-2014. Bethesda (MD): National Cancer Institute; 2017. Based on November 2016 SEER data submission, posted to the SEER web site. Available at: https://seer.cancer.gov.csr.
3. Segelman J, Granath F, Holm T, et al. Incidence, prevalence and risk factors for peritoneal carcinomatosis from colorectal cancer. Br J Surg 2012;99(5):699–705.
4. Bird NC, Mangnall D, Majeed AW. Biology of colorectal liver metastases: a review. J Surg Oncol 2006;94(1):68–80.
5. Tsikitis VL, Malireddy K, Green EA, et al. Postoperative surveillance recommendations for early stage colon cancer based on results from the clinical outcomes of surgical therapy trial. J Clin Oncol 2009;27(22):3671–6.
6. van Gestel Y, Thomassen I, Lemmens VEPP, et al. Metachronous peritoneal carcinomatosis after curative treatment of colorectal cancer. Eur J Surg Oncol 2014; 40(8):963–9.
7. Augestad KM, Bakaki PM, Rose J, et al. Metastatic spread pattern after curative colorectal cancer surgery. A retrospective, longitudinal analysis. Cancer Epidemiol 2015;39(5):734–44.
8. Jayne DG, Fook S, Loi C, et al. Peritoneal carcinomatosis from colorectal cancer. Br J Surg 2002;89(12):1545–50.
9. Dawson LE, Russell AH, Tong D, et al. Adenocarcinoma of the sigmoid colon: sites of initial dissemination and clinical patterns of recurrence following surgery alone. J Surg Oncol 1983;22(2):95–9.
10. Archer AG, Sugarbaker PH, Jelinek JS. Radiology of peritoneal carcinomatosis. Cancer Treat Res 1996;82:263–88. Available at: http://eutils.ncbi.nlm.nih.gov/entrez/eutils/elink.fcgi?dbfrom=pubmed&id=8849956&retmode=ref&cmd=prlinks.
11. de Bree E, Koops W, Kröger R, et al. Peritoneal carcinomatosis from colorectal or appendiceal origin: correlation of preoperative CT with intraoperative findings and evaluation of interobserver agreement. J Surg Oncol 2004;86(2):64–73.
12. Courcoutsakis N, Tentes AA, Astrinakis E, et al. CT-Enteroclysis in the preoperative assessment of the small-bowel involvement in patients with peritoneal carcinomatosis, candidates for cytoreductive surgery and hyperthermic intraperitoneal chemotherapy. Abdom Imaging 2013;38(1):56–63.

13. De Gaetano AM, Calcagni ML, Rufini V, et al. Imaging of peritoneal carcinomatosis with FDG PET-CT: diagnostic patterns, case examples and pitfalls. Abdom Imaging 2009;34(3):391–402.
14. Klumpp BD, Schwenzer N, Aschoff P, et al. Preoperative assessment of peritoneal carcinomatosis: intraindividual comparison of 18F-FDG PET/CT and MRI. Abdom Imaging 2013;38(1):64–71.
15. Low RN, Semelka RC, Worawattanakul S, et al. Extrahepatic abdominal imaging in patients with malignancy: comparison of MR imaging and helical CT in 164 patients. J Magn Reson Imaging 2000;12(2):269–77.
16. Dromain C, Leboulleux S, Auperin A, et al. Staging of peritoneal carcinomatosis: enhanced CT vs. PET/CT. Abdom Imaging 2008;33(1):87–93.
17. Cotte E, Peyrat P, Piaton E, et al. Lack of prognostic significance of conventional peritoneal cytology in colorectal and gastric cancers: results of EVOCAPE 2 multicentre prospective study. Eur J Surg Oncol 2013;39(7):707–14.
18. Sugarbaker PH, Sammartino P, Tentes A-A. Proactive management of peritoneal metastases from colorectal cancer: the next logical step toward optimal locoregional control. Colorectal Cancer 2012;1(2):115–23.
19. Segelman J, Akre O, Gustafsson UO, et al. Individualized prediction of risk of metachronous peritoneal carcinomatosis from colorectal cancer. Colorectal Dis 2014;16(5):359–67.
20. Honoré C, Goere D, Souadka A, et al. Definition of patients presenting a high risk of developing peritoneal carcinomatosis after curative surgery for colorectal cancer: a systematic review. Ann Surg Oncol 2013;20(1):183–92.
21. Elias D, Lefevre JH, Chevalier J, et al. Complete cytoreductive surgery plus intraperitoneal chemohyperthermia with oxaliplatin for peritoneal carcinomatosis of colorectal origin. J Clin Oncol 2009;27(5):681–5.
22. Franko J, Shi Q, Meyers JP, et al. Prognosis of patients with peritoneal metastatic colorectal cancer given systemic therapy: an analysis of individual patient data from prospective randomised trials from the Analysis and Research in Cancers of the Digestive System (ARCAD) database. Lancet Oncol 2016;17(12):1709–19.
23. Klaver YLB, Simkens LHJ, Lemmens VEPP, et al. Outcomes of colorectal cancer patients with peritoneal carcinomatosis treated with chemotherapy with and without targeted therapy. Eur J Surg Oncol 2012;38(7):617–23.
24. Chua TC, Esquivel J, Pelz JOW, et al. Summary of current therapeutic options for peritoneal metastases from colorectal cancer. J Surg Oncol 2013;107(6):566–73.
25. National Comprehensive Cancer Network. Colon Cancer (Version 1.2017). vol. 2017. Available at: http://www.nccn.org/professionals/physician_gls/pdf/colon.pdf.
26. Spratt JS, Adcock RA, Sherrill W, et al. Hyperthermic peritoneal perfusion system in canines. Cancer Res 1980;40(2):253–5. Available at: http://eutils.ncbi.nlm.nih.gov/entrez/eutils/elink.fcgi?dbfrom=pubmed&id=7356508&retmode=ref&cmd=prlinks.
27. Sugarbaker PH. Peritoneal carcinomatosis: natural history and rational therapeutic interventions using intraperitoneal chemotherapy. Cancer Treat Res 1996;81:149–68. Available at: http://eutils.ncbi.nlm.nih.gov/entrez/eutils/elink.fcgi?dbfrom=pubmed&id=8834582&retmode=ref&cmd=prlinks.
28. Elias D, Goere D, Blot F, et al. Optimization of hyperthermic intraperitoneal chemotherapy with oxaliplatin plus irinotecan at 43 degrees C after compete cytoreductive surgery: mortality and morbidity in 106 consecutive patients. Ann Surg Oncol 2007;14(6):1818–24.
29. Prada-Villaverde A, Esquivel J, Lowy AM, et al. The American Society of Peritoneal Surface Malignancies evaluation of HIPEC with Mitomycin C versus

Oxaliplatin in 539 patients with colon cancer undergoing a complete cytoreductive surgery. J Surg Oncol 2014;110(7):779–85.

30. Systemic chemotherapy with or without intraperitoneal chemohyperthermia in treating patients undergoing surgery for peritoneal carcinomatosis from colorectal cancer. ClinicalTrialsgov; 2017. Number NCT00769405. Available at: https://clinicaltrials.gov/ct2/show/NCT00769405.

31. Stephens AD, Alderman R, Chang D, et al. Morbidity and mortality analysis of 200 treatments with cytoreductive surgery and hyperthermic intraoperative intraperitoneal chemotherapy using the coliseum technique. Ann Surg Oncol 1999;6(8): 790–6.

32. Votanopoulos KI, Newman NA, Russell G, et al. Outcomes of cytoreductive surgery (CRS) with hyperthermic intraperitoneal chemotherapy (HIPEC) in patients older than 70 years; survival benefit at considerable morbidity and mortality. Ann Surg Oncol 2013;20(11):3497–503.

33. Dindo D, Demartines N, Clavien P-A. Classification of surgical complications: a new proposal with evaluation in a cohort of 6336 patients and results of a survey. Ann Surg 2004;240(2):205–13.

34. Konstantinidis IT, Chouliaras K, Levine EA, et al. Frailty correlates with postoperative mortality and major morbidity after cytoreductive surgery with hyperthermic intraperitoneal chemotherapy. Ann Surg Oncol 2017;24(13):3825–30.

35. Chemama S, Bayar MA, Lanoy E, et al. Sarcopenia is associated with chemotherapy toxicity in patients undergoing cytoreductive surgery with hyperthermic intraperitoneal chemotherapy for peritoneal carcinomatosis from colorectal cancer. Ann Surg Oncol 2016;23(12):3891–8.

36. Glehen O, Osinsky D, Cotte E, et al. Intraperitoneal chemohyperthermia using a closed abdominal procedure and cytoreductive surgery for the treatment of peritoneal carcinomatosis: morbidity and mortality analysis of 216 consecutive procedures. Ann Surg Oncol 2003;10(8):863–9.

37. Saxena A, Yan TD, Morris DL. Critical assessment of preoperative and operative risk factors for complications after iterative peritonectomy procedures. Eur J Surg Oncol 2010;36(3):309–14.

38. Doud AN, Randle RW, Clark CJ, et al. Impact of distal pancreatectomy on outcomes of peritoneal surface disease treated with cytoreductive surgery and hyperthermic intraperitoneal chemotherapy. Ann Surg Oncol 2015;22(5):1645–50.

39. Dagbert F, Thievenaz R, Decullier E, et al. Splenectomy increases postoperative complications following cytoreductive surgery and hyperthermic intraperitoneal chemotherapy. Ann Surg Oncol 2016;23(6):1980–5.

40. Leapman MS, Jibara G, Tabrizian P, et al. Genitourinary resection at the time of cytoreductive surgery and heated intraperitoneal chemotherapy for peritoneal carcinomatosis is not associated with increased morbidity or worsened oncologic outcomes: a case-matched study. Ann Surg Oncol 2014;21(4):1153–8.

41. Verwaal VJ, van Ruth S, de Bree E, et al. Randomized trial of cytoreduction and hyperthermic intraperitoneal chemotherapy versus systemic chemotherapy and palliative surgery in patients with peritoneal carcinomatosis of colorectal cancer. J Clin Oncol 2003;21(20):3737–43.

42. Verwaal VJ, Bruin S, Boot H, et al. 8-year follow-up of randomized trial: cytoreduction and hyperthermic intraperitoneal chemotherapy versus systemic chemotherapy in patients with peritoneal carcinomatosis of colorectal cancer. Ann Surg Oncol 2008;15(9):2426–32.

43. Goéré D, Malka D, Tzanis D, et al. Is there a possibility of a cure in patients with colorectal peritoneal carcinomatosis amenable to complete cytoreductive surgery and intraperitoneal chemotherapy? Ann Surg 2013;257(6):1065–71.

44. Tomlinson JS, Jarnagin WR, DeMatteo RP, et al. Actual 10-year survival after resection of colorectal liver metastases defines cure. J Clin Oncol 2007;25(29): 4575–80.

45. Elias D, Faron M, Iuga BS, et al. Prognostic similarities and differences in optimally resected liver metastases and peritoneal metastases from colorectal cancers. Ann Surg 2015;261(1):157–63.

46. Elias D, Gilly F, Boutitie F, et al. Peritoneal colorectal carcinomatosis treated with surgery and perioperative intraperitoneal chemotherapy: retrospective analysis of 523 patients from a multicentric French study. J Clin Oncol 2010;28(1):63–8.

47. Kwakman R, Schrama AM, van Olmen JP, et al. Clinicopathological parameters in patient selection for cytoreductive surgery and hyperthermic intraperitoneal chemotherapy for colorectal cancer metastases: a meta-analysis. Ann Surg 2016;263(6):1102–11.

48. Goéré D, Souadka A, Faron M, et al. Extent of colorectal peritoneal carcinomatosis: attempt to define a threshold above which HIPEC does not offer survival benefit: a comparative study. Ann Surg Oncol 2015;22(9):2958–64.

49. Faron M, Macovei R, Goere D, et al. Linear relationship of peritoneal cancer index and survival in patients with peritoneal metastases from colorectal cancer. Ann Surg Oncol 2016;23(1):114–9.

50. Carmignani CP, Ortega-Perez G, Sugarbaker PH. The management of synchronous peritoneal carcinomatosis and hematogenous metastasis from colorectal cancer. Eur J Surg Oncol 2004;30(4):391–8.

51. Chua TC, Yan TD, Zhao J, et al. Peritoneal carcinomatosis and liver metastases from colorectal cancer treated with cytoreductive surgery perioperative intraperitoneal chemotherapy and liver resection. Eur J Surg Oncol 2009; 35(12):1299–305.

52. Maggiori L, Goere D, Viana B, et al. Should patients with peritoneal carcinomatosis of colorectal origin with synchronous liver metastases be treated with a curative intent? A case-control study. Ann Surg 2013;258(1):116–21.

53. Kaibori M, Iwamoto Y, Ishizaki M, et al. Predictors and outcome of early recurrence after resection of hepatic metastases from colorectal cancer. Langenbecks Arch Surg 2012;397(3):373–81.

54. Simkens GA, van Oudheusden TR, Luyer MD, et al. Serious postoperative complications affect early recurrence after cytoreductive surgery and HIPEC for colorectal peritoneal carcinomatosis. Ann Surg Oncol 2015;22(8):2656–62.

55. Baratti D, Kusamura S, Iusco D, et al. Postoperative complications after cytoreductive surgery and hyperthermic intraperitoneal chemotherapy affect long-term outcome of patients with peritoneal metastases from colorectal cancer: a two-center study of 101 patients. Dis Colon Rectum 2014;57(7):858–68.

56. Simkens GA, Razenberg LG, Lemmens VE, et al. Histological subtype and systemic metastases strongly influence treatment and survival in patients with synchronous colorectal peritoneal metastases. Eur J Surg Oncol 2016;42(6): 794–800.

57. Winer J, Zenati M, Ramalingam L, et al. Impact of aggressive histology and location of primary tumor on the efficacy of surgical therapy for peritoneal carcinomatosis of colorectal origin. Ann Surg Oncol 2014;21(5):1456–62.

58. Esquivel J, Elias D, Baratti D, et al. Consensus statement on the loco regional treatment of colorectal cancer with peritoneal dissemination. J Surg Oncol 2008;98(4):263–7.
59. Simkens GA, van Oudheusden TR, Nieboer D, et al. Development of a prognostic nomogram for patients with peritoneally metastasized colorectal cancer treated with cytoreductive surgery and HIPEC. Ann Surg Oncol 2016;23(13):4214–21.
60. Passot G, You B, Boschetti G, et al. Pathological response to neoadjuvant chemotherapy: a new prognosis tool for the curative management of peritoneal colorectal carcinomatosis. Ann Surg Oncol 2014;21(8):2608–14.
61. Passot G, Vaudoyer D, Cotte E, et al. Progression following neoadjuvant systemic chemotherapy may not be a contraindication to a curative approach for colorectal carcinomatosis. Ann Surg 2012;256(1):125–9.
62. Maillet M, Glehen O, Lambert J, et al. Early postoperative chemotherapy after complete cytoreduction and hyperthermic intraperitoneal chemotherapy for isolated peritoneal carcinomatosis of colon cancer: a multicenter study. Ann Surg Oncol 2016;23(3):863–9.
63. Kuijpers AM, Mehta AM, Boot H, et al. Perioperative systemic chemotherapy in peritoneal carcinomatosis of lymph node positive colorectal cancer treated with cytoreductive surgery and hyperthermic intraperitoneal chemotherapy. Ann Oncol 2014;25(4):864–9.
64. Baratti D, Kusamura S, Deraco M. Prevention and early treatment of peritoneal metastases from colorectal cancer: second-look laparotomy or prophylactic HIPEC? J Surg Oncol 2014;109(3):225–6.
65. Sugarbaker PH, Gianola FJ, Speyer JL, et al. Prospective randomized trial of intravenous v intraperitoneal 5-FU in patients with advanced primary colon or rectal cancer. Semin Oncol 1985;12(3 Suppl 4):101–11.
66. Tentes AAK, Spiliotis ID, Korakianitis OS, et al. Adjuvant perioperative intraperitoneal chemotherapy in locally advanced colorectal carcinoma: preliminary results. ISRN Surg 2011;2011(1):529876.
67. Noura S, Ohue M, Shingai T, et al. Effects of intraperitoneal chemotherapy with mitomycin C on the prevention of peritoneal recurrence in colorectal cancer patients with positive peritoneal lavage cytology findings. Ann Surg Oncol 2011; 18(2):396–404.
68. Sammartino P, Sibio S, Biacchi D, et al. Prevention of peritoneal metastases from colon cancer in high-risk patients: preliminary results of surgery plus prophylactic HIPEC. Gastroenterol Res Pract 2012;2012(2):141585–7.
69. Adjuvant HIPEC to prevent colorectal peritoneal metastases in high-risk patients. ClinicalTrialsgov; 2017. https://clinicaltrials.gov/ct2/show/NCT02575859.
70. Klaver CEL, Musters GD, Bemelman WA, et al. Adjuvant hyperthermic intraperitoneal chemotherapy (HIPEC) in patients with colon cancer at high risk of peritoneal carcinomatosis; the COLOPEC randomized multicentre trial. BMC Cancer 2015;15(1):428.
71. Adjuvant HIPEC in high risk colon cancer. ClinicalTrialsgov; 2017. Number NCT02231086. Available at: https://clinicaltrials.gov/ct2/show/NCT02231086.
72. Trial evaluating surgery with hyperthermic intraperitoneal chemotherapy (HIPEC) in treating patients with a high risk of developing colorectal peritoneal carcinomatosis. ClinicalTrialsgov; 2017. Number NCT02179489. Available at: https://clinicaltrials.gov/ct2/show/NCT02179489.
73. Elias D, Goere D, Di Pietrantonio D, et al. Results of systematic second-look surgery in patients at high risk of developing colorectal peritoneal carcinomatosis. Ann Surg 2008;247(3):445–50.

74. Delhorme JB, Triki E, Romain B, et al. Routine second-look after surgical treatment of colonic peritoneal carcinomatosis. J Visc Surg 2015;152(3):149–54.
75. Trial comparing simple follow-up to exploratory laparotomy plus "in principle" (hyperthermic intraperitoneal chemotherapy) HIPEC in colorectal patients (Prophylo-CHIP). ClinicalTrialsgov; 2017. Number NCT01226394. Available at: https://clinicaltrials.gov/ct2/show/NCT01226394.

Palliative Management of Advanced Peritoneal Carcinomatosis

Laura A. Lambert, MD[a],*, Ryan J. Hendrix, MD[b]

KEYWORDS

- Carcinomatosis • Palliative • Ascites • Obstruction • Hospice

KEY POINTS

- Peritoneal carcinomatosis is one of the most challenging oncologic conditions for providers, patients, and families.
- Optimal care of patients with peritoneal carcinomatosis requires knowledge of the natural history of the disease and a multidisciplinary team approach to care.
- Early referral to palliative care is appropriate for any patient with peritoneal carcinomatosis.

INTRODUCTION

From both a therapeutic and palliative perspective, peritoneal carcinomatosis (PC) represents one of the greatest challenges in oncology. Given the advances in surgical techniques, regional therapies, and medications over the past decade, health care providers and patients now have therapeutic modalities to pursue with the hope and intention for cure. However, despite significant advances in the management and treatment of PC, morbidity rates remain high and survival rates remain low. Many patients experience a complex and protracted course after diagnosis plagued by complications such as abdominal pain, mechanical bowel obstruction, symptomatic dysmotility, symptomatic ascites, biliary or ureteral obstruction with end-organ failure, anorexia, tumor cachexia, and fatigue as well as a variety of enteric fistulae. Consequently, knowledge of and experience with managing the clinical manifestations of PC are essential for the optimal delivery of care to this patient population. Furthermore, early referral to a comprehensive palliative care team for supportive management and assistance with goals of care can be extremely helpful

Disclosures: The authors have nothing to disclose.
[a] Surgical Oncology, Huntsman Cancer Institute, 2000 Circle of Hope Drive, Salt Lake City, UT 84112, USA; [b] Division of Surgical Oncology, Department of Surgery, University of Massachusetts Medical School, 55 Lake Avenue N., Worcester, MA 01608, USA
* Corresponding author.
E-mail address: laura.lambert@hci.utah.edu

Surg Oncol Clin N Am 27 (2018) 585–602
https://doi.org/10.1016/j.soc.2018.02.008
1055-3207/18/© 2018 Elsevier Inc. All rights reserved.

surgonc.theclinics.com

in optimizing the care of these complex clinical, emotional, spiritual, social, and existential situations.

This article reviews the multidisciplinary, multimodal options available for the management of PC from a palliative perspective.

PALLIATIVE MANAGEMENT OF BOWEL OBSTRUCTION AND GASTROINTESTINAL DYSMOTILITY FROM PERITONEAL CARCINOMATOSIS

Bowel obstruction is a challenging, ominous, and all too frequent complication of PC. Possibly arising at any point along the gastrointestinal tract, the etiology of a bowel obstruction can be quite diverse and response to nonoperative measures difficult to predict. Regardless, initial management should include appropriate intravenous fluid resuscitation based on the degree of dehydration and correction of any metabolic abnormalities. The patient should be made nil per os to minimize gastrointestinal stimulation and secretions with the placement of a nasogastric tube for gastric decompression if the patient is vomiting. Serial abdominal examinations to monitor for signs or symptoms of peritonitis are essential. Imaging studies such as an abdominal series and/or a computed tomography (CT) scan of the abdomen and pelvis are helpful to determine the level and nature of the obstruction, and also offer insight regarding complications such as ischemic bowel, perforation, or the presence of ascites.

Patients who are hemodynamically stable, without signs of peritonitis, and who have a normal or only mildly elevated white blood cell count (especially in the setting of dehydration), can initially be monitored closely for resolution of their obstruction and return of bowel function This attempt at a nonoperative approach often yields success, but may require a prolonged period of enteric rest. Because patients with PC are often malnourished before an obstruction, health care providers should consider parenteral nutrition while planning additional palliative measures. The clinician can assess the severity of malnutrition and associated indications with assistance from the American Society for Parenteral and Enteral Nutrition guidelines, which recommend screening for insufficient energy intake, weight loss, loss of muscle mass, loss of subcutaneous fat, localized or generalized fluid accumulation, and diminished functional status as measured by handgrip strength.[1]

The development of signs and symptoms of peritonitis or a CT scan suggesting a "closed loop" obstruction (obstruction caused by a loop of intestine twisting around its mesentery) are indications for an urgent surgical intervention (**Fig. 1**). The exact nature of that intervention is ultimately determined at the time of surgery and may involve a simple lysis of adhesions, or segmental bowel resection for a closed loop obstruction, or for a nonclosed loop obstruction, a diverting loop ostomy or end-ostomy (either small or large bowel depending on the location of the obstruction). In more advanced cases, the placement of a decompressive gastrostomy tube for venting the stomach if the obstruction cannot otherwise be relieved may be warranted. From a technical standpoint, these operations are challenging, and pose a high risk for perioperative morbidity and mortality.[2–5] Thus, careful patient selection for a surgical intervention for a malignant bowel obstruction from PC is essential. In an effort to improve outcomes for these patients, the cooperative group, Southwestern Oncology Group (SWOG), is currently conducting a multicenter, prospective clinical trial (SWOG S1316) comparing operative and nonoperative management of malignant bowel obstruction.[6]

For obstructions located in the duodenum, rectum, or at the rectosigmoid junction, it may be reasonable to consider an endoscopic stent placement before, or instead of, surgery. Although the presence of PC has been shown to increase the risk of failure of endoscopic stent placement for colonic obstruction, there is still a reported 77% to

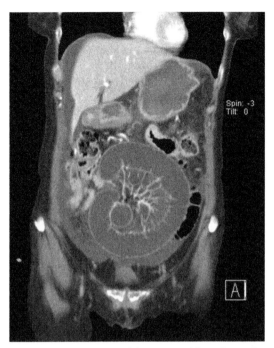

Fig. 1. Closed loop obstruction. A 56-year-old woman with peritoneal carcinomatosis from signet ring cell appendiceal cancer who presented with sudden onset of abdominal pain required emergent exploratory laparotomy and segmental small bowel resection.

85% success rate.[7–10] For patients with a severely limited prognosis, avoiding an operation that would likely involve an intestinal diversion with an ostomy, colonic stents offer a significant palliative option with symptomatic resolution and avoidance of postoperative recovery (**Fig. 2**). For patients in whom surgical or endoscopic relief of the bowel obstruction is not feasible, evaluation for a percutaneous endoscopic gastrostomy tube placement for gastric drainage is a viable palliative option because it will also allow patients to drink liquids and eat some soft foods for comfort.

There are also several medical interventions for patients with bowel obstructions in whom surgery, other than a venting gastrostomy tube, is not an option. Low-dose dexamethasone can help with bowel wall edema and may help to resolve a partial bowel obstruction as well as treat associated nausea.[11,12] Nausea can and should be aggressively treated with combination broad-spectrum antiemetics targeted to the chemoreceptor trigger zone (dopamine receptors), the vomiting center (H1 receptors), and the intestine (cholinergic and 5-HT3 receptors; **Table 1**). Octreotide can be used to decrease intestinal secretions and stretching of the bowel wall, which causes visceral pain.[13,14] The management of medications can be complicated by not having the entire intestinal tract available for absorption necessitating the use of other routes of administration (transdermal, transmucosal, subcutaneous, or intramuscular), especially in the outpatient setting.

PALLIATIVE MANAGEMENT OF GASTRIC OUTLET AND DUODENAL OBSTRUCTIONS FROM PERITONEAL CARCINOMATOSIS

Obstruction of the gastric outlet and/or duodenum is another common indication for palliative surgical consultation. Most patients present with nausea and vomiting of

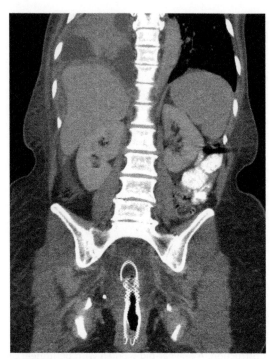

Fig. 2. Rectal stent. A 48-year-old woman with peritoneal carcinomatosis from pancreas cancer who presented with rectal obstruction.

undigested food. Physical examination usually demonstrates upper abdominal distention and tympani. Imaging studies often reveal a distended stomach with retained enteric contents. As with a lower intestinal obstruction, acute symptoms should be managed initially with intravenous resuscitation, aggressive electrolyte repletion, nasogastric decompression, and bowel rest. For patients with chronic gastric outlet

Table 1
Management of nausea

Common Causes of Nausea	Receptors	Site	Drug Class	Drug Example
Opioid induced	D2	CTZ	Butyrephenones	Haloperidol
Gastric stasis	D2	Intestine CTZ	Prokinetics	Metoclopromide domperidone
Intestinal obstruction/ peritoneal irritation	D2 H1 ACHm	CTZ VC Intestine	Phenothiazines Antihistamines Anticholinergics	Prochlorperazine Diphenyhydramine Hyoscine
Chemotherapy/PONV	5-HT3	Intestine CTZ	5-HT3 antagonists	Ondansetron
Late-onset chemotherapy-related	NK1	Widespread	NK1 antagonist	Aprepitant

Abbreviations: 5-HT3, serotonin type 3; ACHm, muscarinic cholinergic; CTZ, chemoreceptor trigger zone; D2, dopamine type 2; H1, histamine type 1; NK1, neurokinin type 1; PNIV, postoperative nausea and vomiting; VC, vomiting center.

obstruction, special attention to chloride repletion is necessary because large quantities can be lost with emesis of gastric secretions. As mentioned, if significant weight loss is present or if there may be a delay in definitive treatment, it may be reasonable to consider parenteral nutrition while planning additional palliative measures.

Options for managing upper gastrointestinal obstructions include intraluminal stenting, surgical bypass, and decompressive gastrostomy with possible feeding jejunostomy. Similar to colonic stenting, the potential benefits of duodenal stenting include immediate palliation of nausea and vomiting with a less invasive procedure than surgical bypass and earlier resumption of enteral nutrition (**Fig. 3**).[15,16] Stents may be particularly useful for patients with advanced and inoperable malignancy, or those who are poor surgical candidates given their high-risk scores. Flexible self-expanding metal stents can be placed using endoscopic or fluoroscopic techniques. Stenting has been shown to provide a comparable survival outcome and equivalent morbidity and mortality to surgical bypass.[17] Ly and colleagues[17] performed a systematic review of the literature from 1990 to 2008 comparing endoscopic stenting with open surgical bypass. They concluded that endoscopic stenting was more likely to result in tolerance of oral intake (odds ratio [OR]. 2.6; $P = .002$) in a shorter period of time (mean difference of 6.9 days; $P<.001$) with a shorter duration of hospital stay (mean difference of 11.8 days; $P<.001$) as compared with open surgical bypass. Similar findings were reported by Zheng and colleagues.[18] Based on these and other findings, it is also likely that stenting is less expensive than surgical bypass.[19–21] The major limitation of the endoscopic approach is the inability to pass the scope distal to the obstruction. The major complications reported are gastric ulceration, bowel perforation, biliary obstruction, stent dysfunction, and stent migration. Stent placement would be contraindicated for patients with multiple levels of intestinal obstruction

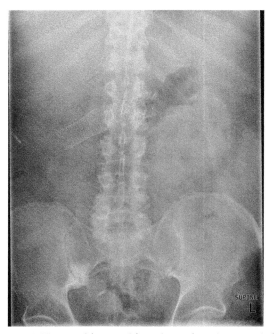

Fig. 3. Duodenal stent. A 50-year-old man with peritoneal carcinomatosis from appendiceal cancer who presented with duodenal obstruction.

and should be considered carefully for patients with PC who are at risk for more distal obstructions.

For patients in whom stenting is not an option, surgical bypass can relieve both the symptoms of the obstruction and allow the patient to resume enteral nutrition. Surgical bypass, most commonly in the form of a gastrojejunostomy, can either be performed laparoscopically or through a relatively small upper midline incision. The estimated risk of morbidity and mortality from these procedures is 25% to 60% and 0% to 25%, respectively.[17,18] Although surgical bypass of the obstructed segment of bowel is usually technically successful, patient selection regarding preoperative nutritional status and life expectancy is imperative to measure its success for palliation. For example, in addition to the general surgical risks such as bleeding, infection, and injury to surrounding structures, a malnourished and cachectic patient with chronic gastric outlet or duodenal obstruction is at significantly increased risk for catastrophic complications, including intestinal anastomotic leak and poor wound healing leading to fascial dehiscence and even evisceration. Other potential complications specific to gastric bypass include dumping syndrome, alkaline reflux gastritis, and delayed gastric emptying.

The placement of a gastrostomy tube for decompression is another option for palliation of gastric outlet, duodenal, and nonoperable small bowel obstruction or profound gastrointestinal dysmotility from carcinomatosis (**Fig. 4**). Gastrostomy tubes can be placed either endoscopically, fluoroscopically, or surgically (either laparoscopic or open). Decompression gastrostomy tubes provide patients the ability to drain the stomach's enteric contents and prevent the progression from mild distention to severe discomfort, nausea, and vomiting. It also provides a significant boost to a patient's quality of life by allowing them to drink liquids and eat small portions of soft foods for pleasure and comfort. Notably, it does not allow for the enteric maintenance of nutrition.

In current practice, many endoscopists, surgeons, and interventional radiologists are leery of placing gastrostomy tubes in the setting of malignant ascites. Concerns highlight the possibly of inducing intraperitoneal leakage from the stomach owing to

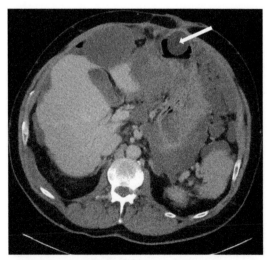

Fig. 4. Venting gastrostomy tube. A 50-year-old man with gastric outlet obstruction owing to peritoneal carcinomatosis from appendiceal cancer managed with venting gastrostomy tube (*arrow* indicates gastrostomy tube balloon in the stomach).

poor apposition to the anterior abdominal wall, leakage of ascites from around the gastrostomy tube, or induction of a contaminating agent into the sterile ascites leading to peritonitis. There is an increasing body of literature demonstrating the feasibility of placing gastrostomy tubes in patients with malignant ascites from a variety of tumors.[22–26] Although ascites may increase the risk of complications, such as leakage at the tube site, reporting on the risk of increased infectious complications is mixed. Paracentesis before or concurrent with gastrostomy placement is advisable. Also, consideration of placing a peritoneal drainage catheter at the time of gastrostomy may also help to lower any risk associated with the ascites. Because gastrostomy may be the only viable palliative option for these patients, all efforts to manage the ascites and increase the safety of gastrostomy placement are warranted.

PALLIATIVE MANAGEMENT OF ENTERIC FISTULAE FROM PERITONEAL CARCINOMATOSIS

Another devastating complication of PC is the development of a fistula from the bowel to either the skin or another organ, most often the bladder, uterus, or vagina. Malignant pelvic fistulae (enterovesicular/colovesicular/rectovesicular/vaginovesicular, entero-vaginal/colovaginal/rectovaginal/uterine) present particularly difficult management challenges because they often develop in the setting of previous pelvic surgery and/or radiation. In addition, owing to the proximity of the anatomic structures of the pelvis, the tumor causing the fistula frequently involves adjacent organs such as the ovaries and ureters. Optimal palliative management of these fistula must be individualized and based on the location, size, and complexity of the fistula, the patient's clinical and nutritional status, the tumor histology, the size and location of the tumor, and the prior treatment history, including surgery and radiation. Cross-sectional imaging including CT scans and MRI have been shown to be superior to fluoroscopic imaging at delineating the location, size, and complexity of the fistula and are essential to patient selection and treatment planning.[27]

Palliative interventions in the management of pelvic fistulae range in complexity from simple urinary drainage for a vesicovaginal fistula to a total pelvic exenteration for an isolated, pelvic tumor recurrence with life-limiting symptoms such as severe pain and incontinence. The more complex cases requiring surgical intervention are optimally managed by a multidisciplinary team led by a surgical oncologist, and consisting of a gynecologic oncologist, a urologist, and a plastic and reconstructive surgeon. In addition to adequate imaging, it is reasonable to perform a diagnostic laparoscopy to determine the true extent of peritoneal tumor dissemination (which can be notoriously underrepresented by both CT scanning or MRI) before embarking on a major abdominal operation such as a pelvic exenteration. Other surgical options for palliation that should be considered include intestinal (ileostomy or colostomy) or urinary (nephrostomy) diversion or stenting. Nonoperative interventions such as bowel rest with intravenous hyperalimentation and the use of somatostatin analogues may also offer symptomatic relief for lower volume fistulae. Although these types of interventions are often assumed to have a negative impact on a patient's quality of life, they can actually often have a salubrious effect with improvement in pain, nutrition, and even facilitate some patients to receive additional palliative chemotherapy.

PALLIATIVE MANAGEMENT OF SYMPTOMATIC ASCITES FROM PERITONEAL CARCINOMATOSIS

Another common complication associated with PC is the development of ascites manifesting as progressive abdominal distention and shortness of breath secondary to mechanical obstruction of the diaphragm (**Fig. 5**). Unfortunately, the efficacy of diuretics for the palliation of malignant ascites in the setting of normal liver function and portal pressure is limited. The use of diuretics poses the additional risk of inducing dehydration and electrolyte abnormalities, and should be used with caution.[28]

Paracentesis affords immediate and significant symptomatic relief to patients suffering from malignant ascites. However, given the pathophysiology, fluid accumulation begins to recur almost instantaneously; thus, the therapeutic effect of each individual paracentesis is temporary, typically on the order of 48 to 72 hours. For patients requiring repetitive paracentesis for refractory ascites, a tunneled intraperitoneal catheter that can be intermittently connected to a self-contained vacuum drainage system is a viable option.[29] These catheters can be placed under local anesthesia either by interventional radiology or surgery.

Another option for the treatment of malignant ascites is hyperthermic intraperitoneal chemoperfusion. A number of studies have demonstrated the efficacy of hyperthermic intraperitoneal chemoperfusion in the treatment of malignant ascites[30–40] (**Table 2**). When the objective is to solely palliate ascites, hyperthermic intraperitoneal chemoperfusion can be performed laparoscopically, sparing patients the morbidity of a larger abdominal incision. However, this modality still requires general anesthesia to maintain pneumoperitoneum and, for this reason, should be reserved for patients with a longer life expectancy and higher performance status.

PALLIATIVE MANAGEMENT OF TUMOR CACHEXIA, FATIGUE, AND ANHEDONIA FROM PERITONEAL CARCINOMATOSIS

Tumor cachexia and fatigue are also frequently seen in patients with PC, and these symptoms are some of the most distressing to the patient and family. To the bystander, an obvious explanation for the weight loss and fatigue is poor nutrition,

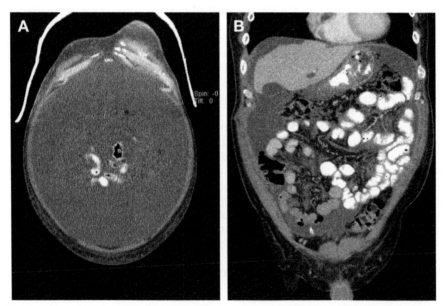

Fig. 5. Large-volume ascites. A 66-year-old man with large-volume ascites (*A*) from appendiceal cancer treated with palliative hyperthermic intraperitoneal chemotherapy (*B*).

Table 2
Outcomes of palliative HIPEC for malignant ascites

Author, Year	N	Tumor	Agent(s)	Technique	Response (%)	Median Survival (Range)
Garofalo et al,[35] 2006	14	Varied	Cisplatin and doxorubicin or mitomycin	Laparoscopic	100	203 d (21–667)
Facchiano et al,[36] 2008	5	Gastric	Mitomycin and cisplatin	Laparoscopic	100	89 d (33–144)
Patriti et al,[32] 2008	1	Mesothelioma	Cisplatin and doxorubicin	Laparoscopic	100	6 mo
Valle et al,[30] 2009	52	Varied	Cisplatin and doxorubicin or mitomycin	Laparoscopic	98	98 d (21–796)
Ba et al,[39] 2010	16	Gastric	5-Fluorouracil and oxaliplatin	Laparoscopic	88	5 mo (2–9)
Antos et al,[40] 2010	8	Varied	Varied	Open	100	6.8 mo (2–23)
Ba, 2013	62	Ovarian	Cisplatin and doxorubicin	Laparoscopic or	93	8 mo (2–20)
		Gastrointestinal	Mitomycin	B-Ultrasound guided	94	9 mo (2–30)
Randle et al,[31] 2014	299	Varied	Mitomycin Carboplatin Oxaliplatin Cisplatin	Open	93	5.3 mo[a]

[a] Incomplete cytoreduction; non–low-grade appendiceal cancers.
(From Ba MC, Long H, Cui SZ, et al. Multivariate comparison of B-ultrasound guided and laparoscopic continuous circulatory hyperthermic intraperitoneal perfusion chemotherapy for malignant ascites. Surg Endosc. Aug 2013;27(8):2735-43; with permission.)

thus prompting the well-intended, natural, reaction to encourage the patient to eat despite his or her anorexia leading to eating-related distress for both the patient and family. Unfortunately, efforts to provide adequate caloric support, either parenterally or enterally, for a patient with advanced cancer have not been shown to improve lean body weight or fatigue. In fact, the lack of improvement with adequate protein nutrition is part of the definition of cancer cachexia, supporting the notion that this is a manifestation of a broader systemic process impacting the entire protein–energy balance and metabolism.[41] Efforts are on-going to better understand and combat cancer cachexia.

Although fatigue and cachexia often occur together, fatigue is not necessarily due to cachexia and seems to be its own complex, multidimensional symptom. In addition to being related to cancer progression, it may also be due to cancer treatments, comorbid conditions, deconditioning, or a product of complex psychosocial factors. There are several assessment approaches for fatigue (performance status, functional capacity, fatigue scales), but there is no current gold standard. Interventions for fatigue can be pharmacologic and nonpharmacologic. Nonpharmacologic approaches include education and counseling, assistance with changing schedules that promote less fatigue, and encourage exercise.[42] Pharmacologic approaches include interventions similar to those for cancer cachexia, namely, corticosteroids, progestins, and psychostimulants. Anhedonia is also a frequent companion of cachexia and fatigue, and may be a sign of unrecognized existential distress. Any evidence of these symptoms in isolation or in combination warrants immediate evaluation and are appropriate indications for both palliative care consult and psychooncology consult.

PALLIATIVE MANAGEMENT OF PERITONEAL CARCINOMATOSIS: THE ROLE OF EMERGENCY SURGERY AT THE END OF LIFE

Emergency surgery at the end of life poses a unique dilemma for patients, family members, and health care providers. Facing an unexpected yet tangible complication, surgical decision making becomes more challenging for patients with PC regarding an emergent operation. It may be argued that this is not a purely palliative surgery consult, because the surgical intervention has the potential to rescue the patient from a life-threatening complication of their life-limiting illness. However, it may also be considered palliative because the intervention will not cure the patient of the underlying disease process. This time is often emotionally charged, even for patients with longstanding illness such as advanced cancer, because they are now faced not with a finite time until death, but with the imminent risk of dying.

A recent study by Cauley and colleagues[43] reported the results of a retrospective cohort study of 875 patients with disseminated cancer undergoing emergency surgery for obstruction (n = 376) or perforation (n = 499). Of the 376 patients who underwent emergency surgery for obstruction, the 30-day mortality rate was 18% with a 41% morbidity rate and 60% were discharged to an institution. Dependent functional status and ascites were independent preoperative predictors of death at 30 days. Postoperative predictors of mortality included respiratory and cardiac complications. Only 4% of patients had do not resuscitate orders in place before surgery.

In the same study by Cauley and colleagues,[43] among the 499 patients who underwent surgery for perforation, the 30-day mortality was 34% with a morbidity rate of 67%, and 52% of patients were discharged to an institution. Independent preoperative predictors of death at 30 days included renal failure, septic shock, ascites, dyspnea at rest, and dependent functional status. Postoperative respiratory complications and advanced age (>75 years) were also predictors of mortality. Similar to the patients who presented with a bowel obstruction, only 4% had a do not resuscitate order in place before surgery despite the advanced nature of their cancer. Further underscoring the dismal prognosis in this particular situation, a study by Pameijer and colleagues[44] showed that patients with metastatic cancer who presented with obstructive symptoms had a median survival of 3 months regardless of operative or nonoperative management.

Although most patients survive the initial operation, a substantial number die soon after surgery and the majority experience a combination of postoperative complications, reoperations, nursing home stays, and hospital readmissions. Such events clearly impact the patient and family experience and their overall quality of life. Generating these types of data provides a framework for surgeons and caregivers to advise patients regarding the risks of surgery, and to set realistic expectations for the postoperative experience, discharge location, and overall survival. However, important data evaluating health care providers' ability to address the goals of patients and families are still lacking, as are assessments of whether the same choice to pursue or forego an emergent operation would be made. Furthermore, in a society in which most people are not prepared for dying, these types of data can often make things more difficult for the surgeon, who is then asked to operate in the face of such overwhelming odds.

PALLIATIVE MANAGEMENT OF PERITONEAL CARCINOMATOSIS AND MORAL DISTRESS

Caught between patients who are suddenly facing their own mortality and families who are not ready to let go, the smallest amount of hope that surgery offers makes even the most daunting risks seem worth taking. In this setting, surgeons and other affiliated providers often experience moral distress. Professionalism demands that the surgeon make a sincere effort to understand, respond with compassion and empathy, and be considerate of all other perspectives, most notably those of the patient and family, without realistic expectation of the same in return. This circumstance can be particularly challenging when the surgeon is busy or when these events occur in the middle of the night. In the name of full disclosure and informed consent, some surgeons paint an exhaustively bleak picture for the patient and family in an effort to dissuade them from choosing surgery. Despite these efforts, when the patient and family are insistent on surgery, some surgeons presume a tacit agreement that the patient will endure to the end irrespective of any additional procedures or maneuvers that may be required—additional surgeries, feeding tubes, tracheotomy, dialysis, rehabilitation, and so on. All too often, this situation culminates in frustration and a sense of betrayal on the part of the surgeon when, within a few days after the index surgery, the family decides to stop any further life-prolonging care. It is for this reason that understanding the perspective of the patient and family is critical for both the outcome of the encounter and the surgeon's well-being.

Tools like the palliative triangle proposed by Miner and colleagues[45] can be helpful for these challenging situations. The palliative triangle is an approach to improving patient selection and patient-acknowledged outcomes specifically for palliative surgery (**Fig. 6**). Through the dynamics of the triangle, the patient's complaints, values, and emotional support are considered while weighing the medical and surgical alternatives. In addition, the triangle offers an opportunity to learn about and address a patient's and/or family's expectations regarding the intent of the proposed procedure helping to moderate any incongruent expectations between surgeon, patient, and family. Miner and colleagues[46] conducted a prospective study to investigate the

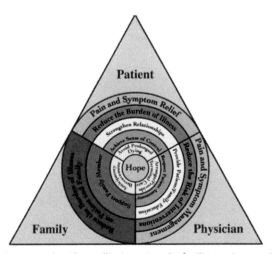

Fig. 6. The palliative triangle. The palliative triangle facilitates interactions between patients, families, and surgeons and helps to guide patients to the best decisions regarding palliative surgery. (*From* Thomay AA, Jaques DP, Miner TJ. Surgical palliation: getting back to our roots. Surg Clin North Am 2009;89(1):27–41; with permission.)

efficacy of the palliative triangle technique during palliative surgery consultation in 227 patients with symptomatic, advanced, incurable cancer. A unique aspect of this study on palliative surgery centered on its inclusion criteria, because patients were analyzed irrespective of their intervention. In total, more than one-half of the patients (53.3%) did not undergo a procedure. Reasons cited included patient preference, low symptom severity, decision for nonoperative palliation, and concerns over possible complications. Of the patients who elected to pursue a palliative procedure (46.7%), 90.7% reported symptom resolution or improvement. The morbidity and mortality associated with these procedures was 20.1% and 3.9%, respectively. The median survival was 212 days. The authors concluded that the use of the palliative triangle facilitates improved patient selection, which translates to better outcomes. Specifically, they noted significantly greater symptom resolution with fewer postoperative complications compared with previously published results. The authors have also postulated that building this strong relationship may explain the observation of high patient satisfaction toward surgeons after palliative operation, even if there is no demonstrable benefit.[45]

As described, the palliative triangle engages all 3 parties in a manner where they are given the chance to express concerns and be heard. It is also significant in that it helps the surgeon to separate the patient's goals and understanding from that of the family's and vice versa. It also gives the surgeon's goals and understanding equal weight in the decision making. However, the success of the palliative triangle approach is predicated on the surgeon's mindset. If the surgeon truly hopes to influence the behavior of the patient and the family in an efficient and professional manner, an outward mindset, in which the patient's and family's objectives matter like the surgeon's objectives matter, is essential. The Arbinger influence pyramid is a proven leadership approach to influencing behavior that is readily applicable to patient–family–physician interactions **(Fig. 7)**.[47]

Starting at the base of the pyramid, the surgeon must adjust his or her mindset to an outward mindset in which the goals and objectives of the patient and family matter

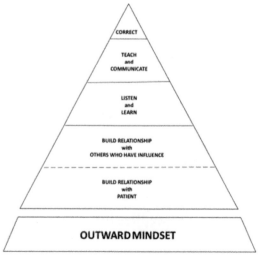

Fig. 7. The Arbinger Influence Pyramid. The influence pyramid is a proven framework designed to help influence behavior and improve results beginning with a shift in mindset. (*Courtesy of* The Arbinger Institute, Farmington, UT; with permission.)

equally with his or hers. The outward mindset will then facilitate building a relationship with the patient and those who have influence on the patient, namely, the family. Building this relationship can happen simply through introductions and a sincere expression of empathy for the challenging situation that the patient and family are facing. Next, the surgeon needs to listen and learn what the patient and family know about the situation and identify their hopes, goals, and objectives. Afterward, the surgeon can teach the patient and family what they need to know, correct any misconceptions, answer questions, and review the risks, benefits, indications, and alternatives to surgery to ultimately make an engaged recommendation that is mindful of the goals of all 3 parties. From there, the surgeon, patient and family can usually come to mutually agreed upon goals and a care plan. There are a few key points about using the influence pyramid. First, the time and effort spent at the lower levels of the pyramid collectively ensures effectiveness at the higher levels. Second, the solution to a problem at one level of the pyramid will be found in spending more time at a lower level of the pyramid. Third, the effectiveness at each level of the pyramid depends on the effectiveness of the level below and ultimately on the deepest level of the pyramid, the mindset.

EARLY REFERRAL TO PALLIATIVE CARE: BETTER CARE FOR THE PATIENT, FAMILY, AND PROVIDERS

Until recently, a diagnosis of PC was uniformly accompanied by a survival prognosis measured in weeks to months. Fortunately, significant recent advancements in the medical and surgical management of PC have altered the natural history of this condition for many patients. However, despite the progress being made in the clinical management and outcomes of PC, it remains a highly lethal condition. Adding insult to injury, PC is also often associated with significant clinical morbidity that can challenge even the most caring and astute clinicians. Furthermore, despite the seemingly obvious state of advanced, incurable disease, an essential part of coping with death anxiety for most patients and their families to continue to hope—either for a cure, more time, or at least a chance to fight. A diagnosis of PC thrusts patients, families, and providers into the vortex of one of the most difficult clinical and emotional situations.

Current American Society of Clinical Oncology and National Comprehensive Cancer Network guidelines recommend early initiation of palliative care for patients with advanced, life-threatening cancers.[48,49] Recent studies in advanced lung cancer have shown that patients who receive an early palliative intervention as part of their treatment actually live longer with better quality of life despite receiving less cancer-directed therapy.[50] It is not unreasonable to expect similar results with other advanced cancers, especially PC.

Many physicians and patients see a palliative care consult and hospice as a sign of giving up. However, this could not be farther from the truth (**Box 1**). Unlike hospice, which is a medical insurance benefit that requires a life expectancy of less than 6 months if the life-threatening disease is untreated and for the patient to forgo disease-directed treatment, any patient with symptoms from an illness or its treatment, are entitled to comprehensive, specialized palliative care. Although most patients' symptoms can be adequately managed by providers who are not board certified in palliative care (such as a primary care physician or other specialist—medical oncologist, surgeon, radiation oncologist), advanced, life-threatening cancers, such as PC, can pose additional challenges in terms of physical, emotional, psychological, spiritual, and social symptomatology. Engaging a palliative care specialist and multidisciplinary team preemptively, before the onset of unmanageable symptoms

---

Box 1
Common misconceptions about hospice

Misconception: Patients will lose contact with their primary physician.

Truth: The referring physician (ie, primary care provider or oncologist) continues to play an important role in the patients' care.

Misconception: Hospice patients cannot go to the hospital.

Truth: Hospice patients can be hospitalized as needed for symptoms that cannot be managed at home or at a hospice house.

Misconception: Patients can use up their hospice eligibility.

Truth: Hospice eligibility does not expire. Patients who live longer than 6 months will continue to receive hospice services provided they still meet the eligibility requirements.

Misconception: Patients cannot come off hospice if a new treatment comes available.

Truth: Hospice is not a one-way street. If a new treatment directed at the patient disease becomes available that may be helpful to the patient, the patient can come off hospice care to receive treatment.

Misconception: Patients enrolling in hospice have to choose not to be resuscitated.

Truth: Although it is typically recommended that patients receiving hospice care choose not to be resuscitated and it is imperative for providers and patients to discuss the role of resuscitation, it is not required for hospice eligibility.

Misconception: Patients on hospice cannot receive parenteral nutrition.

Truth: Although it depends on the benefits covered by an individual's insurance benefit, patients receiving hospice can receive parenteral nutrition, although the actual benefit in terms of symptom control and survival need to be evaluated.

Misconception: Hospice patients cannot participate in research projects.

Truth: Hospice patients can participate in research projects that are consistent with the mission of hospice.

---

and the dire need for the expertise of a palliative medicine provider arises, alleviates the perception among patients and families that one is giving up.

Normalizing the palliative care team's involvement in the multidisciplinary management of patients with advanced cancers is an effective way to improve the timing of referral of patients to palliative care. Many institutions have incorporated palliative care referrals into their cancer center's protocol for all patients with advanced cancer at the time of the initial cancer center visit. This practice helps the palliative care team to quell the fears of patients and their families that their doctors are giving up by informing them that every patient with an advanced cancer is seen by palliative care, and that it is part of the institution's standard, multidisciplinary team effort to care for the patient and family. This also takes the burden off the primary specialist to conduct some of the harder conversations around goals of care and advanced directives, and allows them to focus on the plan of treatment. Having these difficult conversations early is essential in the comprehensive management of advanced cancers such as PC and should not be avoided owing to provider unease. A palliative care specialist who is an expert in communication can be a tremendous help with this aspect of the patient's care.

Earlier palliative care involvement can also help with the transition to hospice when appropriate. Recognition of that time may come first to the oncologist when further cancer-directed treatment is likely to do more harm than good or to the patient and family when they decide that the burden of treatment is not worth the limited potential for more time. Unfortunately, and all too often, both parties do not arrive at this recognition concurrently. The oncologist may find it easier to continue to treat the patient who insists on continuing to fight the cancer even knowing that fighting may take time away from the patient. Similarly, the patient may find it easier to persevere through treatment rather than disappoint the oncologist by stopping. With an early palliative care intervention, conversations about hospice as a potential option can be started early, leaving plenty of time to correct any misconceptions. Patients and families can learn that the mission of hospice is neither to prolong life nor hasten death, but to provide comfort and dignity, and optimize the quality of life that remains. Hospice care is often stigmatized and associated with negative misconceptions; thus, the early involvement of the palliative care team can help to dispel these myths and address other unfounded concerns such as patients on hospice lose contact with their primary physician, hospice patients cannot go to the hospital if necessary, patients cannot come off hospice if a new treatment becomes available, and so on. They will also learn that hospice provides support to both the patient and the family through an interdisciplinary team of providers including physicians, nurses, social workers, chaplains, and volunteers. Hospice also helps to set expectations for families, prepares them for their impending loss, and provides ongoing support after the patient's death via bereavement programs.

REFERENCES

1. White JV, Guenter P, Jensen G, et al. Consensus statement: Academy of Nutrition and Dietetics and American Society for Parenteral and Enteral Nutrition: characteristics recommended for the identification and documentation of adult malnutrition (undernutrition). JPEN J Parenter Enteral Nutr 2012;36(3):275–83.

2. Paul Olson TJ, Pinkerton C, Brasel KJ, et al. Palliative surgery for malignant bowel obstruction from carcinomatosis: a systematic review. JAMA Surg 2014;149(4):383–92.

3. Helyer L, Easson AM. Surgical approaches to malignant bowel obstruction. J Support Oncol 2008;6(3):105–13.

4. Ripamonti C, Twycross R, Baines M, et al. Clinical-practice recommendations for the management of bowel obstruction in patients with end-stage cancer. Support Care Cancer 2001;9(4):223–33.

5. Ripamonti CI, Easson AM, Gerdes H. Management of malignant bowel obstruction. Eur J Cancer 2008;44(8):1105–15.

6. S1316, Surgery or non-surgical management in treating patients with intra-abdominal cancer and bowel obstruction. 2017. Available at: https://clinicaltrials.gov/ct2/show/NCT02270450?term=swog+malignant+bowel+obstruction&rank=1. Accessed September 24, 2017.

7. Yoon JY, Jung YS, Hong SP, et al. Clinical outcomes and risk factors for technical and clinical failures of self-expandable metal stent insertion for malignant colorectal obstruction. Gastrointest Endosc 2011;74(4):858–68.

8. Sagar J. Colorectal stents for the management of malignant colonic obstructions. Cochrane Database Syst Rev 2011;(11):CD007378.

9. Kim JH, Ku YS, Jeon TJ, et al. The efficacy of self-expanding metal stents for malignant colorectal obstruction by noncolonic malignancy with peritoneal carcinomatosis. Dis Colon Rectum 2013;56(11):1228–32.

10. Caceres A, Zhou Q, Iasonos A, et al. Colorectal stents for palliation of large-bowel obstructions in recurrent gynecologic cancer: an updated series. Gynecol Oncol 2008;108(3):482–5.

11. Laval G, Marcelin-Benazech B, Guirimand F, et al. Recommendations for bowel obstruction with peritoneal carcinomatosis. J Pain Symptom Manage 2014; 48(1):75–91.

12. Feuer DJ, Broadley KE. Corticosteroids for the resolution of malignant bowel obstruction in advanced gynaecological and gastrointestinal cancer. Cochrane Database Syst Rev 2000;(2):CD001219.

13. Laval G, Rousselot H, Toussaint-Martel S, et al. SALTO: a randomized, multicenter study assessing octreotide LAR in inoperable bowel obstruction. Bull Cancer 2012;99(2):E1–9.

14. Mariani P, Blumberg J, Landau A, et al. Symptomatic treatment with lanreotide microparticles in inoperable bowel obstruction resulting from peritoneal carcinomatosis: a randomized, double-blind, placebo-controlled phase III study. J Clin Oncol 2012;30(35):4337–43.

15. Mosler P, Mergener KD, Brandabur JJ, et al. Palliation of gastric outlet obstruction and proximal small bowel obstruction with self-expandable metal stents: a single center series. J Clin Gastroenterol 2005;39(2):124–8.

16. Holt AP, Patel M, Ahmed MM. Palliation of patients with malignant gastroduodenal obstruction with self-expanding metallic stents: the treatment of choice? Gastrointest Endosc 2004;60(6):1010–7.

17. Ly J, O'Grady G, Mittal A, et al. A systematic review of methods to palliate malignant gastric outlet obstruction. Surg Endosc 2010;24(2):290–7.

18. Zheng B, Wang X, Ma B, et al. Endoscopic stenting versus gastrojejunostomy for palliation of malignant gastric outlet obstruction. Dig Endosc 2012;24(2):71–8.

19. Fiori E, Lamazza A, Volpino P, et al. Palliative management of malignant antropyloric strictures. Gastroenterostomy vs. endoscopic stenting. A randomized prospective trial. Anticancer Res 2004;24(1):269–71.

20. Jeurnink SM, Steyerberg EW, van Hooft JE, et al. Surgical gastrojejunostomy or endoscopic stent placement for the palliation of malignant gastric outlet obstruction (SUSTENT study): a multicenter randomized trial. Gastrointest Endosc 2010; 71(3):490–9.

21. Mehta S, Hindmarsh A, Cheong E, et al. Prospective randomized trial of laparoscopic gastrojejunostomy versus duodenal stenting for malignant gastric outflow obstruction. Surg Endosc 2006;20(2):239–42.

22. Dittrich A, Schubert B, Kramer M, et al. Benefits and risks of a percutaneous endoscopic gastrostomy (PEG) for decompression in patients with malignant gastrointestinal obstruction. Support Care Cancer 2017;25(9):2849–56.

23. Issaka RB, Shapiro DM, Parikh ND, et al. Palliative venting percutaneous endoscopic gastrostomy tube is safe and effective in patients with malignant obstruction. Surg Endosc 2014;28(5):1668–73.

24. Pothuri B, Montemarano M, Gerardi M, et al. Percutaneous endoscopic gastrostomy tube placement in patients with malignant bowel obstruction due to ovarian carcinoma. Gynecol Oncol 2005;96(2):330–4.

25. Ryan JM, Hahn PF, Mueller PR. Performing radiologic gastrostomy or gastrojejunostomy in patients with malignant ascites. AJR Am J Roentgenol 1998;171(4): 1003–6.

26. Shaw C, Bassett RL, Fox PS, et al. Palliative venting gastrostomy in patients with malignant bowel obstruction and ascites. Ann Surg Oncol 2013;20(2):497–505.

27. Narayanan P, Nobbenhuis M, Reynolds KM, et al. Fistulas in malignant gyneco-logic disease: etiology, imaging, and management. Radiographics 2009;29(4): 1073–83.

28. Sangisetty SL, Miner TJ. Malignant ascites: a review of prognostic factors, path-ophysiology and therapeutic measures. World J Gastrointest Surg 2012;4(4): 87–95.

29. Fleming ND, Alvarez-Secord A, Von Gruenigen V, et al. Indwelling catheters for the management of refractory malignant ascites: a systematic literature overview and retrospective chart review. J Pain Symptom Manage 2009;38(3):341–9.

30. Valle M, Van der Speeten K, Garofalo A. Laparoscopic hyperthermic intraperito-neal peroperative chemotherapy (HIPEC) in the management of refractory malig-nant ascites: a multi-institutional retrospective analysis in 52 patients. J Surg Oncol 2009;100(4):331–4.

31. Randle RW, Swett KR, Swords DS, et al. Efficacy of cytoreductive surgery with hy-perthermic intraperitoneal chemotherapy in the management of malignant asci-tes. Ann Surg Oncol 2014;21(5):1474–9.

32. Patriti A, Cavazzoni E, Graziosi L, et al. Successful palliation of malignant ascites from peritoneal mesothelioma by laparoscopic intraperitoneal hyperthermic chemotherapy. Surg Laparosc Endosc Percutan Tech 2008;18(4):426–8.

33. Ong E, Diven C, Abrams A, et al. Laparoscopic hyperthermic intraperitoneal chemotherapy (HIPEC) for palliative treatment of malignant ascites from gastro-intestinal stromal tumours. J Palliat Care 2012;28(4):293–6.

34. Graziosi L, Bugiantella W, Cavazzoni E, et al. Laparoscopic intraperitoneal hyper-thermic perfusion in palliation of malignant ascites. Case report. G Chir 2009; 30(5):237–9 [in Italian].

35. Garofalo A, Valle M, Garcia J, et al. Laparoscopic intraperitoneal hyperthermic chemotherapy for palliation of debilitating malignant ascites. Eur J Surg Oncol 2006;32(6):682–5.

36. Facchiano E, Scaringi S, Kianmanesh R, et al. Laparoscopic hyperthermic intra-peritoneal chemotherapy (HIPEC) for the treatment of malignant ascites second-ary to unresectable peritoneal carcinomatosis from advanced gastric cancer. Eur J Surg Oncol 2008;34(2):154–8.

37. Facchiano E, Risio D, Kianmanesh R, et al. Laparoscopic hyperthermic intraper-itoneal chemotherapy: indications, aims, and results: a systematic review of the literature. Ann Surg Oncol 2012;19(9):2946–50.

38. de Mestier L, Volet J, Scaglia E, et al. Is palliative laparoscopic hyperthermic intraperitoneal chemotherapy effective in patients with malignant hemorrhagic ascites? Case Rep Gastroenterol 2012;6(1):166–70.

39. Ba MC, Cui SZ, Lin SQ, et al. Chemotherapy with laparoscope-assisted contin-uous circulatory hyperthermic intraperitoneal perfusion for malignant ascites. World J Gastroenterol 2010;16(15):1901–7.

40. Antos F, Dytrych P, Vitek P, et al. Malignant ascites–optional management using hyperthermic peroperative chemotherapy (HIPEC). Rozhl Chir 2010;89(4): 237–41 [in Czech].

41. Strasser F. Weight loss in palliative medicine. In: Hanks G, Cherny NI, Christakis NA, et al, editors. Oxford textbook of palliative medicine. 4th edition. New York: Oxford University Press; 2010. p. 889–900.

42. Mitchell SA, Beck SL, Hood LE, et al. Putting evidence into practice: evidence-based interventions for fatigue during and following cancer and its treatment. Clin J Oncol Nurs 2007;11(1):99–113.

43. Cauley CE, Panizales MT, Reznor G, et al. Outcomes after emergency abdominal surgery in patients with advanced cancer: opportunities to reduce complications and improve palliative care. J Trauma Acute Care Surg 2015;79(3):399–406.

44. Pameijer CR, Mahvi DM, Stewart JA, et al. Bowel obstruction in patients with metastatic cancer: does intervention influence outcome? Int J Gastrointest Cancer 2005;35(2):127–33.

45. Miner TJ, Jaques DP, Shriver CD. A prospective evaluation of patients undergoing surgery for the palliation of an advanced malignancy. Ann Surg Oncol 2002; 9(7):696–703.

46. Miner TJ, Cohen J, Charpentier K, et al. The palliative triangle: improved patient selection and outcomes associated with palliative operations. Arch Surg 2011; 146(5):517–22.

47. The Arbinger Institute. The anatomy of peace - resolving the heart of conflict. Oakland (CA): Berrett-Koehler Publishers, Inc; 2015.

48. Smith TJ, Temin S, Alesi ER, et al. American Society of Clinical Oncology provisional clinical opinion: the integration of palliative care into standard oncology care. J Clin Oncol 2012;30(8):880–7.

49. National Comprehensive Cancer Network. Available at: https://www.nccn.org/professionals/physician_gls/pdf/palliativecare. Accessed September 1, 2017.

50. Temel JS, Greer JA, Muzikansky A, et al. Early palliative care for patients with metastatic non-small-cell lung cancer. N Engl J Med 2012;363(8):733–42.

Moving?

Make sure your subscription moves with you!

To notify us of your new address, find your **Clinics Account Number** (located on your mailing label above your name), and contact customer service at:

Email: journalscustomerservice-usa@elsevier.com

800-654-2452 (subscribers in the U.S. & Canada)
314-447-8871 (subscribers outside of the U.S. & Canada)

Fax number: 314-447-8029

Elsevier Health Sciences Division
Subscription Customer Service
3251 Riverport Lane
Maryland Heights, MO 63043

*To ensure uninterrupted delivery of your subscription, please notify us at least 4 weeks in advance of move.